NEURAL DYNAMICS OF ADAPTIVE SENSORY-MOTOR CONTROL
EXPANDED EDITION

NEURAL NETWORKS: Research and Applications

Pergamon Journal of Related Interest
(Free sample copies available upon request)

NEURAL NETWORKS

NEURAL DYNAMICS OF ADAPTIVE SENSORY-MOTOR CONTROL

EXPANDED EDITION

Stephen Grossberg

Center for Adaptive Systems,
Boston University

Michael Kuperstein

Neurogen, Brookline, MA

PERGAMON PRESS

New York • Oxford • Beijing • Frankfurt • São Paulo • Sydney • Tokyo • Toronto

Pergamon Press Offices:

U.S.A.	Pergamon Press, Inc., Maxwell House, Fairview Park, Elmsford, New York 10523, U.S.A.
U.K.	Pergamon Press plc, Headington Hill Hall, Oxford OX3 0BW, England
PEOPLE'S REPUBLIC OF CHINA	Pergamon Press, Qianmen Hotel, Beijing, People's Republic of China
FEDERAL REPUBLIC OF GERMANY	Pergamon Press GmbH, Hammerweg 6, D-6242 Kronberg, Federal Republic of Germany
BRAZIL	Pergamon Editora Ltda, Rua Eça de Queiros, 346, CEP 04011, São Paulo, Brazil
AUSTRALIA	Pergamon Press Australia Pty Ltd., P.O. Box 544, Potts Point, NSW 2011, Australia
JAPAN	Pergamon Press, 8th Floor, Matsuoka Central Building, 1-7-1 Nishishinjuku, Shinjuku-ku, Tokyo 160, Japan
CANADA	Pergamon Press Canada Ltd., Suite 271, 253 College Street, Toronto, Ontario M5T 1R5, Canada

Library of Congress Cataloging in Publication Data

Grossberg, Stephen, 1939-
  Neural dynamics of adaptive sensory-motor control / Stephen Grossberg, Michael Kuperstein. -- Expanded ed.
     p. cm. -- (Neural networks, research and applications)
  Bibliography: p.
  Includes indexes.
  ISBN 0-08-036828-X -- ISBN 0-08-036827-1 (pbk.)
  1. Saccadic eye movements. 2. Sensorimotor integration.
  3. Neural circuitry. 4. Neuroophthalmology. I. Kuperstein,
  Michael, 1954-   . II. Title. III. Series.
  QP477.5G759   1989
  599'.01823--dc19   88-35605
                                                             CIP

Printed in the United States of America

The paper used in this publication meets the minumum requirements of American National Standard for Information Sciences -- Permanence of Paper for Printed Library Materials, ANSI Z39.48-1984

DEDICATION

To Gail

S.G.

To Rachel, my loving mother

M.K.

TABLE OF CONTENTS

CHAPTER 2: PARALLEL PROCESSING OF MOVEMENT AND ERROR SIGNALS

CHAPTER 3: SACCADIC LEARNING USING VISUAL ERROR SIGNALS: SELF-MOTION VERSUS WORLD-MOTION AND CEREBELLAR DYNAMICS

CHAPTER 10: FORMATION OF AN INVARIANT TARGET POSITION MAP   227

CHAPTER 14: A COMPARATIVE ANALYSIS OF NEURAL MECHANISMS, RECENT DATA, AND ALTERNATIVE MODELS   371

Stephen Grossberg

PREFACE TO THE EXPANDED EDITION

In the four years since the first edition of this book was completed, general interest in computational neuroscience and neural network technology has continued to grow at a phenomenal rate. Scientists from many specialties have become interested in how biological learning systems work, and in how to utilize these insights to design more intelligent machines for technological applications. The results of the first edition, which seemed to be very avant garde when they were first derived, are now rapidly entering the mainstream of scientific interest. This Expanded Edition has been prepared to satisfy this interest.

The results about adaptive visuo-motor control that are found in Chapters 1–11 were derived with the saccadic eye movement system in mind. On the other hand, Chapter 12 made plain our belief that similar principles of organization, with suitable modifications and specializations, would prove to be useful towards understanding other sensory-motor control systems.

Chapter 13 provides one confirmation of this belief. It characterizes a model of arm movement control, developed with Daniel Bullock, that has been called the VITE model. These results clarify how the eye movement system and the arm movement system are joined together in a larger system for adaptive eye-hand coordination.

In Chapter 14, I wrote a unifying essay that ties the preceding chapters together. First it makes a comparative analysis of some of the major results on eye movements and arm movements, notably their use of neural vectors. It also describes a variety of recent data that provide experimental support for a number of our theoretical predictions. Finally, it compares the models presented herein with recent alternative models in the literature, suggests how to further test these models, and points the way towards a new approach to designing self-organizing robots.

During the four years since the first edition was written, our work on adaptive sensory-motor control has been partially supported by the Air Force Office of Scientific Research, the Army Research Office, and the National Science Foundation. I am grateful that sustained support from these agencies has made this type of systematic research possible.

I am also grateful to Cynthia Suchta for, once again, doing such a marvelous job of typing and formatting the text and preparing the illustrations.

Stephen Grossberg
February, 1989
Boston, Massachusetts

PREFACE

This book introduces and develops a quantitative neural theory of a complex sensory-motor system: the saccadic eye movement system. Saccadic eye movements are ballistic movements of great speed and accuracy in humans and many other mammals. The present work describes a number of general functional problems which need to be solved by the saccadic eye movement system, as well as by other sensory-motor systems. Specialized neural circuit solutions of these problems, within the context of ballistic eye movements, are used to unify the discussion of a large behavioral and neural data base concerning this sensory-motor system. A substantial number of new experimental predictions are also made with which to further test the theory.

Many of the functional problems for which we have suggested solutions were identified through a consideration of how the saccadic system can automatically calibrate itself through processes of development and learning. We suggest that an analysis of sensory-motor performance, in the absence of an analysis of self-calibration through learning, does not provide enough constraints to characterize the mechanisms of an entire sensory-motor system.

In addition to unifying and predicting data, the present work suggests new real-time circuit designs for adaptive robots, and thus represents a contribution to artificial intelligence, adaptive control theory, and engineering. All of the neural circuit designs are expressed and analysed using the language of nonlinear systems of differential equations. The work is thus a contribution to applied mathematics and dynamical systems. The interdisciplinary nature of the book may make it useful to scientists in several different fields.

In the six years during which we have developed the results in the book, Stephen Grossberg has been partially supported by the Air Force Office of Scientific Research, the National Science Foundation, and the Office of Naval Research. Michael Kuperstein has been partially supported by the Air Force Office of Scientific Research and the National Institutes of Health. We are grateful to these agencies for making this work possible. Most of the work was carried out at the Center for Adaptive Systems at Boston University.

We are also grateful to Cynthia Suchta for doing a marvelously competent job of typing and formatting the text. Cindy also drew all the figures. Thanks are due also to Jonathan Marshall for preparing the index, and to Beth Sanfield for her clerical support.

May, 1985   Stephen Grossberg
Boston, Massachusetts   Michael Kuperstein

CHAPTER 1
MULTIPLE LEARNING PROBLEMS ARE SOLVED
BY SENSORY-MOTOR SYSTEMS

1.1. Introduction: Brain Designs Are Adaptive Designs

One of the primary facts of life in the study of psychology and neurobiology is the remarkable multiplicity of behaviors, of levels of behavioral and neural organization, and of experimental paradigms and methods. One of the great needs in our science is to find unity behind this diversity.

This book describes a theory that unifies and predicts a large and diverse data base concerning the neural substrates of sensory-motor control. The book also illustrates a theoretical method that has unified other types of brain-related data using a small set of theoretical principles and mechanisms (Grossberg, 1982a, 1985a, 1985b).

The present work focuses upon the design principles and mechanisms whereby a particular type of sensory-motor system is controlled; namely, ballistic, or saccadic, eye movements. Although ballistic eye movements seem to be a relatively simple type of motor behavior, a large number of brain regions are utilized to control them, including retina, superior colliculus, parietal cortex, cerebellum, peripontine reticular formation, visual cortex, frontal cortex, and the oculomotor nuclei. The fact that such a simple type of behavior requires such a massive control structure has made the discovery of quantitative theories of brain dynamics difficult. This fact also raises serious issues concerning the specificity with which brain systems organize different types of behavior. If the brain does use specific types of circuitry, then why are so many different circuits needed to control even simple motor behaviors like ballistic eye movements? Moreover, how can a large number of circuits in a distributed control system coordinate specific and accurate behaviors?

The present approach focuses upon how brain systems are designed to form an adaptive relationship with their environment. Instead of focusing upon a few performance characteristics of a neural system, we consider the types of developmental and learning problems that a brain system *as a whole* must solve before accurate performance can be achieved. We have repeatedly found that an analysis of performance *per se* does not impose sufficiently many constraints to determine underlying control mechanisms. By contrast, an analysis of how development and learning lead to and maintain accurate performance characteristics has, time and again, opened a wide pathway to a rapidly expanding understanding of brain mechanisms. We believe that the unifying power of the theory is due to the fact that principles of adaptation—such as the laws regulating development and learning—are fundamental in determining the design of behavioral mechanisms.

1

Our analysis of ballistic eye movements has identified a set of distinct learning problems that its control system needs to solve in order to achieve accurate performance characteristics. The solutions of these learning problems take the form of real-time circuits that have a natural interpretation as neural networks. Even the simplest, or minimal, circuit solutions have been useful for organizing and predicting data concerning the different brain regions that control ballistic eye movements.

We have translated an anatomical multiplicity of brain regions into a functional multiplicity of learning problems. Behavioral, anatomical, and physiological data have been compared and contrasted with the minimal neural network circuits that are capable of solving these learning problems. We have crossed the conceptual gap between behavioral data and brain data by using these functionally meaningful networks as a bridge. A greatly expanded interdisciplinary data base could then be used to refine our understanding of the functional issues themselves.

With these networks in hand, one can better appreciate that the brain's solutions of its distributed control problems are both specific and efficient. Anatomical and physiological differences between brain regions can be analysed using network solutions of different developmental or learning problems. Using this approach, one can study how different sensory-motor systems solve similar learning problems by using the same functional characteristics that control ballistic eye movements. Different sensory-motor control systems can utilize specific circuits that pass through the same brain regions because these circuits all solve similar functional problems. Each brain region can thus be interpreted as a specialized functional processor that is shared by the many different circuits needing that functional capability. By tracing differences between sensory-motor skills to evolutionary variations on commonly shared functional designs, a significant compression of seemingly unrelated data can be achieved.

1.2. Eye Movements as a Model Sensory-Motor System

We have selected the mammalian eye movement control system to develop our theory because many workers are productively investigating this system as a model system for elaborating general principles and mechanisms of sensory-motor control (Baker and Berthoz, 1977; Fuchs and Becker, 1981; Ito, 1984; Zuber, 1981). Progress in understanding eye movements has been greatly accelerated by a fine tradition of quantitative modeling, inspired by workers like Masao Ito, David Robinson, and Larry Stark, within this field. Models of the eye movement system have rapidly progressed from formal control theory models towards neural network models (Robinson, 1973; van Gisbergen, Robinson, and Gielsen, 1981; Young and Stark, 1963) as the neural data base has expanded. Substantial conceptual progress has hereby been made towards understanding the performance characteristics of the neural components that control eye movements.

Recently it has also been increasingly appreciated that many eye movement characteristics can adaptively change. Robinson (1982) has, for example, reviewed adaptive properties of the control mechanisms of saccades, the vestibulo-ocular reflex (VOR), postural gaze, vergence, and balance behavior. A cerebellar circuit model has also been suggested to explain adaptive properties of the VOR (Fujita, 1982a, 1982b; Ito, 1982, 1984). However, adaptive models of other eye movements, notably saccades, have not been offered.

The present work grew in part out of a parallel development in the neural modelling literature. In Grossberg (1978a), some general principles and mechanisms of sensory-motor learning were articulated. The present work significantly extends this analysis within the specialized problem domain of the saccadic eye movement system. Due to our focus on learning issues, from the start we aimed at deriving a mechanistic understanding of how errors are corrected during saccadic learning. Such an approach rapidly leads to the realization that no individual neuron is able to assess the behavioral accuracy of an eye movement. The neural network as a whole needs to embody self-correcting mechanisms that can generate accurate behavior despite the ignorance of individual cells. Our central concern has been: How can neural networks learn accurate sensory-motor transformations even if the cellular parameters from which they are built may be different across individuals, may change during development, and may be altered by partial injuries throughout life?

One of the most difficult aspects of this work has been, and will continue to be, the identification of the conceptually distinct learning problems that a behaving organism must simultaneously solve in order for accurate reactive and planned movements to occur. The difficulty is due primarily to the one-to-many-to-one nature of behavior-brain relationships. Each individual sensory stimulus often generates an individual motor reaction. Between this ostensibly elementary one-to-one sensory-motor reaction lies a complex one-to-many analysis of the problem into several component parts before a many-to-one synthesis of the parts generates the observable motor reaction. Direct evidence concerning the nature of this one-to-many analysis and many-to-one synthesis can only be partially obtained using present experimental methods. Consequently, several of the basic problems which we have identified have not explicitly been described in the large literature of which we are aware. These component problems were not identified by piecing together the large mass of relevant behavioral and neural data fragments. They came into view through an analysis of the external visual and motor environment in which the eye movement neural system operates, and through actively confronting known eye movement data with known theoretical principles to test for matches and mismatches. As it turned out, in many of our theoretical circuits, known theoretical principles and mechanisms from Grossberg (1981, 1982a) could be developed, adapted, and refined to accomplish the requisite specialized tasks. This fact strengthens our conviction that there do exist general neural design principles and mechanisms, that some of them are already known, and that knowing them can enable a seemingly impossible set of problems to be reduced to a set of difficult but tractable problems.

As we have performed this reduction during the past six years, sensory-motor data and empirical models have been converging towards a greater appreciation of the importance of adaptive constraints upon neural designs. We therefore hope that this monograph will be viewed as a timely stimulus for focusing and amplifying efforts to understand the role which adaptive constraints play on the design of neural circuitry.

The previous discussion indicates why our theoretical analysis has been carried out simultaneously on several levels: behavioral and functional; anatomical; neurophysiological; and mathematical. The remaining sections of this chapter outline in intuitive language some of the major learning problems that need to be solved. Such intuitive language is not powerful enough either to identify or to solve all of the relevant problems. The language and concepts of nonlinear systems of differential equations are needed to do this. An intuitive description is, however, rich enough to clarify the nature of the problems and the scope of their solutions. With this intuitive description clearly in view, the reader can explore our detailed solutions of each separate problem, and its bearing on known and predicted interdisciplinary data, without losing the forest in the trees, or even worse, as we necessarily approach the level of a parametric mechanistic understanding, without losing the forest in the twigs and the leaves.

1.3. Intermodality Circular Reactions: Learning Gated by Comparison of Target Position with Present Position

Our starting point concerns an issue that is not discussed in the traditional eye movement literature (Grossberg, 1978a, Sections 48-51). This issue sets the stage for understanding the types of computations that are carried out within the eye movement system, as well as for understanding how eye movement commands can map onto movement commands for other sensory-motor modalities.

When an observer looks at an object, how does the observer's hand know where to move in order to touch the object? How is a transformation between the parameters of the eye-head system and the hand-arm system learned? Piaget (1963) has provided a deep insight into this learning process using his concept of a *circular reaction*. Imagine that an infant's hand makes a series of unconditional movements, which the infant's eyes unconditionally follow. As the hand occupies a variety of positions that the eye fixates upon, a transformation is learned from the parameters of the hand-arm system to the parameters of the eye-head system. To paraphrase Piaget's concept, we say that a circular reaction occurs when the *inverse transformation* from parameters of the eye-head system to parameters of the hand-arm system is also learned. This inverse map enables an observer to intentionally move its hand to a visually determined position.

How do the eye-head and hand-arm systems know what parameters are the correct ones to map upon one another? Not all positions which the eye-head system or the hand-arm system assume are the correct positions to associate. For example, suppose that the hand momentarily rests at a given position and that the eye quickly moves to foveate the hand. An infinite number of positions are assumed by the eyes as they move to foveate the hand. Only the final or intended position of the eye-head system is a correct position to associate with the position of the hand-arm system.

Learning of a circular reaction must thus be prevented except when the eye-head system and the hand-arm system are near their intended positions. Otherwise, all possible positions of the two systems could be associated with each other, thereby leading to a chaotic result.

How does the eye-head system know when it is close to its intended position? This discrimination can be made if the eye-head system can compute its present position, and can compare its intended position with its present position. The eye-head system has evidence that it is close to its intended position when a good match exists between these two types of information. Several important conclusions follow.

A. *Reciprocal Associative Transformations between Target Position Maps*

The first conclusion recapitulates and emphasizes the main insight of the circular reaction concept. Each adaptive sensory-motor system, such as the eye-head system and the hand-arm system, computes a representation, or map, of target positions. Such target positions may also be called intended positions or terminal motor positions, depending upon one's personal tastes.

B. *Matching of Target Position with Present Position*

Each adaptive sensory-motor system also computes a representation of present position. The target position is matched against the present position. During a movement, a fixed target position may be stored while changing present positions are matched against it. A central problem is to characterize the nature of this matching process. Target positions are *phasic* commands that can be switched on or off through time. For example, at times when a sensory-motor system is at rest, or in a postural mode, no target position whatsoever need be active in the system. By contrast, present position commands are *tonic* commands that are always on, since muscles are always in one or another position. How does one match phasic target position commands with tonic present position commands without causing spurious effects?

C. *Intermodality Map Learning is Gated by Intramodality Matching*

One such spurious effect is prevented by restricting the conditions under which intermodality learning takes place between target position maps (Figure 1.1). We assume that an active target position within the eye-head target position map can be associated with an active target position within the hand-arm system only at times when the target position approximately matches the present position. A *gating* signal is thus controlled by the network that matches target position with present position. This gating signal enables learning to occur when a good match occurs and prevents learning from ocurring when a bad match occurs.

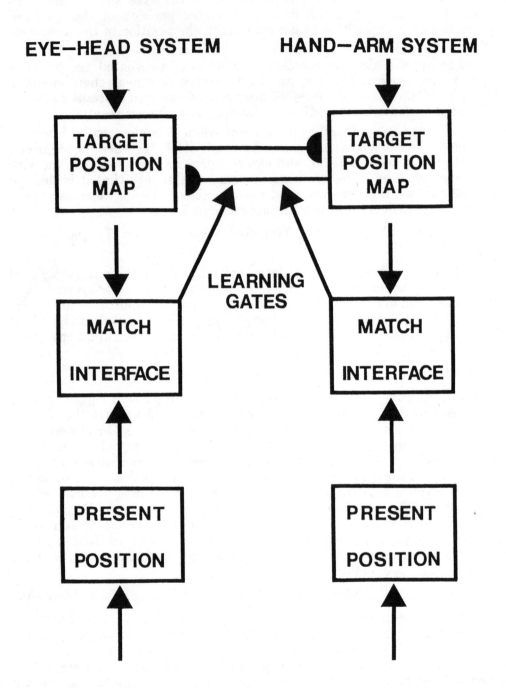

Figure 1.1. Learning intermodal circular reactions: Learning is gated by signals which are sensitive to how well target position matches present position within each modality.

D. *Dimensional Consistency: Head Coordinate Maps*

In order to compare target positions with present positions, both types of data must be computed in the same coordinate system. One cannot compare apples with oranges in neural networks any more than one can in any other scientific endeavor. Within a neural network, what one even means by a coordinate system is a deep issue that requires a systematic analysis. Some of the new problems that we have discovered have arisen from such an analysis. The conclusions of the previous paragraphs were derived without considering the coordinates in which the target positions and present positions are computed. An analysis of possible coordinates supplies important, and surprising, new information.

The present position of the eyes is computed with respect to head coordinates. By head coordinates we mean the following. The eyes rotate in their orbits with respect to the head. The directions in which the eyes point are determined by the amounts of contraction of the extraocular muscles (Figure 1.2). Signals either from the brain to the eye muscles (outflow) or from the eye muscles to the brain (inflow) could, in principle, be used to determine these directions. In either case, the eyes' present positions are computed relative to their position in the head.

As we noted above, in order to compare target positions with present positions, both types of data need to be computed in the same coordinates. Consequently, the target positions of the eye-head system are also computed in head coordinates. This conclusion has far-reaching implications.

1.4. Learning a Target Position Map

An analysis of intermodality circular reactions led to the conclusion that target positions of the eye movement system are computed in head coordinates. This section summarizes issues concerned with building up target position maps in head coordinates. When a light activates a retinal position, we say that it is registered in retinal coordinates. By Section 1.3, the position of a light in retinal coordinates is transformed into a target position computed in head coordinates in order to compute sensory-motor matches. Since this is true for all the possible retinal and target positions that can be activated by lights, we speak of transforming a retinal *map* into a target position *map*.

A. *A Many-To-One Transform*

A target position map is computed from combinations of visual and motor signals; namely, from the position of a light on the retina (visual) and the direction in which the eyeball is pointing in its head-anchored orbit (motor) before a saccade occurs. Many visual and motor positions correspond to a single target position. In other words, this transformation from retinal coordinates to head coordinates is many-to-one. For example, let a light hit the retina at θ degrees to the right of the fovea, and let the fovea point ϕ degrees to the right of its straight-ahead position (Figure 1.3). Many combinations of θ and ϕ correspond to the same target position

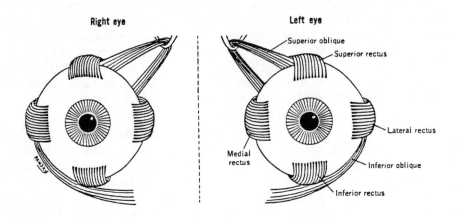

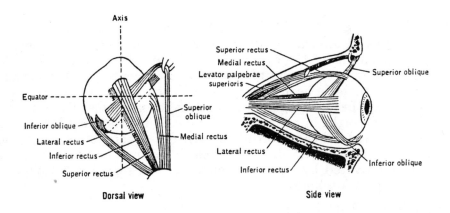

Figure 1.2. Each eye is moved by three agonist-antagonist pairs of extraocular muscles.

μ. A fixed value of μ determines a prescribed egocentric position of the light with respect to the head.

B. *Map Invariance*

This many-to-one relationship raises the general question of *map invariance*: How are command maps built up so that many combinations of input signals can all correspond to a single invariant map position? This question can also be asked in a language that is more familiar in linguistics or artificial intelligence: How can globally consistent *rules* emerge from locally ignorant components?

C. *A Multimodal Map*

Another aspect of the problem derives from the fact that we must transform "apples into oranges" to build up these invariants. That is, the signals to an invariant map often encode different kinds of input information (e.g., visual and motor) into yet another kind of output information (e.g., target position). The problem is to find a common dynamical language into which these diverse informational components can be expressed. Otherwise stated, the problem is to analyze invariant *multimodal* maps or rules.

D. *Error-Tolerance and Map Learning*

How can an *error-tolerant* invariant map get built up from such diverse types of information? The visual and motor systems of living creatures are constructed from many components, each of which may be error-prone. Individual differences in the parameters of these components can also occur due to fluctuations in developmental conditions or due to partial injuries throughout life. In order for an error-tolerant map to be generated from such variable components, some sort of self-organization, notably a self-correcting learning capability, is needed. Thus our problem is to design *self-organizing* invariant multimodal maps.

Invariance means that many combinations of visual and motor inputs can correspond to a single target position output. Expressed slightly differently, a *single* visual input is paired with many motor inputs to sweep out all the target position outputs to which that visual input contributes. A *single* motor input is paired with many visual inputs to sweep out all the target position outputs to which that motor input contributes. Within the context of a self-organizing system, this property of one-many pairing raises two more serious issues.

E. *Self-Consistent Map Learning*

The main issue concerns the possibility of learning a *self-contradictory rule*. A one-many pairing is needed to self-organize an invariant map, but how do each of these pairings encode its own correct invariant position without suffering from interference from all the other pairings in which each input participates?

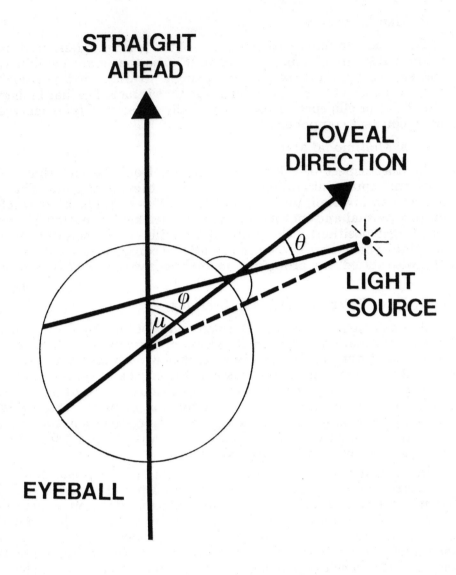

Figure 1.3. Geometry of eye position measured with respect to the head and retinotopic position measured with respect to the fovea: Angle ϕ measures eye position and angle θ measures retinotopic position. Angle μ measures position of the light source with respect to the head.

F. *A Self-Regulating Map*

Another aspect of this one-many issue concerns the question of "how many?". It would be absurd if a map could form in which each motor position is paired with 1000 visual positions, but as soon as it is paired with 1005 visual positions a self-contradiction arises within the system. The map should be able to form in response to a wide range of set sizes from which the inputs are drawn. Varying the set size spanned by the map inputs causes the set size spanned by the map outputs to also vary. Unless map self-organization is an unstable process, the invariant "form" of the map should be independent of its "size". This is the problem of *self-regulation*, which is one of the most important problems of developmental biology. Thus our problem is to understand self-organization of an invariant *self-regulating* multimodal map.

A finer aspect of the self-regulation issue concerns the number, or dimension, of input sources that combine to define a single intended position. We have spoken of a "visual input" and a "motor input". Each of these input channels can, however, be composed of several input pathways, or coordinates. For example, each visual input might be broken up into horizontal and vertical coordinates, or radial and angular coordinates, etc. Each motor input might be broken up into several individual motor inputs that correspond to all the components of the affected motor organ. Thus the self-regulation property includes not only the size of individual input fields, but also the number of input fields that cooperate to define each invariant position.

We will describe several different, but closely related, networks in which an invariant self-regulating multimodal map can form. Each of these networks is compatible with neural data and leads to testable predictions for future experiments. In such an invariant target position map, a single population v_μ can be activated by any of the many pairings of visual positions θ and of motor positions ϕ that correspond to the same target position μ. We will also show how a neural network as a whole can act *as if* it possesses an invariant target position map, whereas in actuality it only possesses maps of visual positions θ and of motor positions ϕ, or of noninvariant pairs (θ, ϕ) of all possible visual and motor positions. In order to understand how these different types of networks work, it is necessary to further analyze how target position commands are transformed into observable movements.

1.5. From Multimodal Target Map to Unimodal Motor Map

Information concerning one stage in this transformation can be acquired by considering the question of coordinates in greater detail. Section 1.3 suggested that target positions are compared with present positions in order to gate the learning of circular reactions. Target positions are partly derived from visual signals due to lights on the retina. By contrast, present positions of the eye within the head are described in motor coordinates. A fundamental calibration problem thus needs to be solved before the network can begin the comparison between target positions and present positions. A visually-derived target position needs to be transformed into motor coordinates so that it can be compared with present position signals that are also computed in motor coordinates. Obviously this transformation must be learned. Otherwise, we would have to conclude that all visual and motor parameters are calibrated with essentially perfect precision by a genetically pre-wired control of all developmental stages.

This learned transformation replaces one representation of target position (the visually-activated one) with another representation of target position (the motor one). Such a transformation involves both a change of map *coordinates* and a change of map *dimension*: The visually activated target position map possesses at least as many topographically distinct populations as there are discriminable lights on the retina. By contrast, the extra-ocular muscles, like many muscle systems, are organized into agonist-antagonist pairs. Each eye is moved by just three pairs of muscles. The present position of each eye can thus be characterized by six quantities. The transformation from visually-activated coordinates to motor coordinates replaces a large number of distinct map locations by arrays, or patterns, of six numbers. Such a transformation replaces complex and abstract combinations of multimodal information by simple and concrete arrays of unimodal motor information.

1.6. Vector Maps from Comparisons of Target Position Maps and Present Position Maps

The previous section noted that visually-derived target position commands need to be transformed into motor coordinates before they can be matched with present position commands that are also computed in motor coordinates. Our theory shows how the *same* network that learns this coordinate change *also* computes the match between target positions and present positions. We call this important network the *head-muscle interface*, or HMI.

The HMI has yet another important property. The degree of mismatch between a target position and a present position generates a motor code that can be used to accurately move the eyes. We conclude that a fundamental calibration problem that is solved through learning automatically generates properties that are necessary for skilled performance.

The degree of mismatch in the HMI represents a "vector difference" that compares the target position of the eye with its present position. This difference between target position and present position encodes how far and in what direction the eyes are to move. When the target position equals its present position, the vector difference equals zero, and no eye movement command is generated. By contrast, large mismatches between target position and present position represent commands to generate large saccadic movements.

1.7. Automatic Compensation for Present Position: Code Compression

The mismatches, or vectors, that are computed within the HMI harmonize two ostensibly conflicting design constraints. An analysis of circular reactions shows that *intermodality* sensory-motor commands are encoded as target positions. Target positions are not, however, sufficient to generate *intramodality* commands. In response to the same target position command, the eye needs to move different distances and directions depending upon its present position when the target position is registered. The HMI vectors automatically compensate for such changes in present position within each modality. They carry out this task in addition to gating associative learning of target position maps between modalities.

Two different types of data are manipulated by the HMI. Target position maps encode motor expectations or intended movements. They represent where the system wants to go. They are encoded and stored by the system long enough to execute the intended movement. They are thus switched on and off with an approximately digital, or logical, characteristic. By contrast, present position signals monitor the present state of the eye. Although they remain on tonically, they change continuously as the eye moves.

Using these two types of information, a *single* target position command can be rapidly transformed into *many* different movement trajectories due to the automatic compensation for present position that is encoded by the HMI vectors. This combination of mechanisms accomplishes a tremendous reduction in the number of commands that need to be stored. The network does not have to store many different movement trajectories with arbitrary initial and terminal positions, as inverse kinematic approaches to movement control would conclude (Brody and Paul, 1984). It does not have to map many different trajectories in one modality into many different trajectories in another modality. Instead, it computes maps of target positions. Such maps do not encode whole trajectories. They encode only the terminal positions of these trajectories. Terminal positions are mapped into terminal positions across modalities. Within each modality, terminal positions are mapped into motor coordinates via a learned transformation. By automatically compensating for present position, this transformation generates a code that can accurately control all possible movement trajectories.

1.8. Outflow versus Inflow in the Registration of Present Position

The need to solve additional learning problems becomes clear by considering possible sources of present position signals to the HMI. Two general types of present position signals have been acknowledged in discussions of motor control: *outflow* signals and *inflow* signals. Figure 1.4 schematizes the difference between these signal sources. An outflow signal carries a command from the brain to a muscle (Figure 1.4a). Signals that

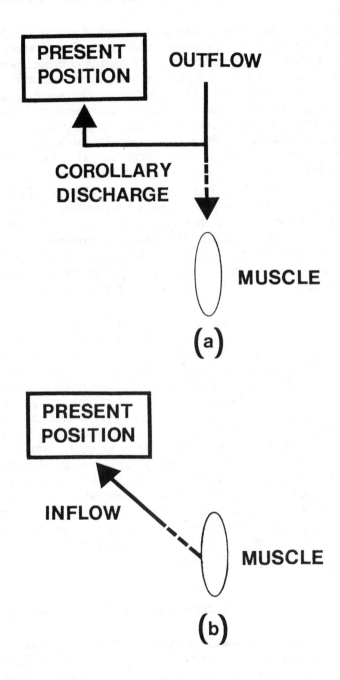

Figure 1.4. Outflow and inflow as sources of present position signals: (a) A source of outflow signals to a muscle branches to give rise to a corollary discharge; (b) A muscle gives rise to proprioceptive inflow signals.

branch off from the direct brain-to-muscle pathway in order to register present position are traditionally called *corollary discharges*. An inflow signal carries a command from a muscle to the brain (Figure 1.4b). Experimental evidence for both outflow and inflow involvement in motor control has accumulated over the years. Many of these tests aim to understand how the visual world achieves its apparent stability despite the fact that an observer's eyes are continually in motion (Epstein, 1977). A primary difference between outflow and inflow is that an outflow signal is triggered only when an observer's brain generates a movement command. By contrast, an inflow signal can be generated by a passive movement of the eye.

Helmholtz (1962) dramatized this difference by recommending that an observer jiggle his eyeball with a finger. The world seems to move due to these externally induced eye movements. By contrast, when an observer generates eye movements using brain-evoked signals, the world does not seem to move, even if an equivalent amount of visual movement is registered on the retina using the two procedures. This demonstration suggests that corollary discharges, rather than inflow signals, are used to compensate for self-induced movements in this situation. This conclusion follows from the fact that, if inflow signals are generated at all, they may be assumed to be generated whether an eye movement is internally or externally caused. Only when the eye movements are internally caused, however, does the brain compensate for the amount of visual movement that is due to the eye movement.

Although this type of demonstration strongly implicates corollary discharges as a source of present position signals, it does not imply that inflow signals play no role in the computation of present position. Since the pioneering works of Ruffini (1898) and Sherrington (1894), a large literature concerning inflow contributions to motor control has accumulated. Disentangling the different roles played by outflow and inflow signals has remained one of the major problems in the sensory-motor field.

1.9. Corollary Discharges and Calibration of Muscle Plant Contractions

Further insight about the roles of outflow and inflow can be achieved by considering the following facts. One role of an outflow signal is to move the eyes by contracting extraocular muscles (Figure 1.4a). However, the laws that govern the muscle plant are not known *a priori* to the outflow source. In particular, it is not known *a priori* how much the muscle will contract in response to an outflow signal of prescribed size. It is also not known how much the eyeball will rotate in response to a prescribed muscle contraction. Moreover, even if the system somehow knew this information at one time, it might turn out to be the wrong information at a later time. The muscle characteristics can change as they grow during development. They can also change as the body ages, or due to partial accidents, such as minor muscle tears or rupture of blood vessel capillaries.

These problems are serious ones even if the muscle contracts as a *linear* function of outflow signal size. A linear muscle plant's contraction is proportional to the size of the outflow signal. Linearity does not, however, guarantee that the proportionality constant, or *gain*, is neither tiny nor huge. What if the largest outflow signals could hardly move the eyes at all? What if even the smallest outflow signals could point the eyes in extreme nasal or temporal directions? A reasonable choice of muscle gain does not solve the problem of calibrating muscle responses if the muscle plant is nonlinear. Then the muscle contraction is not proportional to the outflow signal, so that doubling the outflow signal does not even double the amount of contraction, no matter how the gain is chosen.

These remarks illustrate that the relationship between the size of an outflow command and the amount of muscle contraction is, in principle, undeterminable without some type of additional information. This additional information must, explicitly or implicitly, characterize the muscle plant's response to outflow signals. To accomplish this, the system needs to compute a reliable measure of an outflow command as well as a reliable measure of the muscle's response to that command.

Corollary discharges provide a reliable measure of outflow commands (Figure 1.4a). In particular, corollary discharges are computed using signal sizes that the outflow pathway is capable of generating. The muscle responses to these signals may, however, initially be much too large, much too small, or even nonlinear, due to the characteristics of the muscle plant. In order to convert outflow signals into a full range of linear muscle contractions, somehow the brain needs to eventually adjust the responses of the muscle plant to these outflow signals. Such adjustments have the effect of causing the muscle to respond as if it were a different plant, notably a linear plant with a carefully chosen gain. From the start, outflow signals form a reliable basis on which to compute present position at the HMI. Inflow signals, whose plant characteristics are susceptible to continual change, do not.

1.10. Outflow-Inflow Pattern Matches and Linearization of Muscle Responses: Automatic Gain Control

The use of corollary discharges to compute present position at the HMI does not imply that inflow signals are not used. In fact, we argued in Section 1.9 that some type of information about muscle plant characteristics is needed to calibrate muscle contractions that veridically respond to outflow signals. We suggest that a brain region exists wherein comparisons between outflow and inflow signals are used for this purpose. We call this region the *outflow-inflow interface*, or OII.

The need for inflow data can be appreciated through the following arguments. How does the outflow system determine whether an outflow signal *should* cause a large or a small muscle contraction? Expressed in another way, how does the outflow system determine whether an outflow signal of a fixed size is large or small from a functional viewpoint? How big is "big"? What are the system's computational units?

An answer can be seen by recalling that outflow signals are computed in muscle coordinates, namely in agonist-antagonist coordinates. An outflow signal to its agonist muscle is "big" if the outflow signal to the corresponding antagonist muscle is "small." The *relative* sizes of agonist and antagonist outflow signals, not any absolute quantity, determine the desired size scale. Expressed in another way, the *spatial pattern*, or *normalized motor synergy*, of agonist and antagonist outflow signals determines the functional size scale.

If outflow signal sizes are computed in muscle coordinates, then the information which expresses the muscle plant's responses to these signals must also be computed in muscle coordinates. The simplest way to accomplish this is to use length-sensitive inflow signals from the muscles themselves.

This argument suggests that spatial patterns of outflow signals are matched against spatial patterns of inflow signals at the OII. Good matches imply that the muscles are responding linearly, and with a reasonable gain, to outflow signals. Bad matches must be able to adjust plant gain as well as plant nonlinearities. We will show in Chapter 5 how mismatches within the OII generate error signals that can change the size of the total outflow signal to the muscle plant. The conditionable part of the total outflow signal adds or subtracts the correct amount of signal to make the muscle react *as if* it is a linear muscle plant with a reasonable gain. The muscle plant does not itself change. Rather, automatic gain control signals compensate for its imperfections through learning. If the muscle plant changes due to aging or accidents, mismatches are caused within the OII and trigger new learning. The gain control signals automatically alter the total outflow command until the muscle again reacts linearly. Thus the linearization of the muscle plant is a learning process that takes place on a slower time scale than registration of a corollary discharge.

Throughout all of these learned changes, the corollary discharges to the OII remain intact. The system can compensate for plant changes without disrupting the code whereby present position is internally calibrated. Thus whereas outflow is used to rapidly change present position signals, inflow is used to drive slow recalibrations of the muscle response characteristics to these signals.

1.11. Motor Vectors Calibrated by Visual Error Signals

Linearizing the muscle plant's response to outflow signals does not ensure that the eye can move to accurately foveate a target light. Plant linearization just ensures that *if* outflow commands of correct size can be learned, then the muscles can faithfully execute these commands. Muscle inflow signals are certainly not the type of error signals that can determine whether the eye has foveated a target light.

A light on the retina is transformed by several processing stages before it can generate an outflow command to move the eye. Whether or not the eye successfully moves to foveate the light cannot be decided until the net effect of all these stages actually moves the eye. A reliable test of whether the light is foveated is given by the position of the light on the retina after the movement is over. Visual error signals are thus a reliable basis for modifying the sizes of outflow signals until the eye can successfully foveate target lights.

In Section 1.6, we concluded that a neural vector, by encoding the difference between a target position and the eye's present position, can be used to move the eye the correct distance and direction in order to foveate a retinal light. This conclusion did not specify how these vectors are transformed into correctly calibrated outflow commands. Two aspects of how this is done can now be noted.

The neural vectors within the HMI are encoded in muscle coordinates. Each neural vector is an activity pattern across a fixed set of muscle-coded cell populations. Changing neural vectors does not change *which* populations are activated. It only alters the patterning of this activity. How can a visual error signal *selectively* change the gains of different outflow commands if all of the vectors which generate these commands activate the same HMI populations?

A way is found by noticing that visual error signals are registered in retinotopic coordinates. Should not the HMI vectors be transformed into retinotopic coordinates in order to be dimensionally compatible with the visual error signals? If the HMI vectors are transformed from motor coordinates into retinotopic coordinates, then our problem is greatly simplified. Each motor vector would then excite a different location within a retinotopic map. Different retinotopically coded positions could control different outflow pathways, and their gains could therefore be separately altered by different visual error signals. A deeper reason for this vector transformation from motor coordinates to retinotopic coordinates will be described in Chapter 4.

When we say that a non-foveated light on the retina can act as a visual error signal, we mean that this visual signal somehow changes the outflow command into one that can generate a more accurate movement on the next performance trial. Such an outflow command controls a coordinated reaction, or synergy, of all the eye muscles. To solve this learning problem, one must therefore discover how a single light on the retina can alter an entire motor synergy. We will show in Chapter 3 how this can be accomplished. As mentioned above, a vector command is first transformed from motor coordinates into retinotopic coordinates. Then the vector command and its visual error signal are reconverted into motor coordinates in such a way that the visual error signal can correct the gains of all the relevant motor outflow signals.

1.12. Postural Stability: Separate Calibration of Muscle Length and Tension

The previous discussion suggests that several learning problems must be solved in order for the eyes to accurately foveate visual targets. Later chapters of the book will uncover and suggest solutions for subproblems and related problems that are not easily discerned without using a more mechanistic approach. All of these solutions are needed to understand how the eye moves reactively in response to retinal lights.

After the outflow command that determines a saccadic movement is over, how does the control system guarantee that the eye does not continue to move? What prevents the eye from drifting in its orbit in the absence of active saccadic commands? In other words, after movement is over, how is a stable posture assured?

This is a serious problem because the forces on the eyeball and on the extraocular muscles change rapidly as a saccadic movement terminates. Often the antagonist muscle relaxes while the agonist muscle is contracting (Bahill and Stark, 1979). This arrangement permits rapid motion to occur with a minimum of resistance from the antagonist muscle. By contrast, after the movement is over, the forces exerted by the agonist and antagonist muscles must be balanced in order to prevent large post-saccadic drifts from occurring. A new learning problem must thus be solved. It can be formulated as follows.

Any physically realizable position can be assumed by the eye muscles (Figure 1.5). Thus all possible combinations of agonist-antagonist muscle lengths can correspond to the final positions of saccades. At posture, the tensions of all agonist-antagonist muscle pairs must be equal. For *any* realizable combination of agonist-antagonist muscle *lengths*, how can *equal* tensions of agonist and antagonist muscles be generated in the postural mode?

This problem raises a number of new issues. How does the control system know when it is in the postural mode? How does it know whether the eye is drifting during this mode? If the control system could not tell the difference between the movement mode and the postural mode, then saccadic movements due to correct outflow commands could be misinterpreted as post-saccadic drifts, thereby leading to spurious "corrections" of already correct movement commands. What signals are used as the error signals to correct such a postural drift? How can these error signals balance the tensions of agonist and antagonist muscles without disrupting the correct lengths that were learned using visual error signals? We will conclude in Chapter 8 that visual error signals are also used to correct post-saccadic drifts. These visual error signals are not, however, error signals that compute how far a target light lies from the fovea. They compute the net motion of the eye with respect to the visual world during the postural mode. Visual information is, in fact, used in at least four different ways in our theory.

1.13. Planned versus Reactive Movements: The Rear View Mirror Problem

In Section 1.11, we concluded that visual error signals are used to calibrate the adaptive gains whereby the eyes can accurately foveate retinal lights. In order for this to happen, the saccadic control system must be sensitive to visual signals both before and after a visually reactive saccade occurs. We will now show why a different pattern of visual sensitivity

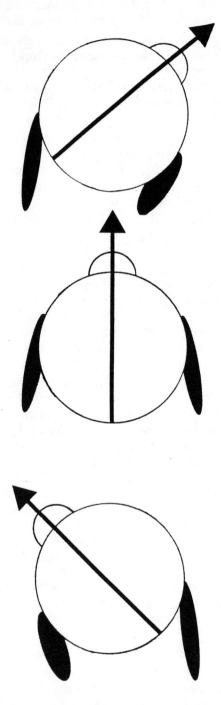

Figure 1.5. Different pairings of agonist-antagonist muscle lengths determine different positions of the eye with respect to the head.

exists when planned, or internally generated, saccades occur. Reconciling these two patterns of visual sensitivity requires additional learning circuits.

To understand this issue, imagine that you are driving your automobile, and that you wish to make a right turn when you reach a familiar corner. In order to determine whether it is safe to turn, you wish to look away from the roadway into your rear view mirror. Suppose that the dimensions of your body and car are such that looking into the rear view mirror can be accomplished by a saccadic eye movement.

Just before you make such a planned eye movement, your eyes are engaged by the flux of visual cues as seen through the windshield. In order to look away from the visual flux, your sensitivity to visual cues needs to be suppressed. Otherwise, the visual cues could command your attention. The initiation of a planned saccade thus requires the suppression of sensitivity to the visual cues that generate reactive saccades.

In order to make an accurate planned saccade, however, the adaptive gains that were learned in response to visual error signals must be used. We can now state the main issue: How do planned movements benefit from parameters that were learned during reactive movements, yet suppress the sensory signals that are needed to learn reactive movements? How can you have your parameters and suppress them too? This issue suggests that the command system which controls planned saccades is not the same as the command system which controls visually reactive saccades, yet that the reactive system can lend its learned parameters to the planned system *at the same time* that visual inputs to the reactive system are suppressed.

1.14. Attentional Gating

The distinction between planned movements and reactive movements raises the more general issue of attentional control. The decision to make a planned movement instead of a visually reactive movement involves a sensitivity shift that may be interpreted as a shift of attention. Even within the visually reactive system, many light sources can compete to be chosen as the targets for a saccadic movement. In order to understand how this occurs, we need to analyse how neural sensitivity can be modulated by sensory and learned factors, how a decision can quickly be made among many possible targets, and how all of these factors can be computed within the same coordinate system.

1.15. Intermodality Interactions in a Head Coordinate Frame

The last question brings us full circle back to the study of head, or egocentric, coordinates. Two types of arguments support the conclusion that attentional decisions take place within a head coordinate frame. The first argument is based upon the observation that sensory cues other than visual cues, notably auditory cues, can compete to be sources of saccadic movements. The second argument is based upon an analysis of the coordinate system within which planned movements are computed.

The first argument arises from a consideration of how intermodality sources of saccadic commands are adaptively calibrated. Section 1.11 pointed out that a retinally activated network for eliciting saccades is needed so that retinal fixation errors can be used to improve future saccadic accuracy via learning. How are accurate saccades in response to a source of sound, or to other nonvisual sources of sensory signals, generated? From what learning mechanisms do these alternative sources of saccadic commands derive their accuracy?

The contrast between visually and auditorily elicited saccades is particularly instructive. In the case of a visually evoked saccade, visual feedback can be used to correct saccadic parameters, because a target light on the retina can act as an error signal after the saccade occurs. This is true even if the head remains stationary throughout the saccade. A saccade to a sound source can also occur while the head remains stationary throughout the saccade. In this situation, however, no obvious source of auditory error signals exists, because the location of the auditory sound source does not change with respect to the head as a result of the saccadic eye movement. If no source of auditory error signals exists in this situation, then how do the eyes learn to accurately saccade towards a sound?

This lack of auditory error signals does not cause a problem if the auditory system can make use of the saccadic command pathways that have been adaptively tuned by visual error signals. Such an intermodality sharing of common pathways not only overcomes a problem of principle, but also significantly reduces the amount of adaptive machinery that is needed to improve the accuracy of intermodality saccades.

Intermodality sharing of retinally activated saccadic command pathways can be achieved if there exists a processing stage at which signals generated by auditory cues feed into visually calibrated saccadic command pathways. Then auditory cues can use the visually learned saccadic parameters by activating these visually calibrated commands. In order for auditory cues to effectively share visually tuned parameters, the overlapping intermodality maps must be dimensionally compatible. That is, if the maps represent coordinate systems with different invariant properties, then no consistent intermodality command structure can be learned. Thus in order to align intermodality coordinate systems, auditory and visual cues must be suitably preprocessed before they are mapped onto retinally activated pathways.

What type of auditory preprocessing is needed? Every auditory cue is registered with respect to head coordinates. An important example of such a head coordinate map has recently been worked out in the barn owl (Knudsen, 1984; Konishi, 1984; Sullivan and Konishi, 1984; Takahashi, Moiseff, and Konishi, 1984). By contrast, a light that is presented to a fixed retinal position determines a different position in head coordinates each time the initial eye position is changed. In order to align the two types of maps, either the auditory cue in head coordinates needs to be transformed into an auditory cue in retinotopic coordinates by compensating for changes in initial eye position, or the visual cue in retinotopic coordinates needs to be transformed into a visual cue in head coordinates. Visual cues are computed both in retinotopic coordinates and in head coordinates, in order to learn circular reactions (Section 1.3). Since auditory cues are directly registered in head coordinates, a learned mapping of auditory signals onto a visually derived head coordinate map would achieve the most parsimonious solution of this problem (Figure 1.6). Considerations other than parsimony will be used to strengthen this conclusion in the next section. However, the possibility cannot be ignored that different animals have evolved according to different evolutionary strategies in order to make intermodality map comparisons dimensionally compatible.

1.16. Head Coordinate Maps Encode Predictive Saccades

In order to ensure dimensional consistency, planned saccades and reactive saccades due to all relevant sensory modalities need to compete with each other within the same coordinate frame.

The need for a head coordinate map is also suggested by considering series of planned saccades, which we call predictive saccades, or the generation of predictive saccades within a more general motor program, such as a dance. A sequence of accurate saccades that occurs in response to the prior occurrence of a spatial or temporal pattern of lights illustrates predictive saccades that are responsive to controllable lights. For example, if a regular pattern of lights is briefly flashed in front of a human observer, the observer's saccadic eye movements can rapidly track the positions of the lights even after the lights are shut off (Kowler, personal communication). Hallett and Lightstone (1976) presented human subjects with two light flashes in sequence: one before a saccade and one during a saccade. In some cases subjects responded with two saccades after the second light presentation; the first to the first flash's spatial position and the second to the second flash's spatial position. Since the second saccade makes allowance for the size of the preceding saccade it cannot be based on retinal position alone. In what coordinate frame are the commands for such predictive saccades encoded and executed?

To clarify the main issues, suppose for the moment that each light in a pattern is encoded in a retinotopic map before the eye moves. After the eye moves in response to the first light, a correct eye movement to the second light can be made only if the eye movement system can compensate for the eye's prior saccade. This type of compensation is not just a matter of computing a new target position by taking into account the eye's new initial position before the second saccade occurs, because the retinal position of the second light is the wrong source to initiate a motion to the desired target position. Suppose, for example, that the eyes are pointing θ degrees to the right of the straight ahead direction when two lights excite the retina at ϕ_1 and ϕ_2 degrees to the right of the fovea (Figure 1.7). Suppose that the eyes somehow move to foveate the light at the ϕ_1 degree position, thereby attaining the eye position μ. No matter how the stored retinal position ϕ_2 and the approximate present eye position μ are juggled, one does not get the desired signal that can tell the

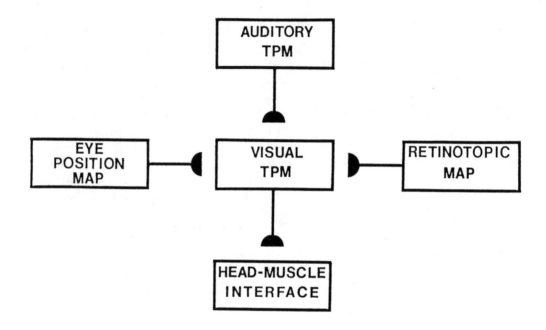

Figure 1.6. A visual target position map (TPM) receives inputs from several types of position maps before recoding its target positions into muscle coordinates at the head-muscle interface (HMI). A retinotopic map and an eye position map combine their signals at the visual TPM to implicitly define target positions there. Each TPM population can receive inputs from many retinotopic positions and eye positions. The auditory TPM can be consistently associated with the visual TPM because both are computed in head coordinates.

eyes how far they must move during the second saccade in order to foveate the second light. Both addition and subtraction of ϕ_2 and μ lead to the wrong answer.

One way to overcome this difficulty is to store the light positions in head coordinates before any saccade occurs. A predictive motion can be accurately made if the stored position of the second light with respect to the head is compared with the present position of the eye with respect to the head after the first saccade is over. The vector difference $\phi_2 - \phi_1$ of these positions determines the correct direction and length of motion that the eye must make to fixate the position of the second light. Then the process repeats itself. The position of the third light with respect to the head is compared with the position of the eye with respect to the head after the second saccade is over. And so on, until all stored saccadic commands are actualized.

In order for this argument to work, all the stored lights that will control a predictive saccade sequence must be stored once and for all in a head coordinate map. After the eye moves *any number of times*, the present eye position in the head can be subtracted from the target position, in head coordinates, that is coded by the next stored command. This "difference vector" represents the motion that will acquire the desired target location, if all possible calibration problems that are tacit in these statements can be solved.

These problems require the consideration of new issues. In addition to being able to simultaneously store all the predictive commands in a head coordinate map, the network that regulates predictive saccades must be able to store the commands in a way that reflects their temporal order, and must eliminate these command sources as their corresponding saccades are executed to make way for the next command in the series. A network that processes these storage, temporal order, reset, and calibration properties is described in Chapter 9.

Another possible way to encode difference vectors is to simultaneously store all retinotopic positions, such as ϕ_1 and ϕ_2, and to compute difference vectors $\phi_2 - \phi_1$ directly from the stored retinotopic values. Such a procedure seems very simple when it is stated without regard to how such vectors are recoded into movement commands expressed in motor coordinates. When such issues of coordinate transformation and calibration are studied, it emerges that a direct mapping from retinotopic values into difference vectors is more difficult to achieve than an indirect mapping from retinotopic values into head coordinates, followed by a comparison with present position. This problem is compounded by the fact that retinotopic coordinates are not invariant under eye movements, and are not suitable for intermodality comparisons, such as those which control eye-head and hand-arm coordination. We will therefore develop transformations from retinotopic into head coordinates, but will also describe in Section 9.10 the problems that need to be solved in order for direct recoding of retinotopic into vector coordinates to be effective.

The above discussion indicates that planned saccadic commands are

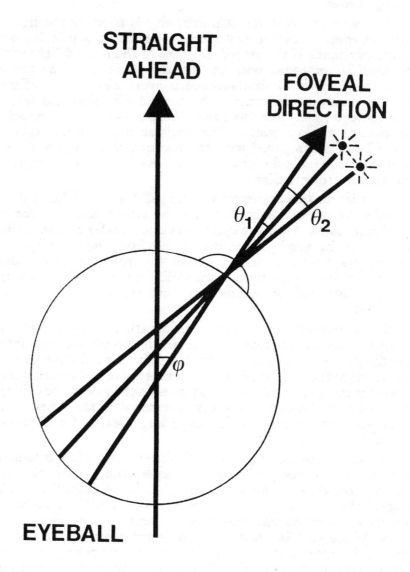

Figure 1.7. Two light sources, at retinotopic positions of θ_1° and θ_2° with respect to the fovea, are encoded in retinotopic coordinates while the eye points ϕ° with respect to the head.

initiated from command maps that are computed in head coordinates. Auditory sources of saccadic commands are directly entered into a head coordinate map due to the fixed positions of the ears in the head. When a saccade is initiated by sources of light, the transformation of retinal coordinates into head coordinates adds onto the retinal coordinates the effects of variable initial eye positions, and is thus analogous to a vector addition. The process whereby a target command in head coordinates is compared with present eye position transforms the head coordinate command into a retinotopic command. This transformation from head coordinates to retinotopic coordinates is analogous to a vector subtraction.

In all, a light that generates a planned saccade undergoes a coordinate transformation from a retinal coordinate map into a target position map in head coordinates before being reconverted into a retinotopic map via operations analogous to vector addition and vector subtraction, respectively. This reciprocal transformation, which seems quite pointless out of context, enables the saccadic system to make the decisions and calibrations that balance between visually reactive, intermodal, intentional, and predictive movement commands.

1.17. The Relationship between Macrotheory and Microtheory

The remainder of the monograph describes three types of information: the functional problems that are solved by an adaptive sensory-motor system such as the ballistic eye movement system; behavioral and neural data that are relevant to these functional problems; and the formal circuits that we propose as neural network solutions of the functional problems. In order to characterize the properties of these formal circuits, we use a combination of mathematical arguments and computer simulations.

The chapters are organized within the goal of maximizing the accessibility of the theoretical ideas. Each chapter therefore begins with a functional analysis and a description of relevant data. Technical details are developed towards the end of each chapter. Thus a feeling for most of the functional arguments can be acquired without the need to follow too many technical details. The mathematical definitions of the circuits are, however, needed to even state some of the concepts. This is true because of the following considerations.

Both the functional and the formal arguments need to be made on two levels: a Macrotheory level and a Microtheory level. These two aspects of the theory coexist in a mutually supportive relationship. The Macrotheory consists of several design principles, dynamical laws, and macrocircuits whose stages compute functionally characterized properties. The Microtheory describes the microcircuits that generate the properties of the various stages. Unlike many artificial intelligence models, the Macrotheory and the Microtheory cannot easily be dissociated. This is because the critical properties at the stages are interactive, or emergent, properties of the Microtheory's processes. Even the apparently local concept of feature detector is the net effect of widespread interactions within a Microtheory network.

The Microtheory thus does not freely invent properties at each macrostage. Each process of the Microtheory generates a formal grouping of interactive properties in response to prescribed external input and internal system constraints. The intrinsic structuring of these groupings defines the Macrotheory properties and is the source of the theory's predictive force. The Macrotheory's general principles and laws severely constrain the types of microprocesses that are allowed to take place at any stage. Only a few principles and laws are used in the entire theory, despite its broad intermodality scope.

A preliminary understanding of Macrotheory circuits can be arrived at from general functional arguments. Consequently, Macrotheory descriptions tend to accompany functional arguments at the beginning of each chapter. The actual transformations that solve the functional problems can, however, only be defined and understood by an analysis of Microtheory mechanisms. Thus an interplay of Macrotheory and Microtheory descriptions will necessarily permeate each chapter.

The macrocircuits that are suggested by this analysis lead to network subdivisions suggestive of such brain regions as retina, superior colliculus, peripontine reticular formation, cerebellum, parietal cortex, frontal eye fields, and oculomotor nuclei. The microcircuits that quantitatively instantiate the designs include analogs of such neuronal components as bursters, pausers, tonic cells, burst tonic cells, quasi-visual cells, Purkinje cells, mossy fibers, parallel fibers, climbing fibers, visuomovement cells, movement cells, light-sensitive cells, saccade cells, and post-saccadic cells. The properties of these circuits are used to suggest explanations of a large behavioral and neural data base in the subsequent chapters.

It remains to describe our strategy for discovering functional problems, and for ordering our exposition of these problems. We have used the *method of minimal anatomies* (Grossberg, 1974, p.69). "Given specific psychological postulates, we derive the *minimal* network...that realizes these postulates. Then we analyse the psychological and neural capabilities of this network. An important part of the analysis is to understand what the network cannot do. This knowledge often suggests what new psychological postulate is needed to derive the next, more complex network. In this way, a hierarchy of networks is derived, corresponding to ever more sophisticated postulates. This hierarchy...leads us closer to realistic anatomies, and provides us with a catalog of mechanisms to use in various situations. Moreover, once the mechanisms of a given minimal anatomy are understood, variations of this anatomy having particular advantages or disadvantages can be readily imagined." The method of minimal anatomies is thus a way to formally conceptualize successive stages in the evolution of a self-organizing system's ability to interact adaptively with different properties of its environment. By testing how simple networks succeed in adaptively solving some environmental problems but not others, a conceptual pressure is generated that points towards the designs which are needed to expand the network's total adaptive competence.

This chapter has provided a top-down view of many of the theoretical issues that the book analyses. In the subsequent chapters, we employ a bottom-up approach which is more suitable to the derivation of rigorous mechanisms. This bottom-up approach begins by considering networks that are much too simple to achieve a realistic competence. As we shall show, even these networks quickly point towards concepts capable of supporting a much more realistic theory.

CHAPTER 2
PARALLEL PROCESSING
OF MOVEMENT AND ERROR SIGNALS

2.1. Sensory-Motor Coordinates: Hemifield Gradients

A neural signal can take on behavioral meaning when it occurs in a network topography that is linked to behavioral consequences. In problems about visually-evoked eye movements, network topographies mediate between the distinct peripheral organizations of retina and extraocular muscles. Many of these topographic features are prewired to create a computational substrate whereby saccades can be initiated, so that saccadic errors can be generated and used to improve future saccadic accuracy. We will begin our discussion by considering the simplest sensory-motor map capable of initiating saccades. Then we will refine this map in several ways to incorporate increasingly sophisticated constraints governing different aspects of saccadic learning.

In the simplest example, lights hit the retina, where they are encoded in retinal coordinates. Eventually some of these lights can selectively activate the six extraocular muscles. These muscles are organized into three agonist-antagonist pairs (Figure 1.2). Thus, even in the simplest examples, a transformation from retinal coordinates to muscle coordinates is required. For definiteness, consider how a retinal signal could influence the pair of muscles controlling horizontal movements, the lateral and medial recti. A simple map that mediates between a two-dimensional retinal array and an agonist-antagonist muscle pair is depicted in Figure 2.1. The "retina" in Figure 2.1 maps topographically into a structure that is subdivided into a right and a left hemifield. A gradient of connections exists from each point of this hemifield map to the muscle pair, such that more eccentric retinal points cause more asymmetric muscle contractions. In particular, more eccentric points in the right hemifield excite the right muscle more and inhibit the left muscle more in a push-pull fashion (van Gisbergen, Robinson, and Gielen, 1981). Edwards (1980) showed evidence for a gradient of projections from superior colliculus of the cat to the oculomotor area. Horseradish peroxidase was injected into the abducens area in order to find its inputs. The results showed that along the rostral-caudal dimension of the superior colliculus the incidence of abducens directed cells gradually increased at successively more caudal levels. More caudal levels of superior colliculus represent more peripheral parts of the visual field.

If each of the three pairs of muscles derives signals from a hemifield map, then each pair determines a different hemifield axis. Figure 2.2 depicts the simplest realization of this idea: a six-sectored map that we call a *sensory-motor sector map*. Such a sector map could be prewired using relatively simple developmental mechanisms: for example, three hemifield gradients of morphogens, in much the same way as tectal coordinates are established (Hunt and Jacobson, 1972, 1973a, 1973b).

31

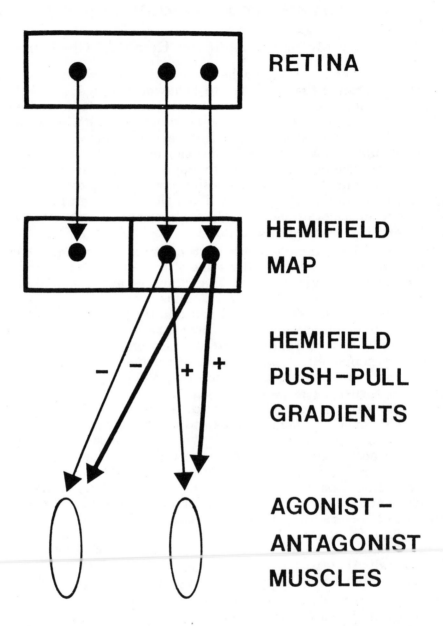

RETINA

HEMIFIELD MAP

HEMIFIELD PUSH−PULL GRADIENTS

AGONIST− ANTAGONIST MUSCLES

Figure 2.1. A scheme for mapping retinal position signals into agonist-antagonist muscle commands: First retinal positions are mapped topographically into a hemifield map. The output signals from the hemifield map increasingly favor one muscle of the pair as a function of retinal eccentricity.

Such a direct link from retina to muscles does not, of course, control saccadic motions *in vivo*. The ensuing theoretical argument shows how intermediate processing stages can be derived from constraints on adaptive saccadic learning and performance. In the complete model, the final stage of the six-sectored map plays the role of the oculomotor nuclei.

2.2. Choice of Fixation Light: Network Competition

A visual scene contains many possible fixation points. One of these points is chosen for fixation from the many possible candidates. Within the computational framework defined in Figure 2.1, such a choice mechanism needs to transform a broad array of lights on the retina into a relatively localized activation of the sector map. The sector map can then, in turn, preferentially contract some muscles more than others. Since broadly distributed lights on the retina activate many pathways to the sector map, a competitive interaction exists between the retina and the sector map that converts a broadly distributed input pattern into a more narrowly focused activity pattern. Section 2.6 describes how to design a competitive network capable of making such a choice across spatially distributed alternatives.

2.3. Correcting Fixation Errors: Competition Precedes Storage in Sensory Short Term Memory

A focal activation of the sector map can elicit eye movements towards the chosen light, but the direction and length of these movements may be inaccurate. We assume that genetic mechanisms are unable to precisely prewire the correct coordination of eye separation and size, muscle inertia, neural signal strengths, and other relevant eye movement parameters. Since several parameters contribute to each motion, the only meaningful test of the collective effect of these parameters is whether or not they generate an accurate fixation. Consequently, we base our saccadic error scheme on the location of the chosen light on the retina after an eye movement takes place. This simple idea imposes several design constraints. To discuss these constraints, we call the chosen light before movement the *first light* and the chosen light after movement the *second light*. This terminology emphasizes the fact that the system does not *a priori* know whether these two lights are due to the same light source.

A. Short Term Memory of the First Light

In order to correct the command due to the first light using information about the position of the second light, the system needs to store an internal marker of the position of the first light until the second light is registered. We call this storage process *short term memory* (STM). Since the command to be stored represents a sensory activation, we call this example of STM *sensory short term memory* (SSTM) to distinguish it from *motor short term memory* (MSTM) processes that will also be needed. Section 2.6 shows how a chosen light position can be stored in STM.

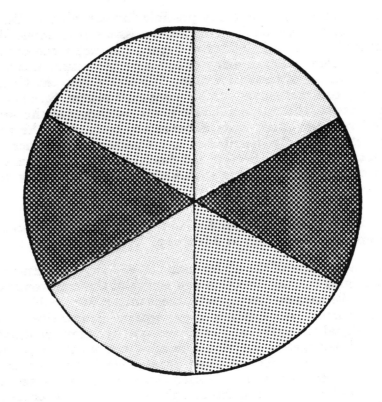

Figure 2.2. A sector map: Each wedge of the circle represents a region that maps preferentially into one of the six extraocular muscles. Pairs of wedges with similar hatching correspond to agonist-antagonist muscle pairs.

B. *Competition Stage Precedes Sensory Short Term Memory Stage*

Another way to say that the first light's position is chosen and stored in SSTM is to say that no other light position can be stored in SSTM while the first light's position is stored there. In particular, the second light cannot be stored in SSTM until the first light is no longer stored there. However, the second light must act as an error signal while the command corresponding to the first light is still being stored. Otherwise there would be no internal trace of which pathways the error signal should correct.

After the movement terminates, many lights will again activate the retina. In order to even define a second light, a competitive process needs to choose a light from among the many retinal lights. This choice process occurs, moreover, while the command corresponding to the first light is still stored in SSTM. Thus the competitive process that chooses among retinal lights, whether the first light or the second light, occurs prior to the stage that stores a light in SSTM (Figure 2.3).

2.4. Parallel Processing of Movement and Error Signals

Activation of a retinal position by a light can elicit signals in two functionally distinct pathways, a movement command pathway and an error signal pathway. To understand why this is so, note that each retinal position can be activated by either the first light or the second light of some saccade. When a retinal position is activated by the second light in a saccade, it can generate an error signal. This error signal is elicited at a stage *subsequent* to the competition that chooses the second light (Figure 2.4). The error signal is elicited at a stage *prior* to the SSTM stage that stores the first light in SSTM, since this stage blocks storage of other lights in SSTM until after the second light error signal is registered.

A second light error signal alters the strength of the conditioned pathway that is activated by the SSTM representation of the first light (Figure 2.4). The role of this learning process is to improve the ability of the first light to elicit correct saccades on future performance trials. Thus the conditioned pathway that is activated by the first light is a source of saccadic movement signals.

We can now draw another conclusion by invoking the fact that every retinal position can be activated by either the first light or the second light of some saccade. This fact implies that the second light provides a source of movement signals for the next saccade, and the first light provides a source of error signals for the previous saccade.

In summary, in order to correct previous errors before helping to generate the next movement, each retinal position gives rise to an error signal pathway as well as a pathway that activates a positional map at the SSTM stage. The SSTM stage, in turn, activates a conditioned pathway which can be altered by these error signals.

Figure 2.4 expands the network to include the new processing stages that are needed to implement these functional requirements. Figure 2.4

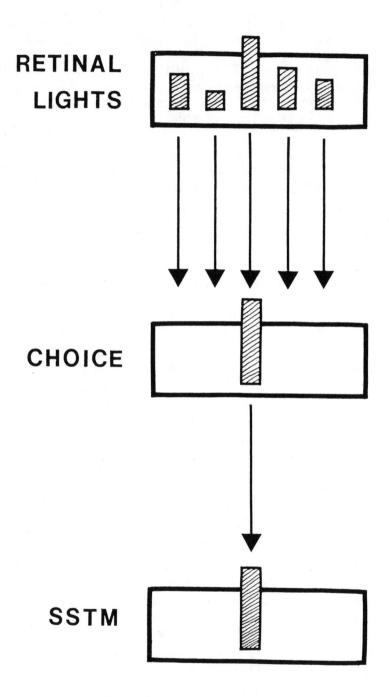

Figure 2.3. A choice among retinal lights occurs before the chosen light is stored in sensory short term memory (SSTM).

includes an unconditioned movement pathway as well as a conditioned movement pathway. The unconditioned pathway enables saccades to be generated by lights even before learning occurs. The error signals that are registered due to these saccades alter the strengths of the conditioned movement pathways. As a result, the total movement signal, which consists of an unconditioned and a conditioned component, generates more accurate movements than the unconditioned component alone. Figure 2.4 thus illustrates an example of a one-to-many analysis of a sensory input that occurs prior to a many-to-one synthesis of a movement (Section 1.4).

2.5. Why Does a Saccade Generator Exist?

In order for an SSTM stage to work well, there must also exist a saccade generator that converts the spatially coded signal within a light-activated retinal map into a temporally coded signal that determines how long and in what direction the eye will move (Keller, 1974; van Gisbergen, Robinson, and Gielen, 1981). To understand why such a spatial-to-temporal conversion is necessary, recall that the SSTM stage activates a conditioned pathway until *after* the eye comes to rest, so that this pathway remains active long enough to sample the second light error signal. The second light error signal cannot, however, be initiated until the eye stops moving. The network needs to convert the sustained output signal from the SSTM stage into a phasic movement signal whose duration is less than that of the SSTM output signal itself. Otherwise the sustained SSTM output signal would keep the eye moving until some muscles maximally contract. The onset of the movement signal that is activated by output from the SSTM stage thus initiates a process that eventually inhibits the movement signal before the SSTM output itself shuts off. The mechanism that initiates, maintains, and terminates the movement signal is called the *saccade generator* (SG).

This argument is important because it shows that the existence and properties of an SG, which have been analysed in the literature entirely from the viewpoint of saccadic performance, take on additional meaning when they are analysed from the perspective of saccadic learning. Indeed, this learning argument is the only one we know which suggests why a saccade generator *must* exist, rather than some other type of mechanism for moving the eyes.

An analysis of SG properties from the viewpoint of saccadic learning places strong constraints on the design of the SG. Two of the more obvious constraints are the following ones. The error signal acts at a stage prior to the SG so that both the unconditioned and conditioned movement pathways can input to the SG. The SG must be designed so that learned changes in the strength of the conditionable pathway can improve saccadic foveation. In particular, changes in the amplitude of the signals in the conditioned pathways must cause changes in the SG output that improve the accuracy of saccadic length and direction. A network synthesis of such an SG circuit will be described in Chapter 7.

To illustrate how our approach supplements earlier work about the SG,

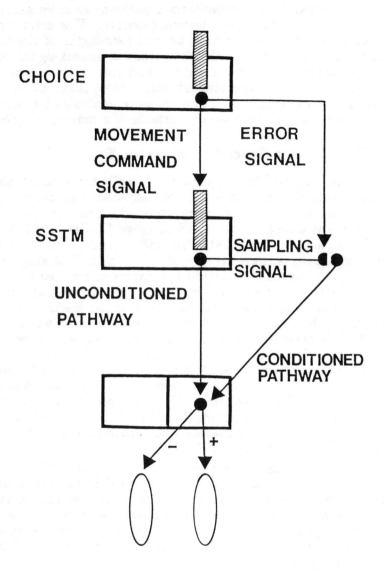

Figure 2.4. The representation of the chosen first light gives rise to an unconditioned movement signal and a conditioned movement signal. The unconditioned signal causes movements that are corrected by the conditioned movement signal via learning. The conditioned pathway carries sampling signals whose strength can be altered by second-light mediated error signals. These sampling signals give rise to the conditioned movement signal. The representation of the first light must be stored until after the end of the saccade, so that the second-light mediated error signal can act.

consider the following quotation from Robinson (1981, p.1302) concerning his important model of the SG: "The output of the neural integrator...is a copy of instantaneous eye position. If higher centers, which selected the target, made available a signal representing the location of the target with respect to the head, the difference between the target and eye signals would be the neurally encoded motor error...If this signal drove the burst neurons, their firing rate would drive the eyes at a high velocity until the error was zero, and at this time the burst would stop. This hypothesis guarantees that all bursts automatically have the correct size for each saccade, because the burst always continues until the eye is on target." For further discussion of Robinson's model, see the summary of Keller (1981, p.57).

We concur with Robinson's concept of an SG in which a difference signal terminates output from burst neurons. Our analysis of this system differs, however, from that of Robinson. This is because, without further mechanisms, a difference signal does not "automatically have the correct size for each saccade." It only achieves the correct size for each saccade after several major problems of calibration are solved. For example: How does the neural network know how a prescribed instantaneous burst activity will be translated into instantaneous eye movement velocity? What if the eye muscle contracts too slowly or too quickly? How does burst activity compensate for possible nonlinearities in muscle response? Each motoneuron cell may have a different threshold and slope of reaction to a given input (Robinson, 1970; Schiller, 1970). How is the total output from a population of such bursters calibrated to produce a linear total response from target muscles? If this is not accomplished, how can "output of the neural integrator" be used to provide "a copy of instantaneous eye position"? In a similar vein, how does the system determine that it has reached the desired target by using a computation wherein a target signal that is calibrated in "higher centers" numerically equals the output from a "neural integrator" in a different part of the brain? Unless these problems of calibration are solved, such a difference computation will not yield the desired behavior. In Robinson's model, it is assumed that these parameters have been correctly chosen. Our theory shows how the model can calibrate its own parameters using only locally computable qualities.

We finish this chapter by illustrating how on-center off-surround feedback interactions among cells which obey membrane equations can be designed to make choices, to store them in STM, and to respond to attentional and motivational signals.

2.6. Competitive Choice and Storage in Short Term Memory

This section reviews basic properties of networks of neurons which obey membrane equations and interact via on-center off-surround anatomies, or related cooperative-competitive anatomies. Then we focus the discussion to consider properties of primary interest such as competitive choice, STM storage, and attentional or motivational modulation. The mathematical theory of such networks began to be developed in Grossberg (1973) and has since undergone rapid development. See, for example, Carpenter and Grossberg (1983, 1984, 1985a, 1985b), Cohen and Grossberg (1983, 1984a, 1984b, 1985), Grossberg (1980, 1981, 1983), Grossberg and Mingolla (1985a, 1985b), and Grossberg and Stone (1985a, 1985b) for some recent contributions.

A. Shunting Interactions

A membrane equation is an equation of the form

$$C\frac{\partial V}{\partial t} = (V^+ - V)g^+ + (V^- - V)g^- + (V^p - V)g^p. \tag{2.1}$$

In equation (2.1), $V(t)$ is the cell's variable voltage. Parameter C is a constant capacitance. The constants V^+, V^-, and V^p are excitatory, inhibitory, and passive saturation points, respectively. Often V^+ and V^- are associated with Na^+, K^+, and Cl^- channels, respectively (Hodgkin, 1964; Katz, 1966). The terms g^+, g^-, and g^p are conductances that can vary through time as a function of input signals. Due to the multiplicative relationship between conductances and voltages in (2.1), a membrane equation is also said to describe a *shunting* interaction. In the next paragraphs, we show how on-center off-surround interactions among cells obeying such shunting interactions can be derived from functional considerations. Then we will indicate how desirable functional properties, such as competitive choice and STM storage, can be achieved by networks of this type whose parameters are appropriately chosen.

B. Ratio Processing and Normalization of Spatial Patterns by Shunting On-Center Off-Surround Networks

Let $x_i(t)$ be the activity, or potential, of the ith cell (population) v_i in a field F of cells v_1, v_2, ..., v_n. Suppose that each v_i has B excitable sites of which $B - x_i$ are unexcited. Let an input pattern $(I_1, I_2, ..., I_n)$ perturb F in such a way that I_i excites v_i's unexcited sites by mass action. Also let excitation x_i spontaneously decay at a constant rate A. Then the net rate $\frac{d}{dt}x_i$ at which sites v_i are activated is

$$\frac{d}{dt}x_i = -Ax_i + (B - x_i)I_i, \tag{2.2}$$

$i = 1, 2, ..., n$.

This law is inadequate because all the activities x_i can saturate at their maximal values B in response to an intensely activated input pattern. To see this, we define a *spatial pattern* to be an input pattern whose relative activities θ_i are constant through time. Then each $I_i(t) = \theta_i I(t)$, where the ratio θ_i is the constant "reflectance" of the input pattern at v_i and $I(t)$ is the total, and possibly variable, background intensity. The convention that $\sum_{i=1}^{n} \theta_i = 1$ implies that $I(t) = \sum_{i=1}^{n} I_i(t)$. Choose a constant background intensity $I(t) = I$ and let the activities equilibrate to their respective inputs. The equilibrium activities of (2.2) are found by setting $\frac{d}{dt}x_i = 0$. We find

$$x_i = \frac{B\theta_i I}{A + \theta_i I}. \tag{2.3}$$

Now set the background intensity I at progressively higher levels without changing the reflectances θ_i. Then each x_i saturates at B no matter how differently the $\theta_i(> 0)$ are chosen.

This saturation problem can be solved by letting lateral inhibitory inputs shut off some sites as excitatory inputs turn on other sites in a feedforward competitive anatomy (Figure 2.5a). In the simplest version of this idea, (2.2) is replaced by

$$\frac{d}{dt}x_i = -Ax_i + (B - x_i)I_i - x_i \sum_{k \neq i} I_k, \tag{2.4}$$

$i = 1, 2, \ldots, n$. The new term $-x_i \sum_{k \neq i} I_k$ says that the lateral inhibitory inputs $\sum_{k \neq i} I_k$ shut off the active sites x_i by mass action. In response to a sustained spatial pattern $I_i = \theta_i I$, the equilibrium activities of (2.4) are

$$x_i = \theta_i \frac{BI}{A + I}. \tag{2.5}$$

By (2.5), each x_i is proportional to θ_i no matter how large the total input I is chosen. The background activity I is factored into the Weber-law modulation term $BI(A + I)^{-1}$, which approaches the constant B as I increases. Thus (2.5) shows that system (2.4) can accurately process the reflectances θ_i no matter how large the total input I is chosen. This property is due to the multiplication, or shunting, of x_i by lateral inhibitory signals in (2.4).

The total coefficient of x_i in (2.4) is called the *gain* of x_i. Thus the saturation problem is solved by automatic gain control due to lateral inhibition. System (2.4) describes the simplest example of a feedforward shunting on-center off-surround network.

System (2.4) also possesses a *normalization* property. The total activity $x = \sum_{i=1}^{n} x_i$ satisfies the equation

$$x = \frac{BI}{A + I} \tag{2.6}$$

because $\sum_{i=1}^{n} \theta_i = 1$. By (2.6), given a fixed total input I, the total activity x is independent of the number of active cells. Shunting competitive networks hereby tend to conserve their total activity. In shunting on-center off-surround feedback networks, the normalization property provides a dynamical explanation of why short term memory is a limited capacity process.

C. Featural Noise Suppression: Adaptation Level and Pattern Matching

In (2.4), activity x_i can fluctuate between 0 and B. *In vivo*, inhibition can often hyperpolarize x_i below its passive equilibrium point 0. To fully understand competitive dynamics requires that we classify other biologically relevant competitive designs than the simplest example (2.4). Hyperpolarization is possible in the following generalization of (2.4):

$$\frac{d}{dt}x_i = -Ax_i + (B - x_i)I_i - (x_i + C)\sum_{k \neq i} I_k, \qquad (2.7)$$

where $-C \leq 0 \leq B$. If $C > 0$ in (2.7), then x_i can be hyperpolarized by inhibitory inputs to any negative value between 0 and $-C$. In response to a sustained spatial pattern $I_i = \theta_i I$, the equilibrium activities of (2.7) are

$$x_i = \frac{(B + C)I}{A + I}\left(\theta_i - \frac{C}{B + C}\right). \qquad (2.8)$$

By (2.8), $x_i > 0$ only if $\theta_i > C/B + C$. Since output signals are generated only by depolarized, or positive, values of x_i. the term $C(B + C)^{-1}$ is called the *adaptation level* of the network. Raising the adaptation level makes output signals harder to generate.

The special choice $B = (n - 1)C$ illustrates how the adaptation level works in its simplest form. Then $C(B + C)^{-1} = 1/n$. In response to any uniform spatial pattern $I_i = 1/n$. Then (2.8) implies that all $x_i = 0$ no matter how large I is chosen. This property is called *featural noise suppression*, or the suppression of zero spatial frequency patterns. Due to this property, the network suppresses input patterns that do not energetically favor any cellular feature detectors.

The featural noise suppression property implies a pattern matching property. For example, let two input patterns $J^* = (J_1, J_2, \ldots, J_n)$ and $K^* = (K_1, K_2, \ldots, K_n)$ add their inputs $I_i = J_i + K_i$ to generate a total input pattern $I^* = (I_1, I_2, \ldots, I_n)$ to the network. If the two patterns J^* and K^* are mismatched so that their peaks and troughs are spatially out-of-phase, then I^* will tend to be approximately uniform and will be suppressed by the adaptation level. By contrast, if J^* and K^* have the same reflectances, say $J_i = \theta_i J$ and $K_i = \theta_i K$, then (2.7) implies that

$$x_i = \frac{(B + C)(J + K)}{A + J + K}\left(\theta_i - \frac{C}{B + C}\right). \qquad (2.9)$$

By (2.9), the network energetically amplifies its response to matched patterns via Weber-law modulation. This type of energetic amplification due

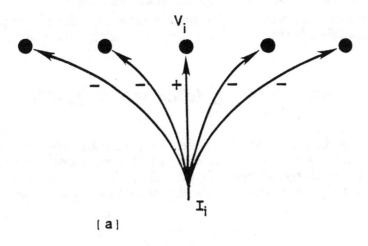

[a]

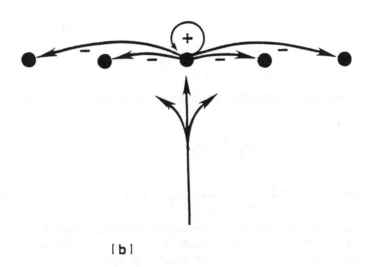

[b]

Figure 2.5. Two types of on-center off-surround networks: (a) A feed-forward network in which the input pathways define the on-center off-surround interactions; (b) A feedback network in which interneurons define the on-center off-surround interactions.

to matching is different from the suppressive matching that occurs when a target position equals a present position (Section 2.6).

D. *Receptive Fields, Spatial Frequencies, and Edges*

In more general feedforward shunting networks, the above properties hold in a modified form. Consider for example the class of feedforward networks

$$\frac{d}{dt}x_i = -Ax_i + (B - x_i) \sum_{k=1}^{n} I_k C_{ki} - (x_i + D) \sum_{k=1}^{n} I_k E_{ki}, \qquad (2.10)$$

$i = 1, 2, \ldots, n$. In (2.10), the coefficients C_{ki} and E_{ki} describe the fall-off with the distance between cells v_k and v_i of the excitatory and inhibitory influences, respectively, of input I_k on cell v_i. In response to a sustained spatial pattern $I_i = \theta_i I$, the equilibrium activities of (2.10) are

$$x_i = \frac{F_i I}{A + G_i I} \qquad (2.11)$$

where

$$F_i = \sum_{k=1}^{n} \theta_k (B C_{ki} - D E_{ki}) \qquad (2.12)$$

and

$$G_i = \sum_{k=1}^{n} \theta_k (C_{ki} + E_{ki}). \qquad (2.13)$$

The featural noise suppression property is implied by the inequalities

$$B \sum_{k=1}^{n} C_{ki} \leq D \sum_{k=1}^{n} E_{ki} \qquad (2.14)$$

since then, by (2.11) and (2.12), all $x_i \leq 0$ in response to a uniform pattern $\theta_i = 1/n$ no matter how large the total input I is chosen.

When the featural noise suppression property holds in a distance-dependent network, the network can, in addition to the other properties cited above, detect edges and other spatially nonuniform gradients in input patterns for the following reason. Inputs are suppressed by all the cells across whose receptive fields the input pattern looks approximately uniform, no matter how intense the input pattern is near these cells. In particular, a rectangular input pattern is suppressed both outside and inside the pattern by this mechanism. Only those cells can respond which occur near input regions where the input intensity changes across space at a rate that is no coarser than the receptive fields.

The responding cells compute input reflectances or relative contrast differences in their vicinity using the ratios that occur in equation (2.11).

Equation (2.11) generalizes the reflectance processing properties of (2.5) and (2.8). The breadth of the edge reflects both the rate of change of the input pattern and of the structural scales of the network. Larger structural scales cause broader edges, other things being equal, and thus make it easier to match a pair of partially out-of-phase edges. Thus both relative contrasts and spatial scaling properties are encoded within the edges extracted by (2.11). Equation (2.11) generalizes the familiar difference-of-Gaussian receptive field model that is broadly used in analyses of spatial vision (Blakemore, Carpenter, and Georgeson, 1970; Ellias and Grossberg, 1975; Enroth-Cugell and Robson, 1966; Levine and Grossberg, 1976; Rodieck and Stone, 1965; Wilson and Bergen, 1979).

E. *Short Term Memory, Feedback Competitive Networks, and Nonlinear Cross-Correlation*

Short term memory (STM) storage of input patterns is possible in networks possessing positive and negative feedback pathways (Figure 2.5b). In order to prevent saturation due to positive feedback signalling, the positive feedback signals are balanced by competitive, or lateral inhibitory, feedback signals that automatically change the network's gain, just as in feedforward competitive networks. The feedback competitive analog of the feedforward competitive system (2.10) is

$$
\frac{d}{dt}x_i = -Ax_i + (B - x_i)[I_i + \sum_{k=1}^{n} f_k(x_k)C_{ki}]
$$

$$
- (x_i + D)[J_i + \sum_{k=1}^{n} g_k(x_k)E_{ki}],
$$

(2.15)

$i = 1, 2, \ldots, n$. In (2.15), I_i is the excitatory input to v_i, J_i is the inhibitory input to v_i, $f_k(x_k)C_{ki}$ is the positive feedback signal from v_k to v_i, and $g_k(x_k)E_{ki}$ is the negative feedback signal from v_k to v_i. Each input term I_i or J_i may itself be a weighted average of distributed inputs from a prior stage of processing. When C_{ki} and E_{ki} are functions of intercellular distances, then the excitatory and inhibitory interaction terms $f_i(x^*) = \sum_{k=1}^{n} f_k(x_k)C_{ki}$ and $g_i(x^*) = \sum_{k=1}^{n} g_k(x_k)E_{ki}$ in (2.15), where $x^* = (x_1, x_2, \ldots, x_n)$, define nonlinear cross-correlations

$$
x^* \rightarrow (f_1(x^*), f_2(x^*), \ldots, f_n(x^*))
$$

(2.16)

and

$$
x^* \rightarrow (g_1(x^*), g_2(x^*), \ldots, g_n(x^*))
$$

(2.17)

of the STM activities x^*. Thus the concepts of feedback signalling and of nonlinear cross-correlation are the same in a distance-dependent network.

F. *Signal Noise Suppression and Nonlinear Signals*

The transformations (2.16) and (2.17) must define *nonlinear* cross-correlators due to a mathematical property of the networks (2.15). The positive feedback signals can amplify small activities into large activities (signals amplify "noise") unless the signal functions $f_k(x_k)$ and $g_k(x_k)$ are nonlinear functions of the STM activities x_k (Grossberg, 1973). Nonlinearity *per se* is not sufficient to prevent this from happening, since a nonlinear signal function such as $f_k(w) = \alpha w(\beta + w)^{-1}$ can cause a pathological STM response in which all STM activities are amplified to equal asymptotes no matter how different, and small, were their initial activities. To avoid such pathologies, the positive feedback signals $f_k(x_k)$ need to be faster-than-linear functions of x_k, such as powers $f_k(x_k) = \alpha x_k^n$ with $n > 1$, at small values of the activities x_k. Sigmoid, or S-shaped, functions of activity are the simplest physically plausible signal functions that solve the signal noise suppression problem (Grossberg, 1973).

G. *Dynamic Control of Network Sensitivity: Quenching Threshold and Attentional Gain Control*

When sigmoid feedback signals are used in a feedback competitive network such as (2.15), the network possesses a parameter that is called the *quenching threshold* (QT): STM activities that start out less than the QT tend to be suppressed, whereas the pattern of STM activities that initially exceeds the QT tends to be contrast enhanced through time (Figure 2.6). The QT is not just the manifest threshold of a signal function. The QT is a parameter that depends on the global structure of the network. For example, consider the following special case of (2.15):

$$\frac{d}{dt}x_i = -Ax_i + (B - x_i)f(x_i) - x_i \sum_{k \neq i} f(x_k), \qquad (2.18)$$

$i = 1, 2, \ldots, n$. In (2.18), all inputs are shut off and the competitive interaction $\sum_{k \neq i}^{n} f(x_k)$ describes long-range lateral inhibition, just like the term $\sum_{k \neq i}^{n} I_k$ in the feedforward network (2.4). Suppose that the feedback signal function $f(w)$ satisfies

$$f(w) = Cwg(w) \qquad (2.19)$$

where $C \geq 0$, $g(w)$ is increasing if $0 \leq w \leq x^{(1)}$, and $g(w) = 1$ if $x^{(1)} \leq w \leq B$. Thus $f(w)$ is faster-than-linear for $0 \leq w \leq x^{(1)}$, linear for $x^{(1)} \leq w \leq B$, and attains a maximum value of BC at $w = B$ within the activity interval from 0 to B. The values of $f(w)$ at activities $w \geq B$ do not affect network dynamics because each $x_i \leq B$ in (2.18). It was proved in Grossberg (1973, pp.238–242) that the QT of this network is

$$QT = \frac{x^{(1)}}{B - AC^{-1}}. \qquad (2.20)$$

By (2.20), the QT is not the manifest threshold of $f(w)$, which occurs where $g(w)$ is increasing. The QT depends on the transition activity $x^{(1)}$ where $f(w)$ changes from faster-than-linear, upon the overall slope C of the

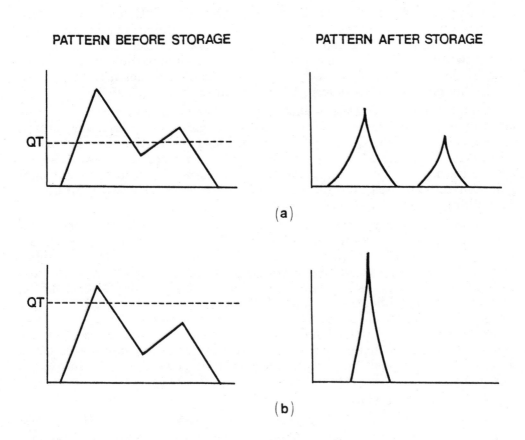

Figure 2.6. The quenching threshold (QT). In Figures 2.6a and 2.6b, the same input pattern is differently transformed and stored in short term memory due to different settings of the network QT.

signal function in the physiological range, upon the number B of excitable sites in each population, and upon the STM decay rate A. Equation (2.20) shows that an increase in C causes a decrease in the QT. Consequently, increasing a shunting signal C that nonspecifically gates all the network's feedback signals facilitates STM storage. Equation (2.20) also shows how using a linear signal function destabilizes network dynamics. If $f(w)$ is linear in (2.19), then $x^{(1)} = 0$. By (2.20), the QT $= 0$. Hence any positive network activity, no matter how small, will be amplified by a linear signal function. From the inception of the theory, it was realized that any of several network parameters can cause the QT to become pathologically small, thereby destabilizing network dynamics and leading to network "seizures" or "hallucinations" (Grossberg, 1973; Traub and Wong, 1983).

Equation (2.20) illustrates that the network's sensitivity can be modulated by dynamical factors. If the nonspecific gain C is chosen very small, for example, then the QT may be so large as to desensitize the network to all inputs. By contrast, a large choice of C can render the network sensitive to its input by decreasing the QT. A nonspecific form of attentional gain control can thus modulate the network's sensitivity to its inputs by controlling the size of the QT through time.

The QT property is not "built into" the network. It is a *mathematical* consequence of using shunting on-center off-surround feedback networks, and was considered surprising when it was first discovered by Grossberg (1973). Thus the network design which prevents saturation by automatically adjusting its gains in response to variable input loads (Section 2.6B), and prevents amplification and STM storage of network noise by using a proper signal function (Section 2.6F) is already prepared to respond adaptively to nonspecific attentional gain control signals. This type of attentional processing will be used to discuss how attention modulates STM storage of target positions within the posterior parietal lobe (Chapters 4 and 11).

H. Competitive Choice

A sigmoid signal function $f(w)$ is composed of a faster-than-linear part at small activity values w, a slower-than-linear part at large activity values w, and an approximately linear part at intermediate activity values w (Figure 2.7). Each of these activity regions transforms input patterns in a different way before storing them as STM activity patterns. If network activities remain within the faster-than-linear range of a sigmoid signal function, then the network is capable of making a competitive choice by contrast-enhancing the input pattern via the network's feedback pathways until only the population with the largest initial activity has positive activity.

A competitive choice can be accomplished in either of two ways: structurally or dynamically. In the structural solution, network parameters are chosen so that all STM activities remain within the faster-than-linear range under all circumstances. In the dynamical solution, a nonspecific attentional gain control signal shifts either STM activities into the faster-than-linear range, or shifts interaction parameters such as inhibitory in-

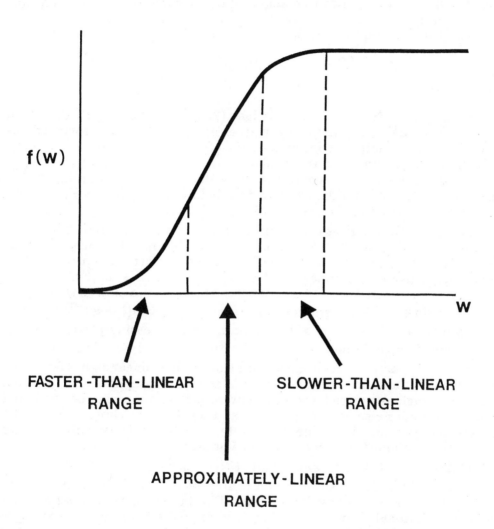

Figure 2.7. A sigmoid signal function: The faster-than-linear part tends to contrast-enhance activity patterns; the linear part tends to preserve activity patterns; the slower-than-linear part tends to uniformize activity patterns, as in Table 2.1. Taken together, these tendencies define the quenching threshold.

teraction strengths into the faster-than-linear range until the choice is made.

A more complete understanding of how the signal function determines the stored STM pattern can be achieved by considering the following special case of (2.15):

$$\frac{d}{dt}x_i = -Ax_i + (B - x_i)[I_i + f(x_i)] - x_i[J_i + \sum_{k \neq i} f(x_k)], \qquad (2.21)$$

$i = 1, 2, \ldots, n$. Network (2.21) is just (2.18) with the inputs I_i and J_i left on. Network (2.21) strips away all extraneous factors to focus on the following issue. After an input pattern $(I_1, I_2, \ldots, I_n, J_1, J_2, \ldots, J_n)$ delivered before time $t = 0$ establishes an initial pattern $(x_1(0), x_2(0), \ldots, x_n(0))$ in the network's activities, how does feedback signalling within the network transform the initial pattern before it is stored in STM? This problem was solved in Grossberg (1973).

Table 2.1 summarizes the main features of the solution. The function $g(w) = w^{-1}f(w)$ is graphed in Table 2.1 because the property that determines the pattern transformation is whether $g(w)$ is an increasing, constant, or decreasing function at prescribed activities w. For example, a linear $f(w) = aw$ determines a constant $g(w) = a$; a slower-than-linear $f(w) = aw(b + w)^{-1}$ determines a decreasing $g(w) = a(b + w)^{-1}$; a faster-than-linear $f(w) = aw^n$, $n > 1$, determines an increasing $g(w) = aw^{n-1}$; and a sigmoid signal function $f(w) = aw^2(b + w^2)^{-1}$ determines a concave $g(w) = aw(b + w^2)^{-1}$. Both linear and slower-than-linear signal functions amplify noise, and are therefore unsatisfactory. Faster-than-linear signal functions, such as power laws with powers greater than one, or threshold rules, suppress noise so vigorously that they make a choice. Table 2.1 shows that sigmoid signal functions determine a QT by mixing together properties of the other types of signal functions.

I. *Attentional Biasing and Competitive Masking*

A suitably designed shunting on-center off-surround feedback network is also capable of biasing its stored STM in response to spatially focussed attentional or developmental factors (Grossberg, 1981; Grossberg and Levine, 1975). Such a spatially delimited attentional bias is not the same process as nonspecific attentional gain control, and it may coexist with attentional gain control (Grossberg, 1978a, 1982b). Both types of mechanism will be used to describe how attention modulates storage of target positions by the posterior parietal lobes (Chapters 4 and 11).

To distinguish focal attentional biasing from nonspecific attentional gain control, we call the focal process competitive *masking*. To illustrate the main properties of masking, we use the simplest possible example. A more sophisticated example, in which masking enables the network to respond in a context-sensitive way to a temporally evolving speech stream, is described in Cohen and Grossberg (1985) and Grossberg (1985c).

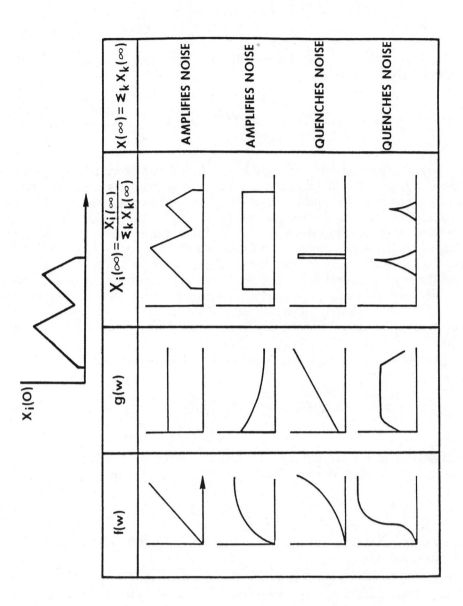

Table 2.1. Influence of signal function $f(w)$ on input pattern transformation and short term memory storage.

Masking occurs in systems

$$\frac{d}{dt}x_i = -Ax_i + (B_i - x_i)f(x_i) - x_i \sum_{k \neq i} f(x_k) \qquad (2.22)$$

in which populations v_i can have different numbers B_i of excitable sites, or equivalently in systems

$$\frac{d}{dt}x_i = -Ax_i + (B - x_i)f(C_i x_i) - x_i \sum_{k \neq i} f(C_k x_k) \qquad (2.23)$$

whose population activities or signals are differentially amplified by shunting factors C_i. System (2.23) can be formally transformed into system (2.22) by a change of variables. Despite this formal equivalence, the physical interpretations of these systems may differ. In (2.22), the different numbers of sites can be interpreted as a developmental bias in which certain input features are coded by more sites B_i than others. In (2.23), the differential amplification of population signals can be interpreted as an attentional shunt that gates all the feedback interneurons, both excitatory and inhibitory, of each population v_i using its own shunting parameter C_i. Such a shunt may, for example, be controlled by a learned incentive motivational signal from a midbrain reinforcement center (Grossberg, 1982b).

If both developmental and attentional biases occur, as in

$$\frac{d}{dt}x_i = -Ax_i + (B_i - x_i)f(C_i x_i) - x_i \sum_{k \neq i} f(C_k x_k), \qquad (2.24)$$

then masking is controlled by the relative sizes of the products $B_1 C_1$, $B_2 C_2$, ..., $B_n C_n$. For definiteness, label the cells so that

$$B_1 C_1 \geq B_2 C_2 \geq \ldots \geq B_n C_n. \qquad (2.25)$$

We now show that the nature of the masking depends upon the choice of signal function $f(w)$.

To start, let the signal function be linear, say $f(w) = Ew$. Then a masking phenomenon occurs such that $x_i(\infty) = 0$ if $B_i C_i < B_1 C_1$, whereas

$$\frac{x_i(\infty)}{x_j(\infty)} = \frac{x_i(0)}{x_j(0)} \qquad (2.26)$$

for all i and j such that $B_1 C_1 = B_i C_i = B_j C_j$. By (2.26), the activity pattern across the subfield of populations v_i with maximal parameters $B_i C_i = B_1 C_1$ is faithfully stored, but all other population activities are competitively masked. This type of masking is inadequate in a sensory processor, because the salience of a feature in an external display, as measured by a large initial $x_i(0)$ value, cannot overcome internal biases $B_i C_i < B_1 C_1$ even if $x_i(0)$ is much larger than $x_1(0)$.

This problem is overcome if a sigmoid signal function $f(w)$ is used. Then a tug-of-war occurs between cue salience $x_i(0)$, developmental biases B_i, and attentional shunts C_i to determine which population activities will be stored in STM (Grossberg and Levine, 1975). Superimposed upon this masking bias is the usual contrast-enhancement that a sigmoid signal function can elicit. Thus the same nonlinear signal function that suppresses noise and contrast-enhances STM activities exceeding the QT automatically generates the type of masking bias that can successfully refocus attention in response to incentive motivational signals.

In summary, the ubiquity in the brain of the shunting on-center off-surround network design can be better appreciated from the mathematical fact that variations of this design imply constellations of formal properties which solve a large number of important functional problems.

CHAPTER 3

SACCADIC LEARNING USING VISUAL ERROR SIGNALS: SELF-MOTION VS. WORLD-MOTION AND CEREBELLAR DYNAMICS

3.1. Compensation for Initial Position in the Movement Signal

An eye can be in different positions with respect to the head before it saccades in response to a light at a fixed position on the retina. Corresponding to each different initial position, the extraocular muscles are in a different state of contraction. The same first light may thus excite the retina while the extraocular muscles are in different states of contraction. In order for a saccade to be correct in response to a first light at a fixed retinal position, it must move the eye a prescribed number of degrees no matter what initial state of muscle contraction prevails before the saccade occurs. Consequently, the total movement signal needs to take into account not only the retinal locus of a light, but also the initial state of the muscles.

Only in the case that the amount of muscle contraction is a linear function of the movement signal can this signal be independent of the initial position of the eye. This fact is illustrated in Figure 3.1. If muscle contraction is not a linear function of the movement signal, then the same movement signal can cause different amounts of contraction if the eye starts out at different initial positions. The movement signal thus cannot depend only on retinal information if the muscle plant is nonlinear, since a retinal command to move the eye ϕ degrees would move the eyes by different amounts depending upon its initial position. Since the muscle plant is nonlinear (Robinson, 1981), both retinal and initial positional information contribute to the total saccadic command.

Neither a retinally activated saccadic command nor a positionally activated saccadic command can possibly have *a priori* knowledge of the muscle plant's characteristics. Thus retinotopic and positional signals must contribute to the *conditionable* components of the total movement signal that activates the muscles. The network in Figure 2.4 must therefore be expanded to include a conditionable movement signal that is activated by a source of information about initial position (Figure 3.2).

3.2. Explicit vs. Implicit Knowledge of Initial Position

Both *explicit* and *implicit* information about initial eye position could, in principle, be used to activate conditionable movement pathways. Explicit information is computed within a network such that retinal maps and eye position maps control separate conditionable pathways that converge before the SG stage (Figure 3.2) or after the SG stage (Figure 3.3). Implicit information is illustrated by a network in which a single invariant

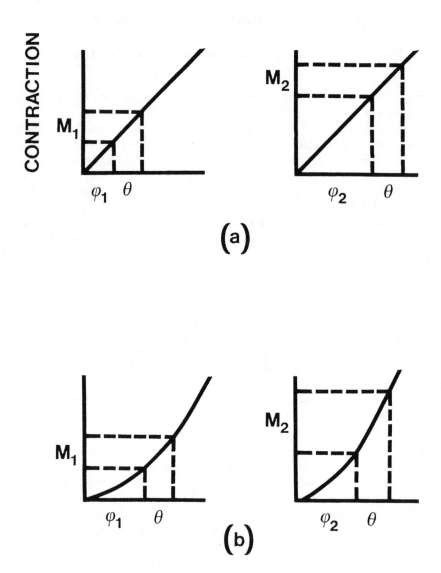

Figure 3.1. Influence of muscle plant on compensation for initial eye position: (a) In a linear plant, the amount of contraction M_1 and M_2 is the same in response to a constant retinotopic position θ given any initial eye position ϕ_1 or ϕ_2; (b) In a nonlinear plant, the amount of contraction can change as a function of initial eye position.

target position map, as described in Section 1.4, controls the conditionable pathways that project to the SG stage (Figure 3.4). A target position map contains only implicit information about eye position because each eye position inputs to many map target positions, and every map target position depends jointly upon eye position and retinal position.

In order to arrive at a complete conceptual understanding of this learning problem, we have numerically analysed how different combinations of eye position sampling maps, retinotopic sampling maps, and target position sampling maps can cooperate to correct saccadic errors due to different types of nonlinear muscle plants using either linear or nonlinear error signals. This type of parametric analysis enables us to infer how the different sampling maps to which we will be led in our subsequent analysis work together. It also shows what types of lesions within the sampling maps can automatically be compensated for by causing error signals which drive new learning within the conditionable pathways of the remaining sampling maps. In Chapter 11, this type of information will be joined to all the other learning constraints of the theory to make a global choice of model.

3.3. Characterization of Correctable Errors

In addition to classifying sampling maps that are capable of compensating for muscle plant nonlinearity, it is also necessary to characterize the error signals that are capable of correcting movement errors due to an imprecise choice of initial parameters. Three types of movement errors to which the network will adapt are:

a) movement errors due to inaccuracies of saccade length or direction; for example, undershoot and overshoot errors;

b) movement errors due to modest lesions of the eye muscles;

c) movement errors due to a contact lens on the eyeball that modestly alters the length and direction (e.g., the curvature) of visual boundaries.

Errors of type (a) can occur due to the normal course of development. Errors of type (b) can occur due to accidents. Errors of type (c) can be due either to alterations in the lens of the eye, or to experimental manipulations.

Not all experimental manipulations that alter the pattern of light reaching the retina will cause adaptation within our network model. As a simple example, no saccadic adaptation will be caused by stationary targets viewed through inverting goggles worn on the head. Such targets do not cause saccadic errors, because the real image of a stationary target is not altered by a saccade. This simple fact raises a number of questions about the types of movements that do cause errors when goggles are worn on the head, and about differences between the adaptations that occur in response to goggles vs. contact lens.

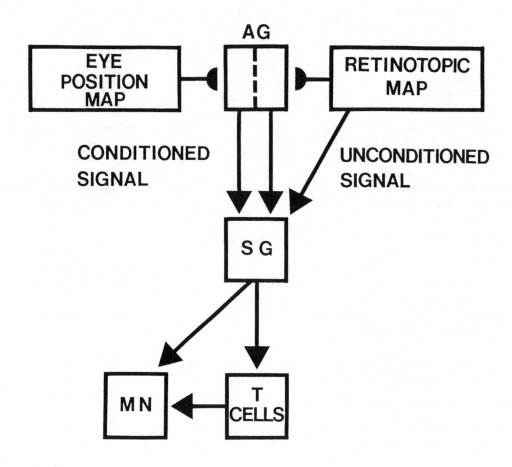

Figure 3.2. Explicit information about eye position and about retinotopic position converge at the saccade generator (SG) either via unconditioned signals or via the adaptive gain (AG) stage at which the conditioned pathways are altered by second-light error signals. T cells are tonic cells and MN cells are motoneurons.

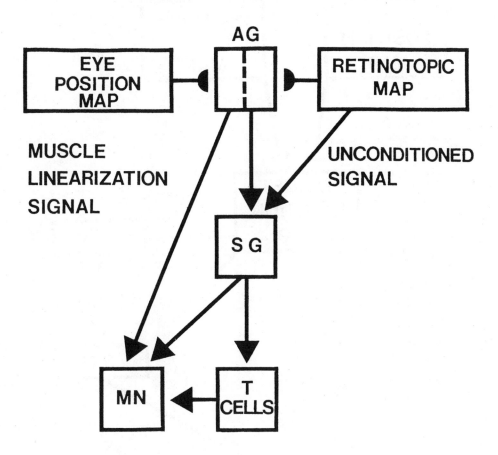

Figure 3.3. Explicit information about eye position and about retinotopic position are registered at different network stages. Retinotopic information converges at the saccade generator (SG). Eye position signals that compensate for muscle nonlinearity are registered at the motoneurons (MN). Chapters 5 and 7 refine these concepts.

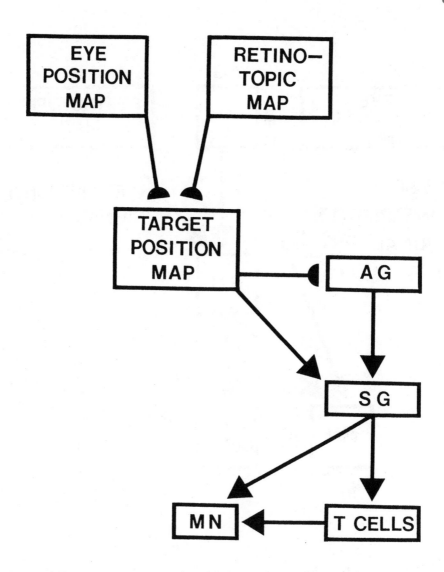

Figure 3.4. Eye position is implicitly encoded at a target position map, which is the source of both conditioned and unconditioned signals at the saccade generator (SG).

Inverting goggles do, for example, cause errors in visually-mediated reaching movements by the arm. This is because the goggles alter the expected relationship between the visual stimulus and a goal-oriented arm movement. Humans and monkeys are capable of adapting their arm movements to compensate for inverting goggles (Epstein, 1977; Welch, 1978). In pioneering experiments Stratton (1897) wore a monocular device that rotated the visual world 180 degrees for up to 8 days. He found nearly complete visuomotor adaptation when he engaged in everyday activities. Foley (1940) first studied visuomotor adaptation in monkeys. He reported that a 9-year-old rhesus monkey acquired significant adaptation after being exposed to binocular inversion for 1 week. Numerous experiments have since verified these results with finer detail and better quantification, but experiments on non-mammals show that they cannot adapt under similar conditions. For excellent reviews on many sensory-motor adaptation experiments see Epstein (1977) and Welch (1978).

Both saccadic eye movements and arm movements are goal-oriented movements that can be initiated by a visual stimulus. One might thus be tempted to conclude that saccadic eye movements can adapt to the same types of visual distortions to which goal-oriented arm movements can adapt. Inverting contact lens worn on the eye alter the visual stimuli that elicit saccades much as inverting goggles worn on the head alter the visual stimuli that elicit arm movements. Can the saccadic system adapt to an inverting contact lens?

The only direct data that we know concerning this issue yields a negative result (Smith, 1966). Our theory is compatible with this result. Our theory and the data also support the idea that adaptation can occur to contact lens which modestly distort visual curvature (Festinger, 1967; Slotnick, 1969; Taylor, 1962). What is the adaptational difference between an arm movement and a saccadic eye movement, and between an inverting contact lens and a curvature-distorting contact lens?

3.4. Self-Movement vs. World-Movement: Ballistic vs. Continuous Movement

We attribute the difference between arm and eye movement results to the different ways in which sensory-motor systems compute answers to the following question: How does the system know whether a change in visual feedback that occurs contingent upon a movement is due to self-movement with respect to a stationary world or to a movement within the world itself (Epstein, 1977)? Unless this distinction is made by an error-correcting mechanism, the mechanism cannot tell the difference between a correctly calibrated motion in a moving world and an incorrectly calibrated motion in a stationary world. An error-correcting mechanism that cannot make this distinction could persistently undo its own correct parametric calibrations in response to adventitious world motions. This destabilizing effect on the calibration of a movement system can be minimized if world-motions are rare during self-motions. The next paragraph comments upon how the rapidity of a saccade may minimize world-motions and thereby compensate for the loss of visual information that occurs during the saccade.

In order for any error correcting mechanism to correlate movement signals and visual signals during movement, it must have access to both types of signals. Saccades differ from arm movements in that the rapidity of a saccade attenuates the registration of visual feedback during a saccadic movement. This is the familiar phenomenon of saccadic suppression (Yarbus, 1967). Due to saccadic suppression, once a given light initiates a saccade, other lights do not strongly influence the saccadic trajectory. Only lights that occur before and after the saccade can be used by the saccadic error correction mechanism. Saccades thus differ from arm movements both in their rapidity and in their approximately all-or-none reactions to light signals. We have constructed our saccadic error correction mechanism to satisfy the hypothesis that the rapidity and all-or-none nature of a saccade prevent the saccadic error mechanism from distinguishing self-motion from world-motion.

Data compatible with this hypothesis have been collected by Optican and Miles (1979). If error correction is based entirely on visual feedback after movement, the saccadic system should not be able to distinguish two different reasons why a second light might not be foveated. One reason is that an incorrect saccade is made because the system's conditionable parameters are incorrectly chosen. The other reason is that a correct saccade is made in response to correctly chosen conditionable parameters, but the light is displaced to another position during the saccade. Optican and Miles (1979) studied how monkeys saccade to lights whose position is moved to the right during saccades to the right. Although these investigators were interested in post-saccadic drift, they found that over many trials the monkeys made systematically longer saccades. Thus although the saccades of the monkeys were correctly calibrated before the experiment began, they became recalibrated by the experiment because the saccadic error correction mechanism of the monkeys could not distinguish self-motion from world-motion.

To prevent misunderstanding of this hypothesis, we emphasize what it does not imply. Compensatory processes that can distinguish self-motion from world-motion can occur in the preprocessing of visual signals before they reach the saccadic system or in the postprocessing of saccadic motor signals before they generate the final motor command. For example, imagine that preprocessing of the retinal light pattern attenuates whole-field motions of the visual field, as would be caused by self-motions in a stationary world. Such preprocessing could also amplify the reactions to relatively localized relative motions within the visual field, as would be caused by an object moving in the world. In fact, localized relative motions excite the superior colliculus with greater efficacy than whole-field motions (Frost and Nakayama, 1983), thereby tending to initiate saccades towards moving targets but not in response to self-motions alone.

Compensation for self-initiated motions can also be accomplished by postprocessing of the saccadic motor command. For example, suppose that head movements are caused by self-motions through the world, such as walking, running, or head turning. Such a head movement can initiate a compensatory eye movement via the vestibulo-ocular reflex (VOR) to maintain the subject's gaze on a prescribed nonfoveal light (Section 3.5). Suppose, for example, that a VOR is initiated by a head movement that occurs while a saccade is being made. Then the VOR motor signal, which independently registers the head movement, can cooperate with the saccadic motor signal to generate a total movement that compensates for the self-initiated head movement (Lanman, Bizzi, and Allum, 1978; Whittington, 1980). A cooperative interaction of the VOR and the saccadic system can compensate for self-initiated head movements, even if the saccadic system by itself cannot distinguish self-motions from world-motions.

A third way to distinguish self-motion from world-motion can exist in the saccadic system as a whole without requiring that the visual error correction mechanism can make this distinction. Suppose, for example, that the eyes move with respect to a stationary light. Then the target position within an invariant target position map does not change (Section 1.4). Consequently the motor representation of this target position within the head-muscle interface (HMI) does not change (Section 1.6). No new saccadic command is therefore generated within this system due to self-motion. By contrast, suppose that a light moves with respect to the stationary eyes. Then a new target position is read into both the invariant target position map and the HMI.

The hypothesis that visual error signals due to saccades do not distinguish self-motion from world-motion implies that saccadic adaptation to inverting prisms should not occur. If saccadic adaptation to an inverting contact lens is eventually reported, then our task would be to show how a preprocessing step in the computation of the saccadic error signal distinguishes between self-motion and world-motion by using corollary discharges (Section 1.8). This preprocessed error signal would be used to alter the conditionable sampling pathways that correct saccadic errors. The data of Smith (1966) and of Optican and Miles (1979) are incompatible with the existence of such an error signal, but further experiments on this matter are needed.

Even if a negative result concerning adaptation to an inverting contact lens is confirmed, the task of explaining adaptation of visually-guided arm motions in response to inverting goggles would still remain. There is no contradiction in expecting corollary discharges to operate in this latter situation but not in response to inverting contact lens. Adaptation to inverting goggles involves intermodality (eye-arm) learning due to continuous movements. Adaptation to inverting contact lens would involve intramodality (eye-eye) learning due to ballistic movements. Thus there is a hierarchy of learning problems whose differences are reflected in the complexity of preprocessing that goes into the computation of their error signals, and in the number of sensory-motor systems that are involved. Despite these differences, all of the problems also share certain basic features in common. The next section focuses on an important shared feature of several movement systems that are capable of adapting to alterations in expected sensory-motor relationships. After that, we begin our analysis of how the saccadic error correction mechanism of our theory works.

3.5. A Universal Adaptive Gain Control Mechanism: Saccades, VOR, Posture, and Muscle Gain

As we noted in Section 3.4, although saccades in response to a stationary visual stimulus are not rendered erroneous by inverting goggles, the eye movements that occur during the vestibulo-ocular reflex (VOR) are rendered erroneous by inverting goggles. Moreover, the VOR can adapt to these errors (Ito, 1984; Welch, 1978). Unlike ballistic saccadic movements, the VOR eye movements are sufficiently slow to permit continuous registration of visual feedback, as in the case of arm movements.

The VOR can be described as follows: a head movement triggers vestibular signals that move the eye in a compensatory way to maintain fixation of a visual target. Successful operation of this system prevents a foveated target from moving with respect to the retina of an animal as it moves with respect to its environment, say as the animal runs towards the target. An inverting goggle changes the expected relationship between head movement and the visual feedback that is caused by a VOR-induced eye movement. Thus the VOR also involves intermodality (head-eye) learning due to continuous movements.

Adaptation of eye-arm coordination and of the VOR are mentioned here to emphasize an important feature of the theory's error correction mechanisms. Adaptation to inverting goggles during the VOR seems to be a very different process from adaptation to curvature-distorting contact lens during saccades. Despite this apparent difference, the same formal network machinery can be used to control adaptive responses in both paradigms. The same formal network machinery can also be used to control adaptation to post-saccadic drift and postural maintenance of gaze (Chapter 8), as well as linearization of muscle responses to outflow signals (Chapter 5). These results support the hypothesis that a single brain region is used as a universal adaptive gain control mechanism, which we have called the *adaptive gain* (AG) *stage*. We identify the AG stage with the cerebellum.

Invoking the cerebellum as part of the adaptive saccadic mechanism is compatible with studies in which ablation of vermis and paraflocculus disrupt adaptive changes in saccadic movements (Optican and Robinson, 1980). Our adaptive gain control model also refines recent cerebellar models of VOR adaptation (Fujita, 1982a, 1982b; Ito, 1982), and sheds new light on the result of Miles, Braitman, and Dow (1980) concerning the anatomical site of VOR adaptation. In the following sections, we build up increasingly precise functional requirements concerning how the AG stage corrects saccadic errors.

3.6. Compatibility of Design Hypotheses

Two major hypotheses concerning the correction of saccadic movement errors have already been made in the preceding sections. Before imposing additional constraints, we note that these requirements are consistent with each other, and that other possible error schemes could lead to serious internal inconsistencies.

A. *Perform and Test*

The saccadic movement system consists of many cellular components. None of these components knows the parameters governing the other components. Moreover, many of these parameters contribute to each saccadic motion. The only way that such a system can decide whether its parameters are correct or not is to test whether or not they lead to accurate foveation of light targets. Consequently, our error correction mechanism uses the position of the light on the retina after a saccade as a source of error signals.

B. *Visual Invariance during Saccades*

Thus to correct a saccade, a mechanism needs to keep track of a first light location that initiates the saccade and a second light location that is registered after the saccade. This need raises the fundamental question: How does the system know that the first and second light positions correspond to the same light source in space? How does the system know whether or not the light itself has moved during the saccade? We have hypothesized that the rapid all-or-none nature of the saccade obviates the need to distinguish world-motion from self-motion in the visual error signal.

Hypothesis (B) that no world-motion compensation occurs is compatible with hypothesis (A) that the second light is the source of light-mediated error signals. It is important to realize that not all plausible hypotheses about error signals are compatible with hypothesis (B). For example, consider a system that uses a sequence of corrective saccades leading to a correct foveation as an aggregate source of error signals. Such a system could correct saccadic errors by integrating all the corrective saccade commands into a total correct saccade command. Such a system could not, however, safely ignore world-motions that occur between successive corrective saccades. This example illustrates that a trade-off can be expected to exist in each sensory-motor system between the system's choice of error signal source and its ability to compute invariants that prevent this error source from undoing correct parameter choices.

3.7. Different Coordinates for Unconditioned and Conditioned Movement Systems

Other trade-offs exist that are capable of reconciling seemingly opposed design constraints. This section refines the conclusion of Chapter 2 that movement and error signals are processing in parallel. It shows that two different coordinate systems, working in parallel, are needed to unconditionally elicit saccades and to register the error signals that can correct these saccades.

A. *Unconditioned Movements due to Prewired Connection Gradients*

A source of unconditioned saccadic commands is needed in order to avoid an infinite regress of the following type. Unless saccades can be elicited at a developmental stage that occurs prior to saccadic learning, no saccadic errors can be generated on which to base the learning process. Since this unconditioned source of movement commands is operative prior to saccadic learning, it must be capable of working without the benefit of finely tuned learned parameters. It does not have to produce completely accurate saccades, because the later learning process will improve saccadic accuracy. On the other hand, some regularity in the transformation from retinal position to unconditioned saccadic motion is needed. For example, if a light that excites a position to the right side of the fovea elicited a movement towards the left, then the task of correcting saccadic errors would be seriously impaired.

To account for these properties of unconditioned movements, we have assumed that asymmetrically distributed pathways, or spatial gradients, are generated during an early stage of development from the retina to the eye muscles (Figure 2.1). Using these spatial gradients, a light to the right hemifield of the retina tends to move the eyes towards the right, and a light to the left hemifield of the retina tends to move the eyes towards the left. A light to an oblique retinal position tends to move the eyes in an oblique direction because the ratio of contractions in the co-contracting agonist muscles determines the net direction of movement (Grossberg, 1970; Sparks and Mays, 1981). Edwards (1980) has reported data which are compatible with such an asymmetric distribution of pathways. He writes that "the incidence of abducens-directed cells gradually increases at successively more caudal levels" of the superior colliculus (p.203).

B. *Conditioned Gain Control due to Visual Error Signals*

We will now show that the coordinates which are needed to learn error-correcting gains within the conditionable pathways are different from the spatial gradients on which unconditioned saccades are based. Thus the spatial gradients and the conditioned gains are computed by two parallel subsystems before these subsystems cooperate to read-out a total saccadic signal. We call this conditionable subsystem the adaptive gain (AG) stage (Section 3.5). Individual error lights to the AG stage must be able to correct whole muscle synergies (Section 1.11) to move the eyes closer to their targets on future performance trials. We now describe how the design of the AG stage solves this problem.

Our first observation about this problem concerns the coordinates in which first light movement signals and second light error signals are registered at the AG stage. A conditionable movement signal that is activated by a first light is registered in retinotopic coordinates, whereas an error signal that is activated by a second light must influence the gains of agonist-antagonist muscle pairs; hence is registered in motor coordinates. Both first lights and second lights arise, however, from lights on the retina. What correspondence between retinal positions and agonist-antagonist muscle pairs enables a light on the retina to be registered as a second light in motor coordinates?

Figure 3.5a suggests an answer to this question. Figure 3.5a depicts a retinal topography that is partitioned into six motor sectors denoted by $\alpha^\pm$, $\beta^\pm$, and $\gamma^\pm$. Each sector corresponds to an agonist muscle $(+)$ or its corresponding antagonist muscle $(-)$. Each light excites the retina in a particular retinal position. As a first light, each light activates a conditionable movement pathway that retains its retinotopic coordinates. As a second light error signal, each light changes the gains of the agonist-antagonist muscle pair that corresponds to the sector in which its retinal position is contained.

C. *Opponent Processing of Visual Error Signals*

For example, suppose that the second light's retinal position falls within the sector corresponding to muscle α^+. We assume that such an error signal *increases* the conditioned gain to the agonist muscle α^+ and *decreases* the conditioned gain to the antagonist muscle α^- in response to the same first light on a later performance trial. In other words, each second light has antagonistic, or opponent, effects on the conditionable gains of its corresponding muscle pair.

To understand why this hypothesis is needed, we consider how it enables the system to correct four different types of saccadic errors.

3.8. Correcting Undershoot, Overshoot, and Skewed Saccadic Errors

Figure 3.5b considers the case of an *undershoot* error in which a first light in sector β^+ generates a second light in the same sector. To correct such an undershoot error, the second light needs to strengthen the total signal to the saccade generator (SG) of muscle β^+ and/or weaken the total signal to the SG muscle of β^-. The following considerations suggest that both a strengthening of the β^+ command and a weakening of the β^- command to the SG simultaneously occur, and help to inactivate the antagonist SG during much of a saccade.

Figure 3.5c describes an *overshoot* error in which a first light in sector β^+ generates a second light in sector β^-. After this error is corrected, a first light in sector β^+ still activates the SG of muscle β^+, but more weakly than it did before error correction. How can an error signal to sector β^- weaken the contraction of the muscle corresponding to sector β^+? The previous case of correcting an undershoot error suggests that a second light in a given sector strengthens the signal to that sector's muscle. Since muscle β^- is antagonistic to muscle β^+, both undershoot and overshoot errors can be corrected by the same mechanism if strengthening within a sector is accompanied by weakening across antagonistic sectors. The strengthening action within a sector is due to excitatory conditioning of the conditionable pathway corresponding to that muscle. The weakening action within the antagonistic sector can be accomplished in either of

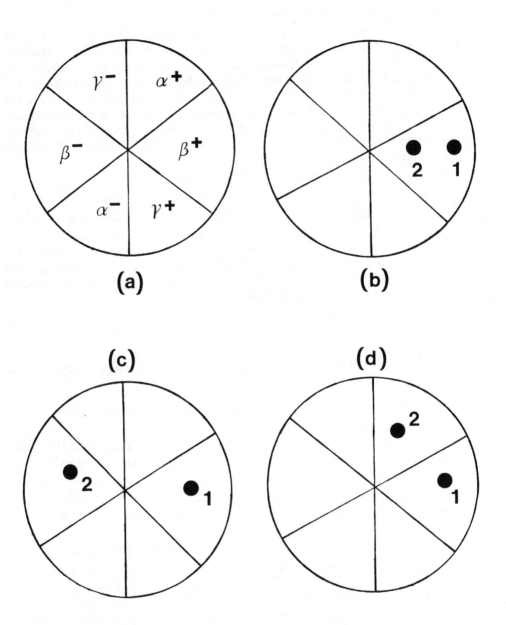

Figure 3.5. (a) Sectors corresponding to agonist muscles $(\alpha^+, \beta^+, \gamma^+)$ and antagonist muscles $(\alpha^-, \beta^-, \gamma^-)$ of one eye. In the text, the sectors represent both the retinotopic coordinates of the sampling signal sources, and the adaptive gain (AG) strips which receive error signals corresponding to the designated muscles. (b) A saccadic undershoot error. Number 1 locates the retinotopic position of the first light whereas number 2 locates the second light. (c) An overshoot error. (d) A skewed undershoot error.

two ways: by inhibitory conditioning of the conditionable pathway corresponding to the antagonist muscle (Figure 3.6a), or by inhibition of the excitatory output to the antagonist muscle (Figure 3.6b). In either case, a second light in sector β^- can weaken the total command controlled by a first light in sector β^+ via inhibitory signals from each sector to the output pathway of its antagonistic muscle. Then, when an agonist muscle contraction causes an overshoot error, the error signal corresponding to the antagonist muscle strip can weaken the conditioned gain of the agonist muscle.

The same rule easily generalizes to other types of errors. Figure 3.5d depicts a *skewed undershoot* error in which a first light in sector β^+ generates a second light in sector α^+ due to a motion of the eye downward and to the right. By the above rules, such a second light strengthens the total signal to muscle α^+ and weakens the total signal to muscle α^-, thereby tending to move the eye more upward on future performance trials to correct the movement error.

3.9. Curvature Distorting Contact Lens vs. Inverting Contact Lens

Given the above error correction mechanism, let us consider how it responds to a curvature distorting contact lens. Suppose for definiteness that the model's parameters are accurately tuned before the contact lens is put on. Let the contact lens transform radially oriented straight lines, such as a radial line in the α^+ sector of the retina, into curved lines, such as a line that crosses retinal sectors α^+, β^+, γ^+ as its retinal eccentricity increases (Figure 3.7). Radial lights placed along a radial line will then cause saccades that terminate along a curved line.

The error correcting mechanism works as follows in this situation. Consider a light that would have fallen in β^+ horizontally to the right of the fovea without the lens on, but which falls on sector γ^+ with the lens on. The eye consequently moves downwards and towards the right. Without the contact lens, the second light caused by this motion would have landed in sector α^+. Due to the contact lens, the second light lands in sector β^+. The error correcting mechanism causes the next saccade to the same first light to move in a more upwards direction to the right. By the same reasoning, the second light falls in β^+, but closer to the fovea than it did before. On successive trials, the second light falls progressively closer to the fovea, thus correcting errors due to curvature of the lens. The ability to correct such errors depends upon the property that the amount of lens distortion increases with the distance from the fovea.

By contrast, consider the effect of a contact lens that reflects the whole visual field with respect to the vertical axis. Consider a light that would have fallen in β^+ horizontally to the right of the fovea without the lens on, but which falls in β^- with the lens on. The eye consequently moves to the left. Without the contact lens on, the second light caused by this

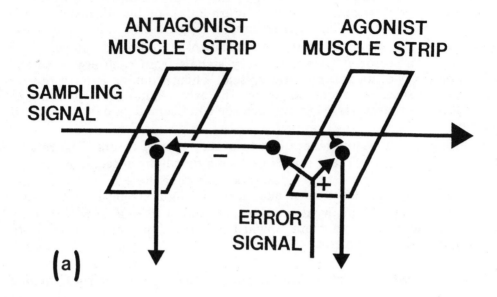

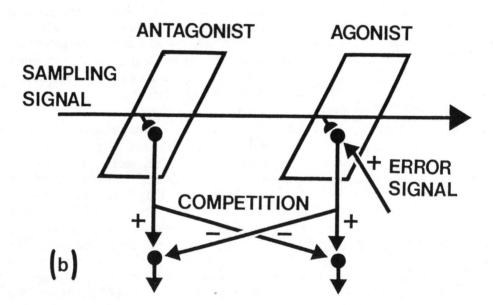

Figure 3.6. Two ways to achieve opponent conditioning of agonist-antagonist muscles: (a) An error signal increases the conditioned gain at the agonist muscle strip and decreases the conditioned gain at the antagonist muscle strip; (b) An error signal increases the conditioned gain at the agonist muscle strip. Competition between agonist and antagonist muscle strip outputs causes the decrease in the net antagonist output.

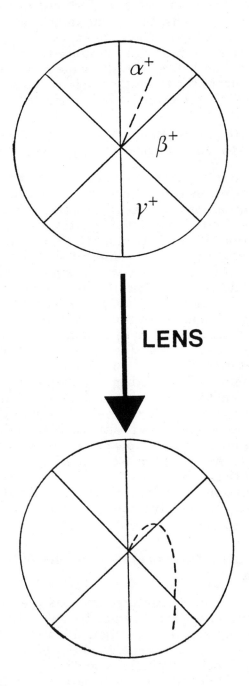

Figure 3.7. A curvature distorting contact lens which converts a linear image in sector α^+ into a curved image that bends across sectors α^+, β^+, and γ^+.

motion would have landed in sector β^+ further to the right than the first light. Due to the contact lens, the second light lands in sector β^- further to the left than the first light. The error correcting mechanism causes the next saccade to the same first light to move to the left again, but with a larger amplitude than before. By the same reasoning, the second light lands further away from the fovea than before. This tendency persists on all trials. Consequently the error is never corrected

3.10. Equal Access to Error Signals: Separate Anatomies for Unconditioned Movements and Conditioned Gain Changes

The above analysis suggests how undershoot, overshoot, skewed, and curvature distorting errors can be corrected no matter where the first light hits the retina In order for this scheme to work, a first light to *any* retinal position must give rise to conditionable pathways that can strengthen or weaken the conditioned signals to the SGs of *all* the eye muscles. Thus the asymmetric retinal-to-motor gradients that are needed to generate unconditioned saccades define the wrong kind of anatomy for saccadic error correction. These asymmetrical retinal-to-motor gradients can work even if each retinal position sends no signals whatever to the SGs of some muscles. All that is required to initiate an unconditioned saccade is a stronger pathway from each retinal position to the muscle corresponding to its sector. By contrast, correcting undershoot, overshoot, and skewed errors requires that every first light position be able to sample second lights in every sector. Expressed in another way, despite the asymmetries in the prewired retinal-to-motor spatial gradients, the mechanism whereby each first light position can adaptively sample all second light positions needs to be unbiased across second light positions. We call the property whereby each first light command can sample error signals due to all second light positions with equal ease the *equal access constraint*. We conclude that the unbiased anatomy that subserves saccadic error correction and the biased retinal-to-motor anatomy that unconditionally initiates saccades are two separate structures. We identify the error correction structure with the adaptive gain (AG) stage.

3.11. Anatomical Interpretation of the Adaptive Gain Stage: The Cerebellum

This equal access constraint suggests that the representations of all second light positions are placed symmetrically with respect to the sampling signals from any first light position. Figure 3.8 depicts the simplest realization of this concept (Grossberg, 1964, 1969a). In Figure 3.8, each first light pathway (labeled 1) gives rise to a branching conditionable pathway that is perpendicular to a series of parallel bands. Each band corresponds to one of the sectors $\alpha^\pm$, $\beta^\pm$, and $\gamma^\pm$. A second light in such a sector delivers an error signal to its *entire band*. Each first light can then sample any such band because its sampling pathway crosses and sends conditionable branches to all bands. The total output from such a band contributes to the conditioned gain of the corresponding muscle.

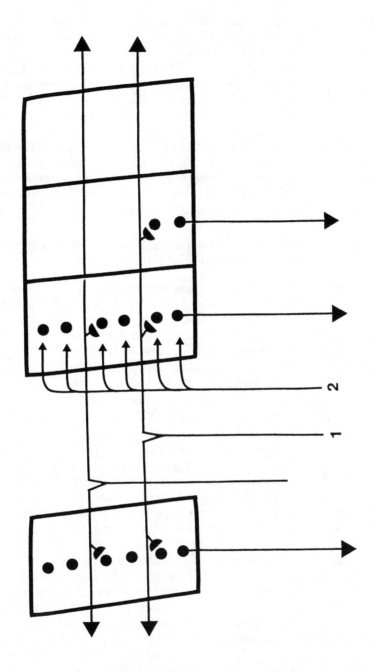

Figure 3.8. Functional diagram of the adaptive gain stage: A perpendicular arrangement of sampling signal pathways (1) and error signals (2) to motor strips enables every retinotopic coordinate to sample all motor strips and to generate output signals to all muscles.

Figure 3.8 is evocative of data on cerebellar circuitry (Eccles, 1977; Eccles, Ito, and Szentágothai, 1967; Llinás, 1969; Oscarsson, 1975) and of cerebellar models of adaptive motor control (Albus, 1971, Brindley, 1964; Fujita, 1982a, 1982b; Grossberg, 1964, 1969a, 1972a; Ito, 1974, 1980; Marr, 1969; McCormick and Thompson, 1984). In this cerebellar interpretation, the sampling pathways are realized by mossy fiber inputs that activate granule cells whose parallel fibers traverse a broad region of cerebellar cortex. The error signal pathways are realized by climbing fiber inputs that activate Purkinje cells (Figure 3.9). The synapses from active parallel fibers to activated Purkinje cells encode the adaptive changes due to the correlation between sampling signal and error signal. Our subsequent discussion will impose increasingly strong design constraints on this error correction circuit and its interaction with the asymmetric gradients of unconditioned retinal-to-motor connections.

3.12. Superposition of Sampling Map and Error Signal Map: Logarithms and Bidirectional Parallel Fibers

Some implications about the macroanatomy of the AG stage can be drawn by comparing Figures 3.5 and 3.8. By Figure 3.5, the set of all first light positions sweeps out the whole retina, as does the set of second light error signals. Thus a *map* of sampling signal sources and a *map* of error signal sources are superimposed within the AG stage. (See Section 3.16 for a discussion of examples in which the sampling signal map is not retinotopic.) The transformation of Figure 3.5a into Figure 3.8 is accomplished by mapping radial sectors into parallel strips. This property suggests that the error signal map is (approximately) logarithmic (Schwartz, 1980).

The existence of such a logarithmic map suggests, in turn, why parallel fibers are emitted by a granule cell in two opposite directions: If each retinal position activates a subset of mossy fiber terminals, then each subset must be able to activate parallel fibers capable of sampling the strips corresponding to all possible second light positions on the retina. The assumption that the parallel fibers form part of the sampling map may help to reconcile the conflicting data concerning whether parallel fibers can activate all Purkinje cells in their path. Bower and Woolston (1983) mapped the spatial organization of somato-sensory fields in the cerebellar cortex. They explored receptive field patterns in Purkinje and granule cell layers with tactile stimuli. Adjacent patches of these cell layers were found to represent widely separated body parts. They also found that Purkinje cells slightly distant from the region of granule cell layer activation occasionally responded with an increment in simple spike activity (parallel fiber excitation) for up to 100 ms. Moreover, their studies indicated that the granule cell to Purkinje cell excitation tended to be colinear with parallel fiber tracts while inhibition was slightly more widely distributed. In apparent contrast to the "parallel fiber beam hypothesis," neighboring Purkinje cells in the direction of parallel fibers often showed variable response characteristics. Only Purkinje cells for which a strong learned parallel fiber→Purkinje cells synapse exists are activated in our

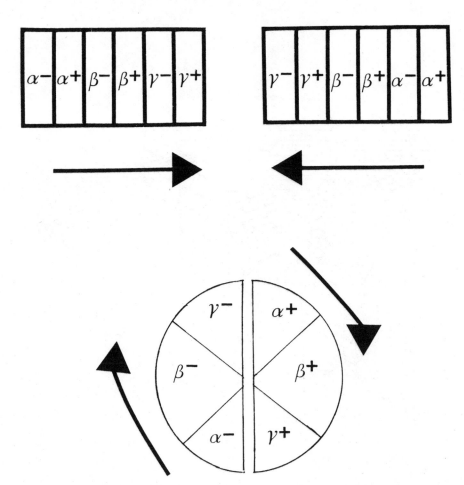

Figure 3.9. Logarithmic map from sensory sectors into motor strips: Each sensory hemifield $(\alpha^+, \beta^+, \gamma^+)$ and $(\alpha^-, \beta^-, \gamma^-)$ maps into a row of parallel motor strips. In this fractured somatotopy, the strips of agonist-antagonist pairs (α^+, α^-), (β^+, β^-), and (γ^+, γ^-) are juxtaposed, much as in the case of ocular dominance columns in the striate cortex. A pair of motor strip maps is depicted, one in each AG stage hemisphere. Outputs from all agonist-antagonist pairs compete before the net outputs perturb the saccade generator (SG). This circuit works even if only agonist muscles $(\alpha^+, \beta^+, \gamma^+)$ receive excitatory error signals in one hemifield and antagonist muscles $(\alpha^-, \beta^-, \gamma^-)$ receive excitatory error signals in the other hemifield. An excitatory error signal to the α^+ strip can weaken the net α^- output of the contiguous strip via competition of the outputs, but cannot strengthen the α^- output signal. An excitatory error signal to the α^- strip of the other hemifield can strengthen the net α^- output.

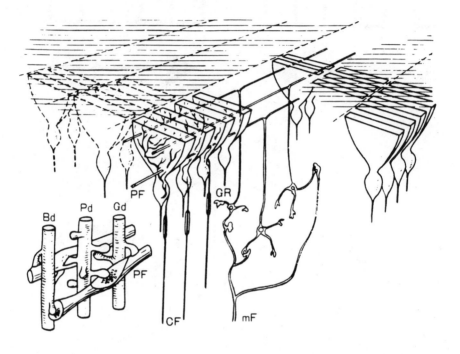

Figure 3.10. Diagram of the cerebellum showing the major cell types and interactions. The sampling signals in Figure 3.8 are assumed to be activated by mossy fibers and parallel fibers. The error signals in Figure 3.8 are assumed to be activated by climbing fibers. From Szentágothai, 1968, modified by Eccles, 1977. Reprinted with permission from **The Cerebellum and Neural Control** by Masao Ito, Raven Press, 1984.

model. Thus the receptive fields of the Purkinje cells can be regularly aligned, yet the synaptic strengths of parallel fiber contacts with these receptive fields can be much more variable.

3.13. Fractured Somatotopy and/or Bilateral Cerebellar Organization

Functional constraints on the microanatomy of the AG stage are also consistent with recent data about the cerebellum. The anatomy in Figure 3.8 can be refined by imposing the functional constraint that strengthening one conditionable pathway corresponding to a prescribed muscle weakens the net effect of the conditionable pathway corresponding to its antagonist muscle (Section 3.7). This constraint leads to the prediction that the cerebellar outputs corresponding to antagonist eye muscles vary in a push-pull, or opponent, fashion. One way to realize this property is to fracture the somatotopy of the cerebellar cortex; that is, to bring the receptive fields of agonist-antagonist muscles into a close antagonistic relationship within the cerebellar cortex, as in Figure 3.9. This type of cerebellar microanatomy has been reported by several investigators (Armstrong and Drew, 1980; Bower and Woolston, 1983; Cody and Richardson, 1979; Coffey, Goodwin-Austen, MacGillivray, and Sears, 1971; Eccles, 1973; Eccles, Faber, Murphy, Sabah, and Táboríková, 1971; Eccles, Sabah, Schmidt, and Táboríková, 1972; Saint-Cyr and Woodward, 1980). For example, a short-latency excitation of a Purkinje cell that is evoked by stimulating the ipsilateral upper lip of a rat can be suppressed by locally stimulating the contralateral upper lip (Bower and Woolston, 1983). Within our theory, such a fractured somatotopy can permit either a learned increase of agonist gain to coexist with a learned decrease of antagonist gain, or a competition to occur between output signals from the agonist and antagonist muscle strips.

Another possible way to realize an inhibitory relationship between the cerebellar pathways corresponding to antagonist eye muscle pairs is to group together the bands of all agonist muscles on one side of the cerebellum, the bands of all antagonist muscles on the other side of the cerebellum, to let each light-activated sampling pathway send parallel fibers bidirectionally across the midline of the cerebellum to sample all these bands, and to let the outputs of antagonistic bands compete across the midline before the net output influences the corresponding SGs.

A combination of these two designs is also possible. In this anatomy, agonist muscles of one eye are brought into a close antagonistic relationship in the cerebellar cortex. Thus strengthening the gain of one agonist muscle via an error signal weakens the gain of the other agonist muscles, thereby shifting the vector direction of agonist contraction in that eye. Somatotopy is fractured by bringing together the agonist representations of corresponding muscles in the two eyes, and letting the error signals that strengthen an agonist muscle command in one eye also strengthen the agonist command of the corresponding muscle in the other eye. At least partial adaptive yoking of the two eyes is hereby achieved. All agonists are represented on one side of the cerebellar cortex, all antagonists are represented on the other side of the cerebellar cortex, and the outputs of agonist-antagonist bands compete across the midline before the net output influences the SGs. We mention all of these anatomical possibilities because, even if one of them is supported in one species, we must still be prepared to understand different versions of this mechanism that may be used by other species.

Eckmiller and Westheimer (1983) have reported data that are consistent with the last two anatomies. These authors show that ablation of the cerebellar cortex on one side in monkeys causes deficits of eye movements on the lesioned side. If future anatomical studies show that fractured somatotopy occurs in the cerebellar vermis, then the third anatomical possibility is favored.

Ebner and Bloedel (1981) have reported cerebellar data that are compatible with the third possibility, albeit not in a cerebellar circuit that subserves saccadic control. These authors described the correlations of spontaneous climbing fiber inputs with mossy fiber activations due to flexions of the forepaw. They found that if a mossy fiber tended to enhance activity of a Purkinje cell before being paired with climbing fiber activity, then this enhancing effect was amplified after termination of climbing fiber activity. They also found that if a mossy fiber tended to depress activity of a Purkinje cell before being paired with climbing fiber activity, then this depressive effect was amplified after termination of climbing fiber activity. Gilbert and Thach (1977) also described compatible cerebellar data. They showed that if a known extensor load is increased to a novel load level, then an increase in climbing fiber activity is caused that leads to a decrease in later Purkinje cell activity in response to mossy fiber inputs. The climbing fiber input frequency to a known flexor load did not change, but the Purkinje cell activity caused by mossy fiber input decreased. These results during the known flexor motion are compatible with the existence of an agonist-antagonist fractured somatotopy, and also suggest that learning can cause a decrease in synaptic strength. The ratio of gains across agonist-antagonist pathways can also be changed by such a learning mechanism.

As part of their studies of the VOR, Ito and his colleagues (Ito, 1982; Ito, Sakurai, and Tongroach, 1982) have also reported data indicating that climbing fiber inputs that are correlated with mossy fiber activity can depress the responsiveness of target Purkinje cells to later mossy fiber inputs. This depression was caused by conjunctive stimulation of a vestibular nerve (mossy fiber) and of the inferior olive (climbing fiber). Llinás and Wolfe (1977) have recorded from saccade related Purkinje cells in the cerebellar vermis. They found some Purkinje cells that fired at a rate inversely proportional to the amplitude of concurrent saccadic eye movements. They attributed this Purkinje cell activity to "the highly stereotyped spike burst characteristics of climbing fiber induced activity" (p.4). Such an effect could be produced by changes in the ratio of agonist-antagonist activation recorded at the antagonist motor strip of the saccadic command.

Such cerebellar results are consistent with our model, but do not un-equivocally support or reject it, primarily because these data do not di-rectly measure cerebellar effects on antagonistic muscle pairs as a result of learning. The functional constraints that our theory imposes on cerebel-lar design are consistent with many evolutionary variations. If our theory is correct, however, then all of these variations must embody a form of agonist-antagonist opponency whose balance can be regulated by learning.

3.14. More Constraints on Cerebellar Learning

Further constraints on the saccadic learning mechanisms will now be derived and shown to be realizable by several related mechanisms. The physiological data do not yet seem to decide between these alternatives ei-ther. Part of the ensuing discussion applies only to the problem of saccadic error correction. For example, the saccadic learning problem under con-sideration is a case of temporally discrete sampling wherein both sampling and error signals can be activated by the same modality, namely vision. By contrast, the VOR describes a continuous sampling problem wherein the sampling signal is vestibular and the error signal is visual. Differ-ences therefore exist in the types of sampling signals and sampled signals that are used for saccadic vs. VOR adaptation. Part of the discussion nevertheless has general implications for cerebellar design. Although each learning circuit, whether mediating saccades or VORs, may preprocess its inputs in different ways, we believe that the same internal cerebellar machinery is used in all cases.

The following hypotheses about cerebellar learning will be explored below:

A. The dual action of each light.
B. The incremental effect of error signals on performance.
C. The attenuation of error signals by prior learning trials.

3.15. Dual Action, Incremental Learning, and Error Signal Attenuation

By the dual action of each light, we mean that each light is a source of an error signal for correcting a previous saccade, as well as a source of a movement command for the next saccade By the incremental effect of error signals on performance, we mean that the effect of error signals is to progressively improve the accuracy of saccades. In particular, as learning progressively increases the conditioned gain of an agonist muscle, it progressively decreases the conditioned gain of its antagonist muscle. This opponent learning process biases which of the saccade generators corresponding to the two muscles will be activated. By the attenuation of error signals due to prior learning trials, we mean that saccadic error correction tends to undermine its own source of error signals by caus-ing more accurate saccades. This last property is the main justification for calling the second light a source of error signals. This property implies that the size of the error signal generated by a second light decreases as the second light approaches the fovea.

These three properties imply further constraints upon the microscopic design of the AG stage. The main constraints arise from a consideration of how sampling signals and error signals are allowed to overlap in network space and time in order to realize these three functional properties.

The dual action of each light constrains the possible onset times and durations of sampling signals and error signals. To see why this is so, suppose that the eyes make a sequence of inaccurate saccades in response to a single unmoving light in the outside world. These saccadic movements generate a series of lights on the retina. Denote the sampling signal due to the ith light in such a saccadic sequence by S_i and its error signal by E_i, $i = 1, 2, \ldots$. Several possible cases may arise, and our goal is to indicate which cases are consistent with functional requirements. If inconsistent cases are found *in vivo*, then our model of cerebellar learning needs correction.

Case 1: Suppose that the onset time of E_i precedes that of S_i and that E_i terminates before S_i begins (Figure 3.11a). Since S_{i-1} must sample E_i, the offset time of S_{i-1} is later than the onset time of E_i. In this situation, E_i can alter the effect of S_{i-1} on future performance without altering the effect of S_i on future performance, even though both S_i and E_i are elicited by the same light.

Case 2: Suppose that the onset time of E_i is subsequent to the onset time of S_i (Figure 3.11b). Since S_{i-1} must be able to sample E_i, S_{i-1} is still active in SSTM at the onset time of S_i. The timing configuration in Figure 3.10b can create the following difficulty.

The effect of an error signal such as E_i on the sampling signal S_{i-1} of a prior light is to progressively improve the accuracy of the saccade that corresponds to S_{i-1}. Thus after sufficiently many learning trials take place, S_{i-1} will read-out conditioned signals leading to accurate foveations which generate zero error signals. In order for E_i's to correct an S_{i-1} in this way, the effect of successive E_i's on the conditionable pathway sampled by S_{i-1} must be incremental, so that each successive saccade foveates better in response to the same first light. When this incremental learning effect ultimately causes accurate foveations, no further error signals are registered until parameter changes elsewhere in the system cause fixation errors anew.

Given these learning properties, an S_i that overlaps its own E_i on every trial, as in Figure 3.11b, can create a serious learning anomaly. If a given nonfoveal light increments its S_i-activated sampling pathway with its own nonzero E_i on every saccadic trial, then the error signal never terminates even if the saccade becomes more accurate. Unless precautions are taken, every saccade will eventually overshoot due to the persistent action of its own error signal. Can this problem be prevented if the timing relationships of Figure 3.11b prevail?

This problem cannot be escaped just by claiming that S_i is insensitive to E_i because S_i's onset time precedes that of E_i. Such a sensitivity-

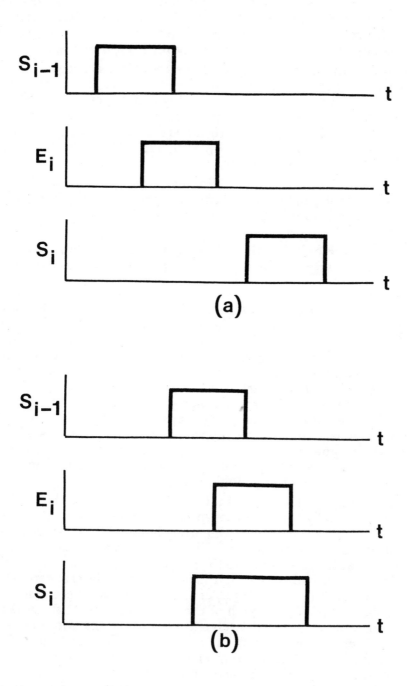

Figure 3.11. Two possible configurations of sampling signals and error signals: S_j is the sampling signal and E_j is the error signal on the jth trial, plotted through time.

timing argument fails because S_{i-1} must be sensitive to E_i even though the onset time of S_{i-1} precedes that of S_i. If S_i were already insensitive to E_i when E_i occurred, then surely S_{i-1} would also be insensitive, thereby preventing any saccadic learning whatsoever from occurring.

This self-sampling problem can be overcome if a preprocessing stage exists at which both the sampling map and the error map are topographically superimposed. Suppose at this stage that the source of sampling signals due to a given light topographically inhibits the source of error signals due to the same light before the error signals reach the AG stage. Then no S_i could sample its own E_i, although any active $S_{i-1} \neq S_i$ could sample E_i.

Cases 1 and 2 show that two different timing rules can, in principle, govern cerebellar learning if these rules are joined to suitable topographic restrictions on self-sampling of error signals.

3.16. Numerical Studies of Adaptive Foveation due to Cerebellar Gain Changes: Learned Compensation for System Nonlinearities

We have numerically analyzed the formal learning capabilities of several types of AG stage models to achieve a quantitative understanding of the AG stage concept. We have sought the type of understanding that can meet the challenge of species-specific variations of several conceivable types. We have paid particular attention to the issue of muscle nonlinearity. To this end, we have carried out computer simulations wherein different combinations of eye position sampling maps, retinotopic sampling maps, and target position sampling maps are used with two varieties of agonist-antagonist competitive interactions to learn accurate foveations using different types of nonlinear muscle plants and error signals. This type of parametric analysis provides a conceptual understanding that transcends the limitations of any single model.

In this spirit, we have systematically analyzed how thirty-six related models learn visually reactive (non-predictive) sequences of saccades, and have studied the stability of learning in each model given several numerical choices of important parameters. Eighteen of the models use a learning rule that instantiates a fractured cerebellar somatotopy and eighteen of the models use a learning rule that instantiates a bilateral cerebellar organization (Section 3.7). Both types of anatomy use an incremental learning rule (Section 3.15). Within each of these learning types, six of the models use a linear error signal and twelve use two different nonlinear error signals. All the error signal functions increase with the distance of a second light from the fovea. The different error signal functions embody different spatial gradient rules that transform a second light in retinotopic coordinates into an error signal in motor coordinates. The six model choices corresponding to each choice of error signal embody different strategies for compensating for initial eye position. These strategies will be described in the following paragraphs.

In all cases, saccades converge to the correct target position, on the average, with increasing numbers of learning trials. However, the errors fluctuate around the correct target position in a manner that depends in a systematic way on the design of the system. Given a nonlinear muscle, a significant damping of errors occurs only if initial position is taken into account in the learning rule. The following empirical rule has been derived from our studies of these thirty-six models.

The Nonlinear Dimension Rule: An extra degree of freedom in the sampling maps is needed to compensate for each nonlinearity in the muscle response.

The remainder of this section describes the results of these computer simulations in an intuitive language. Section 3.18 defines the learning models mathematically.

A. *Purely Retinotopic Sampling*

To see that compensating for a nonlinear muscle plant is a real problem, consider Figure 3.12. In Figure 3.12A, only a retinotopic sampling map can be conditioned by error signals. Figure 3.12A shows that, although saccades become more accurate on the average due to learning, the mean error rate never becomes smaller than approximately ±6.7% of the total visual field. The negative result holds even if the error function increases linearly with distance of the second light from the fovea, and if the relationship between muscle contraction and motion of the light on the retina is equal and opposite.

The cause of this learning difficulty is the nonlinear relationship between the total saccadic signal and the amount of muscle contraction. In the system of Figure 3.12A, this nonlinearity is a slower-than-linear one: The amount of contraction is proportional to the saccadic command at small values of the command, and gradually begins to decrease, or to saturate, at larger values of the command. In this example, a half-maximal muscle signal causes a 4/5-maximal muscle contraction. Thus the nonlinearity has a significant effect on system performance.

Figure 3.12B shows that the nonlinear muscle function is the cause of this difficulty. When a linear muscle function is used, essentially perfect learning occurs. This occurs even though a demanding rule is imposed governing the amount of muscle contraction and the corresponding motion of the light on the retina: an increment of ΔL in muscle contraction is assumed to cause a change $-2\Delta L$ in the position of the light on the retina.

In order to learn well using a nonlinear muscle plant, the learning system needs somehow to compensate for the different contractions that are caused by fixed movement signals when the muscle starts out in different initial positions. A retinotopic sampling map contains no information whatsoever about initial position. The remaining simulations include information about initial position in several different forms. In the computer studies that are summarized below, we considered a mean error rate to be unacceptable unless it was less than about 4 percent of the visual field. This approximates the accuracy of human saccades (Weber and Daroff, 1972).

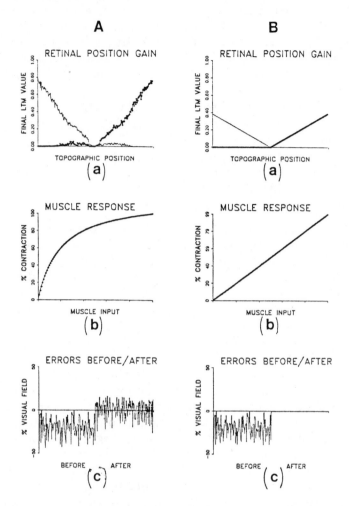

Figure 3.12. Computer simulation of saccadic error correction model with sampling from retinal position map using a linear learning function $L(w) = \epsilon w$: **(A)** Slower-than-Linear Muscle Function: The following parameters were used in the simulation: $m = 1$, $\alpha = .2$, $\gamma = 1$, $\delta = 1$, $\epsilon = .01$, and $n = 100,000$. (a) Topographic distribution of LTM trace values after learning. Bold curve indicates values in the right adaptive gain (AG) stage hemifield. Thin curve indicates values in the left AG stage hemifield. (b) Muscle response function used in the simulation. (c) Errors in 100 trials before learning begins and 100 trials after learning ends. Negative values correspond to undershoots and positive values correspond to overshoots. Learning was poor. **(B)** Linear Muscle Function: The following parameters were used: $\gamma = 2$, $\delta = 1$, $\epsilon = .01$, and $n = 100,000$. Learning was perfect.

B. *Invariant Target Position Map*

One way to take the initial eye position into account without increasing the total number of long-term memory (LTM) traces in the sampling maps is to let a single LTM trace multiply a composite signal that is the sum of two signals. Let one signal code a retinotopic light position, the other signal code an initial eye position, and the two signals add to influence a single LTM trace only if their sum represents a fixed target position. A different LTM trace exists corresponding to each target position that is computed within the spatial resolution of the network. Such a sampling map is called an invariant target position map because a single LTM trace corresponds to each target position independent of how that position is synthesized from its component signals (Section 1.4).

In this system, a single LTM trace must compensate for all the initial eye positions that can correspond to a fixed target position. Each of these initial eye positions corresponds to a different part of the nonlinear muscle function. Despite this fact, a significant reduction in the mean error rate occurs compared to the case of purely retinotopic sampling. Figure 3.13 depicts a simulation in which the mean error rate eventually becomes 1.8% of the visual field. Thus if a single sampling map implicitly embodies two degrees of freedom (one retinotopic position plus one initial eye position), then excellent learning occurs (Section 3.2).

C. *Invariant Target Position Map Plus Retinotopic Map*

Increasing the number of adaptive degrees of freedom causes a further improvement in error rate, even if no more LTM traces correspond to initial eye position information *per se*. These additional degrees of freedom enable part of the burden of adaptation to be absorbed by a different sampling map. In Figure 3.14A, both an invariant target position map and a retinotopic map separately send sampling signals to the AG stage. Each of these maps undergoes independent learning within the AG stage. The two sampling maps then add their conditioned movement signals to unconditioned movement signals at the SG. The LTM traces of the independent retinotopic map and invariant target position map embody three degrees of freedom. The retinotopic map explicitly embodies one degree of freedom and the invariant target position map implicitly embodies two degrees of freedom. In these simulations, a mean error rate of 1.5% of the visual field was attained using a nonlinear S-shaped muscle function. Thus if three degrees of freedom are used and at least one degree of freedom incorporates initial eye position signals, then excellent learning takes place. This is true even if the learning function is nonlinear; for example, if error signals grow as a cubic function of error size.

D. *Retinotopic Map Plus Eye Position Map*

Better learning than with purely retinotopic sampling (Figure 3.12A) occurs using two degrees of freedom in which the first map is a retinotopic map and the second map is a map of initial eye position. In these simulations, the network takes into account the target position of the eye (initial position plus retinal light position), but does not compute a map whose individual cells represent target position (Figure 3.14B). In these

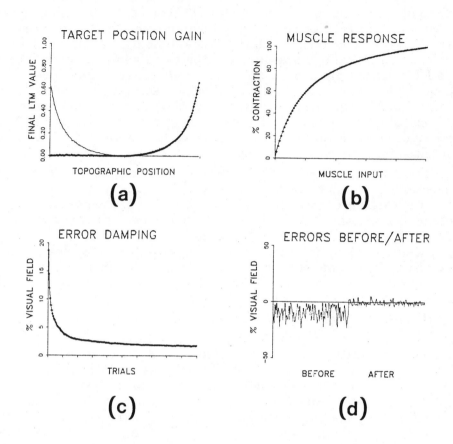

Figure 3.13. Computer simulation of saccadic error correction model with sampling from an invariant target postion map using a slower-than-linear muscle function and a linear learning function. The following parameters were used in the simulation: $m = 1$, $\alpha = .2$, $\gamma = 1$, $\delta = 1$, $\epsilon = .01$, and $n = 100,000$. (a) Topographic distribution of LTM trace values after learning. Bold curve indicates values in the right adaptive gain (AG) stage hemifield. Thin curve indicates values in the left AG stage hemifield. (b) Slower-than-linear muscle response function used in the simulation. (c) Error damping over 100,000 trials. Error damping value D_n at trial n approximates the average error via the equation $D_{n+1} = (999D_n + |E_n|)/1000$, where $D_0 = 25$. (d) Errors in 100 trials before learning begins and 100 trials after learning ends. Negative values correspond to undershoots and positve values correspond to overshoots.

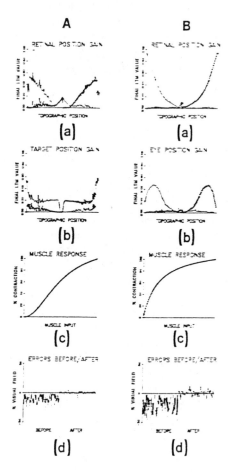

Figure 3.14. Computer simulation of saccadic error correction model with two sampling signal maps. (A) Sampling from an invariant target position map and a retinal position map using an S-shaped muscle function and a cubic learning function. The following parameters were used in the simulation: $m = 2$, $\alpha = .5$, $\gamma = 1$, $\delta = 1$, $\epsilon = 1$, and $n = 1,000,000$. (a) and (b) Topographic distribution of LTM trace values after learning. Bold curves indicate values in the right adaptive gain (AG) hemifields while the thin curves indicate values in the left AG hemifields. (c) Sigmoid muscle response characteristic used in the simulation. (d) Errors in 100 trials before learning begins and 100 trials after learning ends. Negative values correspond to undershoots and positive values correspond to overshoots. (B) Sampling from a retinal position map and an initial eye position map using a slower-than-linear muscle function and a linear learning function. The following parameters were used in the simulation: $m = 1$, $\alpha = .2$, $\gamma = 1$, $\delta = 1$, $\epsilon = .01$, and $n = 1,000,000$.

simulations, a mean error rate of 3.5% of the visual field was attained using a nonlinear slower-than-linear muscle function. Note that, although both Figures 3.14A and 3.14B use two sampling maps, their final error rates and spatial distributions of LTM traces are different due to their different sampling maps and the different nonlinear muscle plants to which they are adapting. In other words, different sampling maps automatically learn different LTM patterns to compensate for the initial position errors that are caused by different nonlinear muscle functions.

E. *Noninvariant Target Position Map*

Two degrees of freedom can also be realized by allowing every possible pair of retinotopic positions and initial eye positions, up to some finite spatial resolution, to have its own sampling pathway and LTM trace. Figure 3.15 shows that this model can achieve arbitrarily good mean error rates. Because each unique pair of positions has its own LTM trace, learning by this model is very stable. The model has the disadvantage that a given LTM trace will not be tuned until its unique pair of positions is activated on learning trials. By contrast, when an invariant target position map is used, learning occurs at a retinotopic or initial eye position whenever this position is a component of any target position. Thus there exists a tradeoff between convergence rate, stability, and the number of independent sampling sources. The expected interval between successive learning increments at each LTM trace of a noninvariant target position map can be decreased by expanding the receptive fields of positions in the sampling map. Then positions near to a fixed position can induce some learning at that position. The LTM traces then attain limiting values that are averages of the gains appropriate to nearby map positions. Given sufficiently symmetric and localized receptive fields, these average LTM values approximate the values that occur without any receptive field spread, but at a faster rate.

F. *Retinotopic Map Plus Initial Eye Position Map Plus Invariant Target Position Map*

If three independent sampling maps send sampling signals to the AG stage, then learning is again very accurate and stable. Figure 3.16 depicts an example in which a muscle contraction of ΔL causes a change of $-2\Delta L$ in the retinal position of the light. Despite this distortion, the system quickly achieves error rates of .3% of the visual field.

3.17. Shared Processing Load and Recovery from Lesions

Inspection of Figures 3.12–3.16 shows that the spatial maps of LTM traces that arise due to learning in different models need not be the same. For example, the retinotopic LTM map or the invariant target position LTM map may differ due to the existence of other sampling maps in the network. These results illustrate that the adaptive behavior of each region of the network is influenced by the design of the network as a whole. Each region automatically assumes a different share of the processing load depending upon how many other regions exist to share this load. This type of insight helps to explain experiments wherein behavioral losses right after

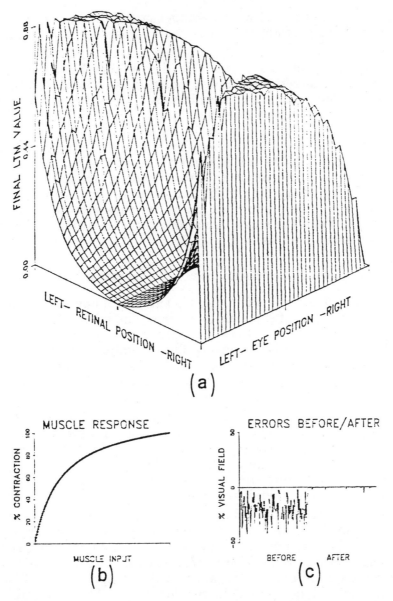

(a)

(b)

(c)

Figure 3.15. Computer simulation of saccadic error correction model with sampling from a non-invariant target position map using a slower-than-linear muscle function and a linear learning function. The following parameters were used in the simulation: $m = 1$, $\alpha = .2$, $\gamma = 1$, $\delta = 1$, $\epsilon = .1$, and $n = 100,000$. (a) Topographic distribution of LTM trace values after learning. (b) Muscle response function used in the simulation. (c) Errors in 100 trials before learning begins and 100 trials after learning ends. Negative values correspond to undershoots and positive values correspond to overshoots.

certain lesions are eventually fully compensated whereas losses after other lesions are at best partially compensated by spared neural subsystems.

An example of how lesions can change learning LTM maps can be developed from the simulation described in Figure 3.16. In this simulation, LTM traces of retinotopic, eye position, and invariant target position sampling maps share the learning load. If the target position map is destroyed, then the remaining retinotopic and eye position LTM traces can absorb the processing load, as in Figure 3.14B. By contrast, if both the target position and the eye position map are destroyed, then the remaining retinotopic LTM traces cannot absorb the full processing load, although they can keep the mean errors centered around the fovea, as in Figure 3.12A. Two sampling maps can be destroyed without preventing full adaptation, if these sampling maps are the retinotopic and the eye position maps. Then the single remaining target position map can absorb the full processing load, as in Figure 3.13.

3.18. Models of Saccadic Error Correction

This section describes the numerical analysis of how 36 network models learn to correct errors of saccadic foveation. The task of the networks is to produce accurate foveations to retinal lights starting from any eye position, even if the muscle plant is nonlinear. The simulations describe learning by one pair of agonist-antagonist muscles. The same mechanism generalizes to any number of independent agonist-antagonist pairs using the sampling anatomy of the AG stage in Figure 3.8.

For definiteness, let the agonist-antagonist muscle pair control horizontal eye movements, and let a one-dimensional strip of cells receive the retinal inputs that drive these muscles. Divide the strip into a right hemifield and a left hemifield. A row of 100 nonfoveal cells form each hemifield in the following simulations. The mechanisms work using any spatial resolution in one and two spatial dimensions.

The simulations are carried out using a discrete time variable as well as a discrete mesh of cells for two reasons: The saccade is a ballistic motion that is initiated by commands set up before it begins, and that is corrected by error signals that are registered after it ends. Use of a continuous time variable can only increase the stability of the computations. This discrete approximation will be refined in Section 3.19. There we will consider effects of inertial properties which develop continuously during a saccade, and will discuss how these tendencies towards dynamic overshoot may be controlled. The results in the present section provide a foundation for these later analyses.

Let the index i, $-100 \leq i \leq 100$, denote the spatial location of a light input on the retina, and the index n, $n \geq 1$, denote the learning trial. A randomly chosen light is assumed to activate the retina, unless the prior saccade was incorrect. In this latter case, the retinal position at which the nonfoveated light is registered after a saccade gets activated on the next trial. This procedure formalizes the idea that a second light position on trial n is the first light position on trial $n + 1$, except when an

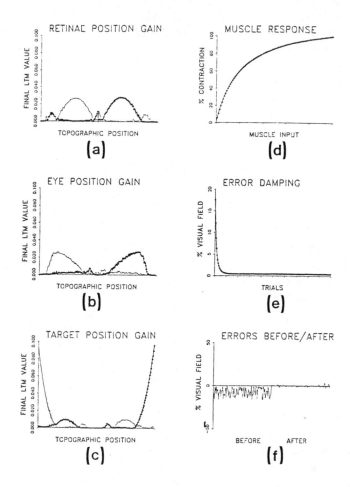

Figure 3.16. Computer simulation of saccadic error correction model with simultaneous sampling from retinal position, invariant target position, and eye position maps using a slower-than-linear muscle function and a linear learning function. The following parameters were used in the simulation: $m = 1$, $\alpha = .2$, $\gamma = 2$, $\delta = 1$, $\epsilon = .01$, and $n = 100,000$. (a), (b), and (c) Topographic distribution of LTM trace values after learning. Bold curves indicate values in the right adaptive gain (AG) hemifields while thin curves indicate values in the left AG hemifields. (d) Slower-than-linear muscle response function used in the simulation. (e) Error damping over 100,000 trials. Error damping value D_n at trial n approximates the average error via the equation $D_{n+1} = (999D_n + \mid E_n \mid)/1000$, where $D_0 = 25$. (f) Errors in 100 trials before learning begins and 100 trials after learning ends. Negative values correspond to undershoots and positive values correspond to overshoots.

accurate foveation occurs. To express this rule formally, let $i = i_n$ be the position of the retinal light on trial n, where $-100 \leq i_n \leq 100$. Position $i_n = 0$ corresponds to a light at the fovea. Let E_n be the second light position that is caused by a saccade to a first light at position i_n. The function E_n also represents the size of the error caused by the nth saccade, since $E_n = 0$ corresponds to a correct saccade. In order to restrict the computation to a discrete array of cells, we also define an error tolerance E, which was chosen equal to .1 in the simulations. In terms of these definitions, let

$$i_{n+1} = \begin{cases} \text{random } i, -100 \leq i \leq 100 \text{ and } i \neq 0 & \text{if } \left| E_n \right| \leq E \\ E_n & \text{if } \left| E_n \right| > E. \end{cases} \quad (3.1)$$

In order to define a complete model, several rules need to be specified.

A. *The Light-Motoneuron Transform*: the rule whereby a light at position $i = i_n$ generates outputs from the motoneurons.

B. *The Motoneuron-Muscle Transform*: the rule whereby outputs from the motoneurons determine prescribed lengths of their target muscles before and after saccades.

C. *The Muscle-Retina Transform*: the rule whereby changes in muscle length cause changes in the position of the light on the retina.

D. *The Retina-Learning Transform*: the rule whereby the new second light position acts as an error signal that alters the sizes of LTM traces at the AG stage.

In order to state these rules clearly, we need to introduce some notation. Since the same Motoneuron-Muscle Transform is used in all models, we start by defining this transform. Let O_{Rn} (O_{Ln}) equal the total motoneuron output to the right (left) muscle after the saccade on trial n, and let M_{Rn} (M_{Ln}) equal the total muscle contraction of the right (left) muscle after the saccade on trial n. In order to relate these two types of functions, we define a *contraction function* $C(w)$ that converts motoneuron signals into muscle contractions. The computation is scaled so that

$$M_{Rn} + M_{Ln} = C(1) \quad (3.2)$$

for all $n \geq 1$. The left and right muscles are assumed to contract and relax in a push-pull fashion.

Motoneuron-Muscle Transform and Push-Pull

Let

$$M_{Rn} = \begin{cases} C(O_{Rn}) & \text{if } i_n > 0 \\ C(1) - C(O_{Ln}) & \text{if } i_n < 0, \end{cases} \quad (3.3)$$

$$M_{Ln} = \begin{cases} C(1) - C(O_{Rn}) & \text{if } i_n > 0 \\ C(O_{Ln}) & \text{if } i_n < 0, \end{cases} \quad (3.4)$$

for $n \geq 1$, and

$$M_{RO} = M_{LO} = 1/2 C(1). \quad (3.5)$$

Equation (3.3) says that the right muscle contracts if the right hemifield received a light, and relaxes if the left hemifield receives a light. In case $i_n < 0$ of (3.3), O_{Rn} can be defined by the relation

$$O_{Rn} = C^{-1}[C(1) - C(O_{Ln})].$$ (3.6)

Equation (3.4) makes the analogous statements about control of the left muscle. Equation (3.5) says that the eye starts out in a head-in-center position before learning trials begin. Contraction functions of the form

$$C(w) = \frac{w^m}{\alpha^m + w^m}$$ (3.7)

were used in the simulations, where $m = 1$, 2, or 4 and $\alpha = .1, .2$, or $.5$. Parameter m determines the nature of the muscle plant nonlinearity. The choosing $m = 1$ defines a slower-than-linear nonlinearity. Choosing $m = 2$ or 4 defines an S-shaped, or sigmoidal, nonlinearity. Choice $m = 4$ defines a more nonlinear muscle plant than does choice $m = 2$. Parameter α also controls the nonlinearity of the muscle. A smaller α determines a steeper increase in muscle contraction as a function of w because $C(\alpha) = 1/2$. Different choices of α thus correspond to different thresholds of muscle contraction and different sensitivities of the muscle plant to motoneuron signals. Equation (3.2) shows that the maximal total contraction is scaled to equal $C(1)$, which by (3.7) is less than 1.

We can now define the Muscle-Retina Transform. This amounts to defining the second light position E_n on trial n as a function of the amount of muscle contraction due to the nth saccade. To do so, it is necessary to keep two spatial scales clearly in view. Retinal lights can fall on any position i such that $-100 \leq i \leq 100$, whereas muscles can contract no more than an amount $C(1) < 1$. We assume that the change in retinal position of a fixed light on trial n is proportional to the amount by which the muscles contract or relax on that trial. The proportionality constant need not equal 1 for some of the models to learn accurate foveations. To define E_n, we use the notation

$$[[\xi]] = \begin{cases} \text{largest integer} \leq \xi & \text{if } \xi > 0 \\ \text{smallest integer} \geq \xi & \text{if } \xi \leq 0. \end{cases}$$ (3.8)

Muscle-Retina Transform
Let

$$E_n = \begin{cases} \max\{-100, [[i_n + \beta(M_{R,n-1} - M_{Rn})]]\} & \text{if } i_n > 0 \\ \min\{100, [[i_n + \beta(M_{Ln} - M_{L,n-1})]]\} & \text{if } i_n < 0, \end{cases}$$ (3.9)

where

$$\beta = \frac{100\gamma}{C(1)}.$$ (3.10)

To understand this definition, consider the case where $i_n > 0$. Then a light hits the right hemifield on trial n. This event causes a saccade towards the right. This saccade cannot move the eye farther than the right muscle can maximally contract. For simplicity, we assume that such a maximal contraction causes the light to fall on the leftmost cell of the array, namely $E_n = -100$. This property explains the use of the function $\max\{-100, \cdot\}$ in this case. All saccadic motions cause the light to excite a definite new cell in the array. This property explains the use of the function $[[\cdot]]$, which causes every motion to excite the cell nearest to the light's new position. Term $i_n + \beta(M_{R,n-1} - M_{Rn})$ says that the new position of the light is determined by the light's initial position i_n plus the amount $\beta(M_{R,n-1} - M_{Rn})$ by which the light moves across the retina. The term $\beta(M_{R,n-1} - M_{Rn})$ says that the amount of retinal motion is proportional to the amount of muscle contraction $M_{Rn} - M_{R,n-1}$ caused by the light. Since the light moves to the left when the right muscle contracts, the change in retinal position is $\beta(M_{R,n-1} - M_{Rn})$ rather than $\beta(M_{Rn} - M_{R,n-1})$. Parameter β in (3.10) scales amount of muscle contraction into amount of retinal motion as follows. By (3.2), term $C(1)$ is the maximal amount of muscle contraction. Dividing $M_{R,n-1} - M_{Rn}$ by $C(1)$ defines a function that stays between -1 and 1. Multiplying this ratio by 100 defines a function that stays between -100 and 100. The extra term γ calibrates the gain of the Muscle-to-Retina Transform. In our simulations, gain values of $\gamma = 1, 2$, or 3 were studied. The equation for saccades to the left in (3.9) (case $i_n < 0$) has a similar interpretation.

We are now ready to define the Retina-Learning Transform. Different learning models use different combinations of sampling maps. Each sampling map sends conditionable signals to the AG stage and then on to the saccade generator (SG) or the motoneuron (MN) stages. To define rules for LTM change, let $z_{Rin}(z_{Lin})$ be the value of the LTM trace from the ith population of a sampling map to the AG strip corresponding to the right (left) muscle at the beginning of trial n. Learning by each LTM trace is assumed to alter the production rate of the chemical transmitter in its synapse (Eccles, 1953; Hebb, 1949; Grossberg, 1968a, 1969b, 1969c; Kandel and Schwartz, 1982). Each LTM trace, in turn, controls the net rate of release of its transmitter in response to its sampling signal. Two types of learning rules have been simulated. In both rules, a *learning function* $L(w)$ converts the position E_n of the light after the nth saccade into the size $L(E_n)$ of a learning signal. We physically interpret $L(E_n)$ as an error signal that is carried by pathways from a retinal map to cerebellar climbing fibers that project to the motor strips of the right and left muscles (Figure 3.8). Since no learning occurs when $E_n = 0$, we choose $L(0) = 0$. Since learning rate should increase, or at least not decrease, as E_n increases, we assumed that $L(w)$ is an increasing function of $w \geq 0$. Since an increase in $z_{Ri,n+1}$ should occur if $E_n > 0$, whereas an increase in $z_{Li,n+1}$ should occur if $E_n < 0$, we assume that $L(w)$ is an odd function of w; viz.,

$$L(w) = -L(-w). \tag{3.11}$$

The two types of learning rules that we have studied can now be stated using the notation $[\xi]^+ = \max(\xi, 0)$.

Hemifield Gradient Learning Rule

Let

$$z_{Ri,n+1} = \delta z_{Rin} + [L(E_n)]^+ \qquad (3.12)$$

and

$$z_{Li,n+1} = \delta z_{Lin} + [-L(E_n)]^+, \qquad (3.13)$$

where $0 < \delta \leq 1$.

Fractured Somatotopy Learning Rule

Let

$$z_{Ri,n+1} = [\delta z_{Rin} + L(E_n)]^+ \qquad (3.14)$$

and

$$z_{Li,n+1} = [\delta z_{Lin} - L(E_n)]^+, \qquad (3.15)$$

where $0 < \delta \leq 1$.

A difference equation such as (3.12) is a discrete approximation to a related differential equation. Rewriting (3.12) as

$$z_{Ri,n+1} - z_{Rin} = -(1 - \delta)z_{Rin} + [L(E_n)]^+, \qquad (3.16)$$

the corresponding differential equation is seen to be

$$\frac{d}{dt}z_{Ri} = -(1 - \delta)z_{Ri} + [L(E_n)]^+. \qquad (3.17)$$

In (3.17), z_{Ri} is a time average of the error signal $[L(E)]^+$. The averaging rate is $1 - \delta$. If $\delta = 1$, then no forgetting occurs.

The Hemifield Gradient Learning Rule says that at most one of the LTM traces $z_{Ri,n+1}$ and $z_{Li,n+1}$ can grow due to E_n on trial n, since by (3.11), $[L(E_n)]^+ > 0$ only if $E_n > 0$ and $[-L(E_n)]^+ > 0$ only if $E_n < 0$. By contrast, the Fractured Somatotopy Learning Rule says that $z_{Ri,n+1}$ increases by the same amount that $z_{Li,n+1}$ decreases, and conversely, until one of the LTM traces becomes zero. Consequently the sum $z_{Rin} + z_{Lin}$ is constant until one of the LTM traces vanishes.

In the simulations, the learning functions $L(w) = \epsilon w$, $L(w) = \epsilon w^3$, and $L(w) = \{\epsilon$ if $w > 0$, $-\epsilon$ if $w < 0$, and 0 if $w = 0\}$ were used. These choices permitted a comparison of the effects of linear and nonlinear error signals on the learning process. In order to guarantee an incremental effect of error signals on learning and performance, the forgetting rate $1 - \delta$ was chosen small. The values used in the simulations were $\delta = 1, .999$, and .998. We also chose the learning rate ϵ to be larger than the forgetting rate $1 - \delta$. The choices $\epsilon = .002, .005, .01, .1$, and 1 were studied. Too large a choice of ϵ destabilizes the system by amplifying the LTM traces too much on a single trial.

It remains to define the Light-Motoneuron Transform. This transform was chosen differently in different models because the sampling maps that were used vary across models. In every model, prewired light-activated pathways elicit unconditioned saccades even before learning occurs, and competition occurs between agonist-antagonist muscle commands (Section 3.7). The agonist-antagonist competition can occur at any of several anatomical stages. If the Fractured Somatotopy Learning Rule (3.14)-(3.15) holds, then competition between agonist-antagonist LTM traces already occurs within the AG stage. A subsequent stage of competition is nonetheless still necessary to guarantee the push-pull Motoneuron-Muscle Transform (3.3)-(3.4). If both the left and the right saccade generators receive positive signals from the AG stage, then their outputs must compete before the muscles receive the net signal, so that the motoneurons whose SG has the larger output will receive a positive signal, and the other motoneurons will receive a negative signal, thereby realizing push-pull. In such a network, two agonist-antagonist competition stages occur: intracerebellar competition and competition at a stage between the SG and the MN stages. In an alternative scheme to achieve muscle push-pull, right and left hemifield outputs from the AG stage compete after the AG stage but before the SG stage. Then only one SG can generate an output signal. This output signal must then excite its own motoneurons and inhibit the antagonist motoneurons to achieve push-pull. In this network, there are three, rather than two, agonist-antagonist competition stages: intracerebellar, pre-SG, and post-SG competition.

If the Hemifield Gradient Learning Rule (3.12)-(3.13) is used, then agonist-antagonist competition must occur at some post-SG stage to realize LTM competition, as well as push-pull competition.. The pre-SG and post-SG competitive anatomies described above achieve these properties with this learning rule. For definiteness, we write down only equations for the pre-SG competitive anatomy. Post-SG competition gives rise to similar learning properties, but the push-pull equations (3.3)-(3.4) must then be redefined in an obvious way.

The input to the motoneurons in all the simulations is a sum of an unconditioned retinotopic signal plus conditionable signals from one or more sampling maps. The unconditioned signal U_{Rin} (U_{Lin}) from retinotopic cell i to the right (left) MN at the end of trial n is

$$U_{Rin} = S_{in}^{(r)} G_{Ri} \tag{3.18}$$

and

$$U_{Lin} = S_{in}^{(r)} G_{Li}. \tag{3.19}$$

Term $S_{in}^{(r)}$ is the signal emitted by the ith retinotopic cell, and G_{Ri} (G_{Li}) is the path strength of the ith pathway to the right (left) MN. For simplicity, let

$$S_{in}^{(r)} = \begin{cases} 1 & \text{if } i = i_n, \\ 0 & \text{otherwise,} \end{cases} \tag{3.20}$$

where i_n is defined by (3.1). In a similar fashion, sampling signals will be chosen equal to 1 or 0 depending upon whether or not the corresponding sampling map population is activated on a given trial. The definitions of the *spatial gradient functions* G_{Ri} and G_{Li} embody the intuition that prewired connections tend to cause larger contractions in response to more eccentric retinal inputs (Figure 2.1). The networks can learn to foveate in response to a wide variety of such spatial gradient functions G_{Ri} and G_{Li}. For definiteness, we let the strength of these gradient connections increase as a linear function of retinal eccentricity; namely,

$$G_{Ri} = G[i]^+ \tag{3.21}$$

and

$$G_{Li} = G[-i]^+. \tag{3.22}$$

In the simulations described in Figures 3.11-3.15, we chose $G = .1$. Other things being equal, smaller G values induce learning of larger LTM traces at the AG stage.

We can now define the combined effects of unconditioned and conditioned movement signals on the Light-Motoneuron Transform given different combinations of sampling maps.

A. Purely Retinotopic Sampling

In order to describe the motoneuron outputs O_{Rn} and O_{Ln} that correspond to a retinotopic sampling map, we use a superscript "(r)", as in the notations $S_{in}^{(r)}$ and $z_{Rin}^{(r)}$ for sampling signals and LTM traces, respectively. The total output signal from the right MN stage after the nth saccade terminates is defined to be

$$O_{Rn} = \max\{1, [\sum_{i \in R} S_{in}^{(r)}(z_{Rin}^{(r)} - z_{Lin}^{(r)}) + \sum_{i \in R} P_{Rin} + O_{R,n-1}]^+\}. \tag{3.23}$$

The expression $\max\{1, \cdot\}$ in (3.23) says that the right muscle contracts maximally when it receives a unit signal, as in (3.2). This expression, which forms part of all subsequent O_{Rn} and O_{Ln} equations, will henceforth be omitted for notational convenience.

The sums $\sum_{i \in R}$ in (3.23) are taken over all cells in the retinotopic sampling map. Since on trial n, the active sampling position is $i = i_n$, (3.20) implies that all terms in the sum vanish except term $i = i_n$. Thus (3.23) simplifies to

$$O_{Rn} = [S_{i_n n}^{(r)}(z_{Ri_n n}^{(r)} - z_{Li_n n}^{(r)}) + S_{i_n n}^{(r)} G[i_n]^+ + O_{R,n-1}]^+. \tag{3.24}$$

In (3.24), term $S_{i_n n}^{(r)} z_{Ri_n n}^{(r)}$ says that the (i_n)th retinotopic population reads out a movement signal from the AG motor strip corresponding to the right muscle R. This signal is the product of the retinotopic sampling signal $S_{i_n n}^{(r)}$

times the LTM trace $z_{Ri_n n}^{(r)}$ from retinotopic position i_n to muscle strip R. Due to the multiplicative form of this relationship, we say that the LTM trace *gates* the sampling signal. Term $-S_{i_n n}^{(r)} z_{Li_n n}^{(r)}$ says that a similar LTM-gated read-out occurs from the AG strip corresponding to the left muscle strip L. Due to the minus sign in front of this expression, the left-muscle signal competes with the right-muscle signal before the net signal can reach the right MN. Term $S_{i_n n}^{(r)} G[i_n]^+$ says that an unconditioned movement signal is also read-out by the (i_n)th retinotopic signal. The total, unconditioned plus conditioned, signal adds onto the previous MN activity $O_{R,n-1}$. If the updated total activity is positive, then the $[\cdots]^+$ enables a signal to be emitted to the right muscle.

Equation (3.24) can be further simplified. Using (3.20) again, we can write

$$O_{Rn} = [z_{Ri_n n}^{(r)} - z_{Li_n n}^{(r)} + G[i_n]^+ + O_{R,n-1}]^+. \qquad (3.25)$$

The subscripts in this formula are unwieldly. Henceforth we write subscripts i instead of i_n to simplify the notation. Then (3.25) becomes

$$O_{Rn} = [z_{Rin}^{(r)} - z_{Lin}^{(r)} + G[i_n]^+ + O_{R,n-1}]^+. \qquad (3.26)$$

A similar analysis shows that

$$O_{Ln} = [z_{Lin}^{(r)} - z_{Rin}^{(r)} + G[-i_n]^+ + O_{L,n-1}]^+. \qquad (3.27)$$

B. Invariant Target Position Map

Using the same simplified notation as in (3.27), we can recursively define the motoneuron output corresponding to the right muscle by

$$O_{Rn} = [z_{Rkn}^{(t)} - z_{Lkn}^{(t)} + G[i_n]^+ + O_{R,n-1}]^+, \qquad (3.28)$$

where $z_{Rkn}^{(t)}$ and $z_{Lkn}^{(t)}$ are the target position map LTM traces. In (3.28), the target position on the kth trial is denoted by $k = k_n$. It is necessary to define k_n in terms of the retinotopic position i_n and the initial eye position j_n at the beginning of trial n. We find that

$$k_n = \begin{cases} i_n + i_j & \text{if } -100 \le i_n + j_n \le 100 \\ \text{undefined} & \text{if } | i_n + j_n | > 100 \end{cases} \qquad (3.29)$$

and

$$\dot{j}_n = \begin{cases} \beta M_{R,n-1} & \text{if } i_n > 0 \text{ and } \beta M_{R,n-1} \le 100 \\ \beta M_{L,n-1} & \text{if } i_n < 0 \text{ and } \beta M_{L,n-1} \ge -100 \\ \text{undefined otherwise.} \end{cases} \qquad (3.30)$$

Function j_n in (3.30) defines the initial eye position at the beginning of trial n, in terms of the amount of muscle interaction in (3.3) and (3.4) due to the previous saccade. Then function k_n in (3.29) determines the target position arising from retinotopic position i_n and initial eye position j_n. In cases when k_n is undefined, the next retinotopic position i_{n+1} is chosen randomly. In a similar fashion, the motoneuron output corresponding to the left muscle is defined by

$$O_{Ln} = [z_{Lkn}^{(t)} - z_{Rkn}^{(t)} + G[-i_n]^+ + O_{L,n-1}]^+. \tag{3.31}$$

Two other combinations of sampling maps can be defined by using these definitions.

C. Invariant Target Position Map Plus Retinotopic Map
Let

$$O_{Rn} = [(z_{Rkn}^{(t)} - z_{Lkn}^{(t)}) + (z_{Rin}^{(r)} - z_{Lin}^{(r)}) + G[i_n]^+ + O_{R,n-1}]^+ \tag{3.32}$$

and

$$O_{Ln} = [(z_{Lkn}^{(t)} - z_{Rkn}^{(t)}) + (z_{Lin}^{(r)} - z_{Rin}^{(r)}) + G[-i_n]^+ + O_{L,n-1}]^+. \tag{3.33}$$

D. Retinotopic Map Plus Eye Position Map
Let

$$O_{Rn} = [(z_{Rin}^{(r)} - z_{Lin}^{(r)}) + (z_{Rjn}^{(p)} - z_{Ljn}^{(p)}) + G[i_n]^+ + O_{R,n-1}]^+ \tag{3.34}$$

and

$$O_{Ln} = [(z_{Lin}^{(r)} - z_{Rin}^{(r)}) + (z_{Ljn}^{(p)} - z_{Rjn}^{(p)}) + G[-i_n]^+ + O_{L,n-1}]^+. \tag{3.35}$$

In (3.34) and (3.35), $z_{Rjn}^{(p)}$ and $z_{Ljn}^{(p)}$ are the eye position map LTM traces. The subscript $j = j_n$ is defined by (3.30).

E. Noninvariant Target Position Map
A similar definition of MN output signal can be given for the case wherein each pair (i, j) of retinotopic positions and initial eye positions activates its own sampling map population. Essentially perfect learning can rapidly occur in this case even if no LTM agonist-antagonist competition occurs. This is due to the fact that each (i, j) pair controls an LTM trace z_{ij} that is unique to its position. For example, the learning simulation described in Figure 3.15 used the MN signals

$$O_{Rn} = [z_{ijn} + G[i_n]^+ + O_{R,n-1}]^+ \tag{3.36}$$

and
$$O_{Ln} = [z_{ijn} + G[-i_n]^+ + O_{L,n-1}]^+ \qquad (3.37)$$

where
$$z_{ij,n+1} = [z_{ijn} + L(E_n)]^+. \qquad (3.38)$$

In these simulations, $1 \le i, j \le 40$, thereby generating 1600 sampling populations.

F. Retinotopic Map Plus Initial Eye Position Map Plus Invariant Target Position Map

Let
$$\begin{aligned}
O_{Rn} = &[(z^{(r)}_{Rin} - z^{(r)}_{Lin}) + (z^{(p)}_{Rjn} - z^{(p)}_{Ljn}) \\
&+ (z^{(t)}_{Rkn} - z^{(t)}_{Lkn}) + G[i_n]^+ + O_{R,n-1}]^+
\end{aligned} \qquad (3.39)$$

and
$$\begin{aligned}
O_{Ln} = &[(z^{(r)}_{Lin} - z^{(r)}_{Rin}) + (z^{(p)}_{Ljn} - z^{(p)}_{Rjn}) \\
&+ (z^{(t)}_{Lkn} - z^{(t)}_{Rkn}) + G[-i_n]^+ + O_{L,n-1}]^+
\end{aligned} \qquad (3.40)$$

The formal lesions describes in Section 3.17 can be carried out on equations (3.39) and (3.40) by deleting the LTM traces with superscripts (t), then (t) and (p), and then (r) and (p).

3.19. Dynamic Coasting

In the preceding sections, we have analysed examples in which the final position of the eye is a function $C(O_{Rn})$ or $C(O_{Ln})$ of the total movement signals O_{Rn} and O_{Ln} to an agonist-antagonist pair of eye muscles. *In vivo*, the eye may continue moving for awhile after the saccade generator shuts off. Van Gisbergen, Robinson, and Gielen (1981) have noted that "after the main pulse the eye requires time to coast to a stop" (p.427). The duration of an agonist saccadic command may be "only 82.2% of saccade duration on the average, indicating that the saccade does outlast [the agonist command] by about 18%" (p.427).

Dynamic coasting is due to the fact that the eyeball builds up inertia during the saccade. This inertia enables the eyeball to keep moving after the saccadic command terminates. Dynamic coasting does not imply that the saccade must overshoot its target. Indeed, second light error signals are registered only after a saccade terminates, and are indifferent to whether or not part of the saccade was due to eyeball inertia.

On the other hand, the question remains concerning what types of sampling maps can use second light error signals to generate accurate saccades even if these saccades include an interval of dynamic coasting. A deeper question must also be considered: Why are not the adaptive gain mechanisms of the saccadic movement system sufficient to compensate for dynamic coasting? Why cannot these adaptive mechanisms terminate a saccade more quickly after the saccade generator shuts off?

We will suggest a simple, albeit tentative, answer to both questions. This answer is consistent with the computer simulations that are summarized in the preceding and ensuing sections. A more complete answer must await an analysis of how the AG stage controls a complete mechanical model of an eyeball and its extraocular muscles.

3.20. Outflow-Inflow Comparisons: A Large Movement as a Series of Small Movement Segments

In Section 1.10, we noted that comparisons between outflow signals and inflow signals are used to linearize the response of the muscle plant to outflow movement signals. This mechanism enables the brain to use outflow-generated corollary discharges as a measure of eye position, since the actual eye position will then tend to covary with the size of the outflow signals. This mechanism works by letting mismatches of outflow and inflow signals generate error signals that can change the size of the total outflow signal to the muscle plant. The conditioned part of the outflow signal adds or subtracts the correct amount to make the muscle react approximately linearly to the total outflow signal. In effect, this conditioned signal automatically changes the gain of the total outflow signal through learning.

In Chapter 5, this linearization mechanism will be described in detail. We will argue that matches and mismatches between outflow and inflow are registered throughout a saccade. The gain of the movement command can hereby be learned and updated sequentially as a saccade proceeds. We suggest that its takes anywhere from 10–20 msec for this learning circuit to encode an outflow-inflow mismatch, register it as a error signal, and then reset the circuit to encode the next possible mismatch. In this way. the circuit breaks up a total movement into small movement segments. The circuit learns and reads-out a temporal series of gains, each one of which is capable of approximately linearizing one segment of the total movement.

3.21. Mismatch due to Plant Nonlinearity or to Dynamic Coasting?

The outflow-inflow interface, or OII, at which mismatches are registered cannot distinguish between mismatches due to plant nonlinearity and mismatches due to dynamic coasting. The question thus arises: If the OII can linearize the muscle response, then why cannot the OII prevent dynamic coasting? We suggest that the OII performs both tasks equally well, but that the 10–20 msec delay in the learning circuit enables a certain amount of nonlinear muscle response *and* of dynamic coasting to occur.

In particular, the conditioned gain corresponding to a particular eye position tends to be an average of all the gains that are appropriate for saccades passing through that position. This average gain will tend to be smaller than the gain needed to prevent coasting during saccades which reach their maximal velocity through that position. Hence some coasting must be expected. This argument suggests that the amount of coasting should increase with the cycle time of the learning circuit. The amount of coasting should also increase if the average speed of saccades passing through prescribed eye positions is much less than the speed required by a suddenly imposed experimental manipulation.

3.22. Adaptive Control of Dynamic Coasting

Given that some dynamic coasting is to be expected, it remains to explain how accurate foveations can nonetheless be learned. In the following analysis, we consider several approximate rules to express the effects of dynamic coasting, and describe computer simulations which demonstrate how well the resultant network learns to foveate.

First, we need a rule to replace equations (3.3) and (3.4). To replace (3.3), we considered the following rule.

Dynamic Coasting Rule

$$M_{Rn} = \begin{cases} C(O_{Rn}) + D(C(O_{Rn}) - M_{R,n-1}) & \text{if } i_n > 0 \\ C(1) - C(O_{Ln}) & \text{if } i_n < 0. \end{cases} \tag{3.41}$$

A similar rule is defined for M_{Ln}. Equation (3.41) differs from (3.3) by the term

$$D(C(O_{Rn}) - M_{R,n-1}), \tag{3.42}$$

where $D(\xi)$ may be a linear or nonlinear function of the difference $\xi = C(O_{Rn}) - M_{R,n-1}$. This term expresses the amount of coasting that occurs over and beyond the movement due directly to the saccadic command $C(O_{Rn})$. Term (3.42) makes rigorous the hypothesis that the amount of coasting increases as a function of how much the new saccadic command $C(O_{Rn})$ exceeds the previous eye position, as expressed by $M_{R,n-1}$. In other words, more coasting can occur if the eye movement is bigger, other things being equal.

It is also necessary to consider more sophisticated rules for O_{Rn} and O_{Ln}. Consider, for example, the old rule (3.34) for combining a retinotopic sampling map with an eye position sampling map; namely, the

Static Command Rule

$$O_{Rn} = [S_n + O_{R,n-1}]^+, \tag{3.43}$$

where

$$S_n = (z_{Rin}^{(r)} - z_{Lin}^{(r)}) + (z_{Rjn}^{(p)} - z_{Ljn}^{(p)}) + G[i_n]^+. \tag{3.44}$$

This rule does not provide an adequate summary of the total output signal in situations where part of this signal may be due to a conditioned gain that is sensitive to the amount of dynamic coasting. In order to partially overcome this deficiency, we compared computer simulations using (3.43) with computer simulations using the

Dynamic Command Rule

$$O_{Rn} = \left[S_n + C^{-1}(M_{R,n-1}) \right]^+. \qquad (3.45)$$

Rule (3.45) acknowledges that the initial position $C^{-1}(M_{R,n-1})$ of the eye before the nth saccade begins may be due to the combined effects of the saccade command $C(O_{R,n-1})$ and of the dynamic coast $D(C(O_{R,n-1}) - M_{R,n-1})$ in (3.41). Rules (3.43) and (3.45) are identical in cases where no dynamic coasting occurs, since then $M_{R,n-1} = C(O_{R,n-1})$. The present discussion thus generalizes the analysis of Section 3.19 to the case where dynamic coasting can occur.

In the computer simulation summarized by Figure 3.17, we chose a linear dynamic coast function

$$D(\xi) = \frac{\xi}{C(1)} \qquad (3.46)$$

and the static command rule (3.43). Despite the linearity of $D(\xi)$, the system's ability to learn accurate foveations deteriorated relative to the situation depicted in Figure 3.14. By contrast, in Figure 3.18, the same linear dynamic coast function (3.46) was paired with the dynamic command rule (3.45). Learning significantly improved.

In Figure 3.18, a nonlinear dynamic coast function

$$D(\xi) = C\!\left(\frac{\xi}{C(1)}\right) \qquad (3.47)$$

was used where, as in all these simulations,

$$C(w) = \frac{w}{.2 + w}. \qquad (3.48)$$

When this slower-than-linear signal function was paired with the static command rule (3.43), an even more serious breakdown of saccadic learning occurred. In Figure 3.20, by contrast, (3.47) was paired with the dynamic command rule (3.45), and learning was again greatly improved.

Figures 3.21 and 3.22 show that a change of the nonlinearity which defines the dynamic coast function can alter the details of learning, but not the qualitative conclusion drawn from Figures 3.19 and 3.20. In both Figure 3.21 and 3.22, we chose

$$D(w) = \frac{\left(\frac{w}{C(1)}\right)^2}{.2^2 + \left(\frac{w}{C(1)}\right)^2} \qquad (3.49)$$

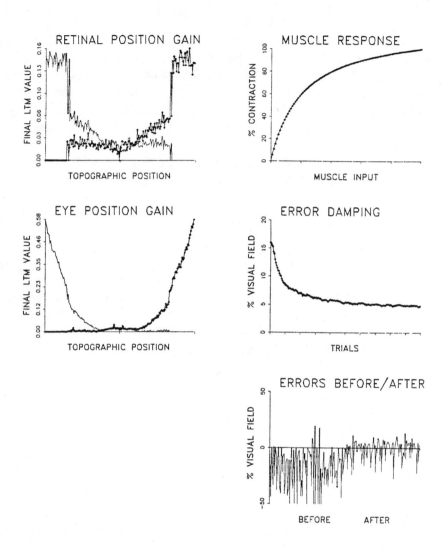

Figure 3.17. Computer simulation of learning using a linear dynamic coast function, a static command rule, and a slower-than-linear muscle response. See text for details.

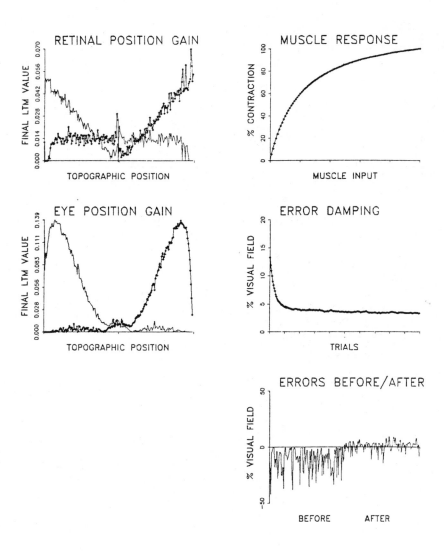

Figure 3.18. Computer simulation of learning using a linear dynamic coast function, a dynamic command rule, and a slower-than-linear muscle response. Learning is much better than in Figure 3.17.

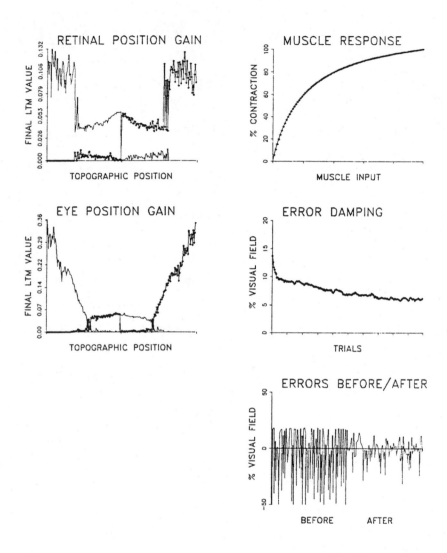

Figure 3.19. Computer simulation of learning using a slower-than-linear dynamic coast function, a static command rule, and a slower-than-linear muscle response.

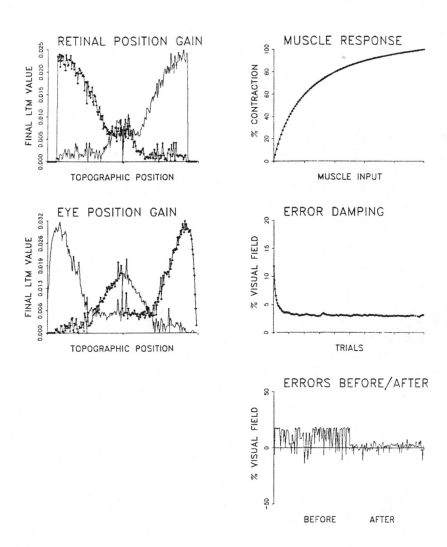

Figure 3.20. Computer simulation of learning with a slower-than-linear coast function, a dynamic command rule, and a slower-than-linear muscle response. Learning is much better than in Figure 3.19.

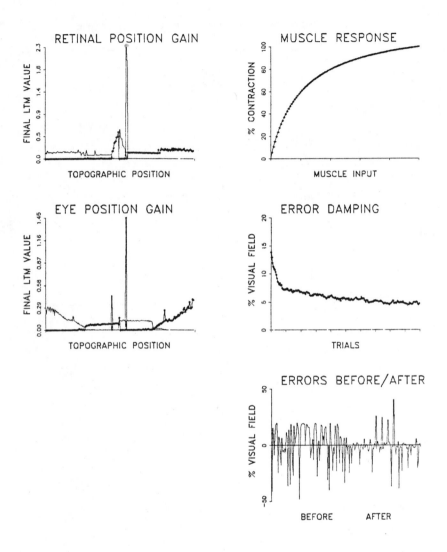

Figure 3.21. Computer simulation of a sigmoid coast function, a static command rule, and a slower-than-linear muscle response.

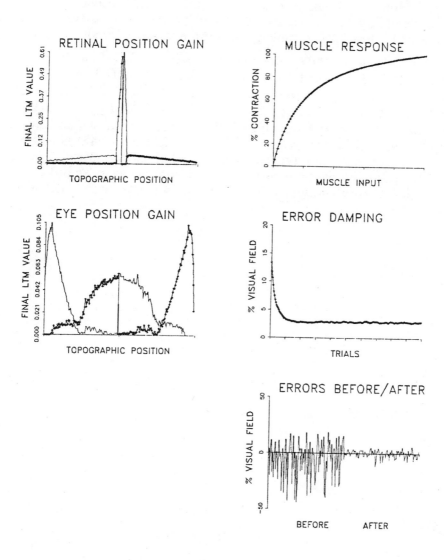

Figure 3.22. Computer simulation of a sigmoid coast function, a dynamic command rule, and a slower-than-linear muscle response. Learning is much better than in Figure 3.21.

instead of (3.47). Function $D(w)$ in (3.49) is a sigmoidal signal function which is quadratically nonlinear at the small w values where (3.47) is approximately linear. When paired with a static command rule in Figure 3.21, poor learning again occurred. When paired with a dynamic command rule in Figure 3.22, excellent learning again occurred.

It remains to physically interpret term $C^{-1}(M_{R,n-1})$ in the dynamic command rule (3.45). Until a complete eyeball and muscle plant is simulated, our interpretation of this term must be cautious. The critical issue is: What circuit can realize commands such as $C^{-1}(M_{R,n-1})$ during the nth saccade? The most likely possibility is the circuit which linearizes the muscle plant. If this interpretation is correct, then (3.45) is just a discrete approximation to the dynamic process whereby the muscle linearization circuit updates movement segments in a somewhat loose but effective fashion, at least from the viewpoint of enabling accurate foveations to be learned.

CHAPTER 4
COMPARING TARGET POSITION WITH
PRESENT POSITION: NEURAL VECTORS

4.1. Reconciling Visually Reactive and Intentional Computations

In Chapter 1, we outlined several basic reasons why the positions of light on the retina need to be recoded as target positions in a head coordinate map. The calibration of intermodality movement signals, the attentional selection of a target position for an intentional movement, and the encoding of sequences of predictive saccades can all be carried out using a target position map. In Chapter 3, we described how retinotopically encoded light positions can be used to correct visually reactive saccades. In this chapter, we begin to show how these two types of processing requirements, which on the surface may seem to be contradictory, can be reconciled. Indeed, we will argue that both types of processing are essential. The visually reactive system provides a way to learn accurate saccades. The attentional, intentional, and predictive systems can then make use of the movement parameters that were learned in the visually reactive mode. We will argue in Chapter 11 that the learned parameters of the visually reactive system provide a foundation without which the attentional, intentional, and predictive systems could never learn to operate well. This claim does not imply that accurate intentional movements cannot be made in an adult organism after large parts of the visually reactive system are extirpated. The suggested nature of the dependence between these two systems is more subtle than that, and is based upon an analysis of neuronal development rather than upon performance characteristics of an adult network.

In this chapter, we will focus on a core problem in the construction of the intentional system: the design of the *Head-Muscle Interface*, or HMI (Section 1.6). The HMI mediates between target position computations and retinotopic computations. It does so by comparing target positions with present positions to compute vector differences in motor coordinates. By describing first our solution of this problem, our solutions of a number of other problems become easier to motivate, such as how to design an invariant target position map, how to transform vector differences from motor coordinates into retinotopic coordinates, and how to attentionally modulate which movement commands will finally be expressed in observable saccades. These problems become easier to understand because we can then see how to constrain their solutions to be compatible with input-output constraints that are imposed by HMI design.

4.2. Experimental Evidence for Vector Inputs to the Superior Colliculus

Before describing our formal solution to this problem, we review some relevant experimental data. A number of experiments on saccadic performance have suggested that vector differences are somehow computed by the saccadic control system (Hallett and Lightstone, 1976; Mays and Sparks, 1980; Schiller and Sandell, 1983; Zee *et al.*, 1976). All of these experiments test how the saccadic system responds to two or more inputs that are delivered to the saccadic system in rapid succession. The experiments of Mays and Sparks (1980) are particularly notable.

Mays and Sparks (1980) have ingeniously tested whether the nervous system computes transformations analogous to vector operations by recording from quasi-visual (QV) cells of the superior colliculus (SC). The SC is a structure that receives inputs from the retina and the visual cortex, among other neural regions. The SC plays an important role in generating saccades, but this role is not easy to characterize despite the facts that the SC is a phylogenetically old structure that receives inputs directly from the retina.

The Mays and Sparks (1980) experiments illustrate the subtlety of SC architecture. The SC is divided into a succession of functionally distinct stages. The superficial layer reacts rather directly to retinotopically coded information. The final stages react to information that is attentionally modulated and encoded in motor coordinates (Huerta and Harting, 1984; Schiller and Stryker, 1972). The QV cells from which Mays and Sparks (1980) recorded lie between these processing extremes.

Mays and Sparks isolated QV cells that fired before the eye saccaded from position O to a light flash at position C (Figure 4.1). They then studied how these cells responded to a light at position B followed by direct electrical stimulation of the superior colliculus. The direct electrical stimulation caused the eye to move from O to A before it could saccade to the light at position B. Both positions A and B fall within the right hemifield of the retina while the eye fixates position O. By contrast, a light to position C excited the left retinal hemifield while the eye fixated position O. Consequently, if the QV cell that fired before the motion $O{\rightarrow}C$ encoded retinal position, then this cell should not fire before the eye saccaded from A to B. Note, however, that the vectors $\vec{OC}$ and $\vec{AB}$ encode the same direction and length of motion. Thus if the QV cell encoded vector differences, then it should fire both before the eye moved from O to C and before the eye moved from A to B. This is, in fact, what Mays and Sparks (190) observed. Schiller and Sandell (1983) have replicated these findings, in addition to showing that the frontal eye fields can also compute a similar compensatory "vector". These data suggest that vector differences between a target position map and an eye position map influence the firing of QV cells in the superior colliculus, as well as a subset of cells in the frontal eye fields. In an attempt to localize the compensatory "vector" mechanism, Schiller and Sandell (1983) performed a bilateral ablation of the frontal eye field or superior colliculus. Monkeys could still accurately compensate for ocular perturbations caused by electrical stimulation. This suggests that neither the frontal eye field nor the superior colliculus alone is uniquely responsible for corrective saccade computation. In contrast, even normal monkeys could not accurately compensate for ocular perturbations caused by stimulation of the motoneurons within the abducens nucleus.

4.3. Adaptive Inhibitory Efference Copy in Motor Control

Mays and Sparks (1980) described this vector operation as one that compares an expected position with an actual position of the eye. We use the terms target position and head coordinate map instead of expected position. We prefer this terminology because there are several senses in which expectations are computed within the nervous system. The present computation differs both qualitatively and quantitatively from the types of sensory expectation that help to complete ambiguous visual forms, as in perceptual switches between ambiguous figures (Grossberg, 1980); to regulate motivational decisions using templates formed by patterns of conditioned reinforcer signals (Grossberg, 1982b); to focus attention on motivationally valued cues (Grossberg, 1982b); or to control phonemic restoration, word superiority effects, and priming of lexical decisions during processing of speech or printed text (Grossberg, 1985c; Grossberg and Stone, 1985a). In all these cases, input patterns that match the expected pattern are selectively amplified (Section 2.6). In the present instance, an eye position that matches the target position causes an attenuation, rather than an enhancement, of activity, due to the property that the difference of two equal vectors is zero. A suppressive effect of a target controlled motor template on feedback signals has also been reported in the electric eel (Bell, 1981), where an efference copy exists that is opposite in sign to the efferent input from ampullary electroreceptors. This efference copy is adaptive, as is the motor template that exists in our model network. Taken together, these results suggest that many sensory expectancies, when matched, cause selective pattern amplification, whereas many motor commands, when matched, cause selective pattern attenuation.

Another reason for refining the language used to describe "expected position" is to explain how the "expected position" is computed. To compare a target position that is computed in head coordinates with a present eye position that is computed in agonist-antagonist motor coordinates, it is necessary to first convert both types of information into the same coordinate system (Section 1.6). We show how a learning process converts target positions in head coordinates into target positions in motor coordinates. This transformation is designed so that differences between target position motor coordinates and present position motor coordinates can be used to generate the correct "vector difference" command in retinotopic coordinates (Section 1.11). All of these computations use dynamical neural network operations rather than algebraic vector calculus operations. We hereby explicate the vector metaphor and develop terminology that includes the distinctions necessary to do so. These nonlinear neural network computations provide an alternative to the linear tensor computations of Pellionisz and Llinás (1980, 1982).

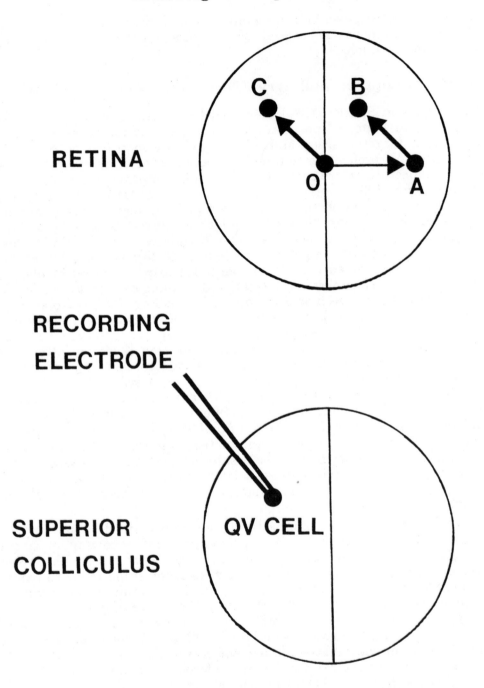

Figure 4.1. The Mays and Sparks (1980) paradigm. Motions from O to C and from A to B represent the same vector length and direction. A quasi-visual (QV) cell that fires before a $\overrightarrow{OC}$ saccade also fires before a $\overrightarrow{AB}$ saccade.

4.4. Multistage Elaboration of a Vector Map

Mays and Sparks (1981) interpreted their data in the manner depicted in Figure 4.2, which represents the vector model of Zee *et al.* (1976). In Figure 4.2, eye position and retinal position are first combined by a vector addition process before a vector subtraction process compensates for eye position. The vector subtraction process is delayed in time relative to the vector addition process. This property is needed because the vector addition that computes the target position of the light uses the position of the eye before the eye saccaded to the electrical stimulus. The vector subtraction that converts the target position of the light into a vector command uses the eye position after this saccade occurs. Then the vector command generates a second saccade to the correct target position of the light. It is not clear from Figure 4.2 why such a long delay should exist between the first and second registrations of eye position or how the nervous system computes a vector difference operation. Figure 4.3 describes a macrocircuit that suggests a resolution of the time delay problem. Variations on the stages in Figure 4.3 may occur in different species.

Stage 1 in Figure 4.3 is computed in retinal coordinates. A retinal light that excites a region of stage 1 transfers this excitation to stage 2, at which retinally induced signals and initial eye position signals are joined to compute a target position map in head coordinates. In monkeys, this target position map is computed outside the SC (Schiller and Koerner, 1971). We suggest that these computations take place in a circuit within the parietal cortex (Goldberg, 1980; Hyvärinen, 1982; Lynch, 1980; Motter and Mountcastle, 1981; Mountcastle, Anderson, and Motter, 1981; Sakata, Shibutani, and Kawano, 1980) and/or the internal medullary lamina of the thalamus (Schlag and Schlag-Rey, 1981; Schlag, Schlag-Rey, Peck, and Joseph, 1980; Schlag-Rey and Schlag, 1983). A target position map has, however, been found alongside a retintotopic map in the SC of cats (Guitton, Crommelinck, and Roucoux, 1980; Peck, Schlag-Rey, and Schlag, 1980). Thus the location of the target position map may vary from species to species. Behaviors due to unilateral ablation of the parietal cortex are consistent with the hypothesis that parietal cortex includes a target position map in egocentric coordinates. Such an ablation leads to hemifield neglect, or a lack of goal-oriented behaviors to one side (Motter and Mountcastle, 1981).

Stage 3 computes a vector map by combining signals from the target position map with signals that register present eye position. Stage 3 is the HMI. This vector map relays its signals to stage 4, which is interpreted to be a retinotopic map within the SC. These SC cells are identified with the quasi-visual (QV) cells in the intermediate layers of the SC (Mays and Sparks, 1980). Then the retinotopic map projects to stage 5, which is interpreted as the deep layers of the SC.

This anatomical interpretation of the stages that occur within the SC is compatible with the results of Schiller and Koerner (1971). These authors found retinally coded cells throughout the depth of the monkey SC. Although all of the cells in the model SC are "retinally coded", some of them should be interpreted as retinotopically recoded vectors, as the data of Mays and Sparks suggest.

In this macrocircuit, competition between visually reactive, intermodality, and intentional sources of saccadic commands is assumed to occur within the target position maps of stage 2. The projection from stage 2 to stage 3 (the HMI) is adaptive, as we will show in Section 4.6. It transforms target positions from head coordinates into motor coordinates. The projection from stage 3 to stage 4 is also adaptive. It transforms vectors from motor coordinates into retinotopic coordinates. This adaptive process enables the HMI vectors to make use of visually reactive movement commands that can be corrected using second light visual error signals (Chapter 3). Competitive interactions within stage 4 are used to help choose the map locations that will engage in this learning process (Chapter 11). Thus competitive interactions are assumed to occur within at least two stages of the macrocircuit: stages 2 and 4. Both of these competitive stages play a role in choosing between different sources of saccadic commands. In the experiments of Mays and Sparks (1980), the electrode input and the HMI vector take precedence over the direct light-activated retinal signal.

The hypothesis that a direct visually reactive, retinotopically encoded pathway exists suggests that total ablation of all target position maps that contribute to saccadic commands may disinhibit the direct retinotopic pathway. The data of Schiller, Sandell, and Maunsell (1984) on express saccades in the monkey are consistent with this hypothesis. Such a test may be confounded by secondary effects if destruction of a target position map also alters the gating of cell responsiveness in the deeper layers of the SC (Hikosaka and Wurtz, 1983) in the manner described within the next section. Chapter 11 describes in greater detail the processing stages and the types of behavioral effects that lesions of these stages would be expected to have.

4.5. Attention Modulation in Parietal Cortex and Inhibitory Gating of SC Signals: The Delay in Vector Subtraction

Given that many, possibly conflicting, sources of saccadic commands exist in the several target position maps, a mechanism is needed to decide which of these commands will elicit a saccade. Attentional factors obviously influence this choice. We assume that attentional processing occurs at stage 2, which is interpreted to be a neocortical region, such as the posterior parietal cortex, or a subcortical region that is intimately connected with neocortex (Mountcastle, Anderson, and Motter, 1981; Wurtz, Goldberg, and Robinson, 1982).

We can now physically interpret the formal delay of vector subtraction in Figure 4.2 by noting that the neocortical attentional computation which is hypothesized to occur in stage 2 of Figure 4.3 takes time. Thus the eye position information that is used to compute target positions at stage 2 is earlier eye position information than is used to compute vectors at stage 3. Given that the attentional processing within stage 2 is relatively

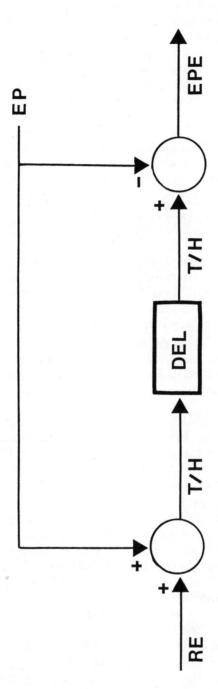

Figure 4.2. The Zee *et al.* (1976) vector model. See the text for a description. The abbreviations mean: RE = retinal error signal; EP = eye position signal; T/H = position of the target with respect to the head; DEL = delay; EPE = eye position error signal.

slow, we are confronted with a new design problem. The direct light-reactive retinotopic pathway between stages 1→4→5 does not necessarily pass through stage 2, or in any case could be expected to react quickly to retinal lights (Chapter 11). Somehow this light-reactive pathway must be prevented from automatically eliciting a saccade until the outcome of the attentional competition in stage 2 is completed. Otherwise visually reactive saccades would always preempt the occurrence of other types of saccades. The excitability of the direct light-reactive retinotopic pathway must therefore be modulated by attentional factors. Given our suggestion that the formal stages 4 and 5 have analogs within the SC, this argument implies that a surprisingly long delay should occur between activation of the superficial and deep layers of the SC. Such a delay between activation of the superficial and deep SC layers does, in fact, occur.

Schiller and Stryker (1972) and Sparks (1978) have shown that the delay between activation of the deep SC layers and saccade initiation is approximately 20 msec. The delay between onset of the visual stimulus and activation of the superficial SC layers is approximately 50–60 msec. For a typical saccade, it therefore takes approximately 120 msec. for activation of the superficial SC layers to reach the deep SC layers (Sparks and Mays, 1981). This is a surprisingly long time, but it provides a physical basis for the delay postulated in Figure 4.2.

The hypothesis that this delay is due to attentional interactions within cortical target position maps of stage 2 can be used to clarify the results of Mays and Sparks (1980). In particular, the target position of light B (Figure 4.1) can be computed at stage 2 shortly after the light occurs using pre-saccadic eye position signals. Ordinarily, the delay within stage 2 is used to select the particular target whose head coordinates will be used as a basis for a saccade. In the Mays and Sparks experiment, this delay enables the eye position signals that obtain after the electrode-induced saccade occurs to be used in computing the vector command at stage 3 that gives rise to the second saccade.

It remains to say how the direct visually reactive retinotopic pathway is prevented from activating the SC deep layers much sooner than 120 msec. after the SC superficial layers are activated. Hikosaka and Wurtz (1983) have shown that the excitability of the deeper layers of the SC is gated by inhibitory signals from the substantia nigra (SN). Disinhibition of the SN is one factor that enables the deep layers of the SC to generate saccadic commands. Inhibitory gating by the SN of the SC may be jointly controlled both by visually reactive and intentional mechanisms. Hikosaka and Wurtz (1983) have, for example, studied monkeys who were rewarded if they could delay their saccades to a light source until after the light was turned off. Although the light itself did cause some SN cells to be inhibited, the monkeys successfully performed the task. We will describe this type of gating mechanism in greater detail when we discuss attentional processing in Chapters 10 and 11.

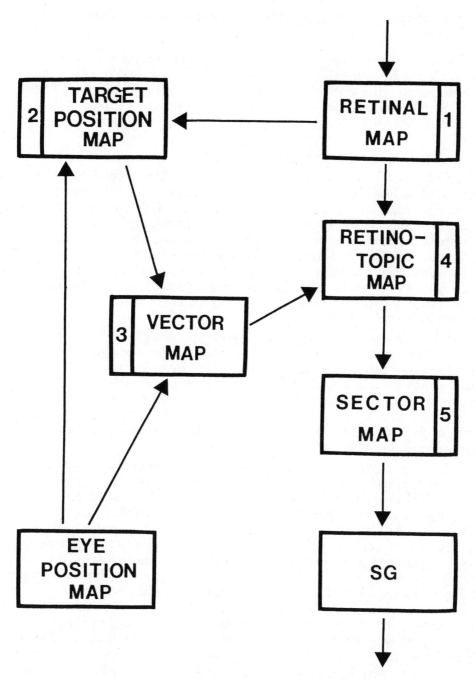

Figure 4.3. The functional stages and coordinate systems needed to neurally compute vector additions and subtractions. The delay between registering the target positions of competing sensory signals at stage 2 and reading the chosen target position into stage 3 is assumed to explain the formal delay in Figure 4.2.

4.6. Stages in the Adaptive Neural Computation of a Vector Difference

This section outlines how the computation of vector differences can be accomplished by self-calibrating neural mechanisms. We call a network capable of carrying out such a computation Vector Command Network, or VCN. A visually-reactive network is, by contrast, called a Retinotopic Command Network, or RCN. The following four problems are solved by a VCN.

A. Head-to-Muscle Coordinate Transform

To compare a target position computed in head coordinates with an eye position computed in agonist-antagonist motor coordinates, the target position is transformed into motor coordinates. The transforming mechanism that we use works even if the target position map, or TPM, possesses a complex internal structure. The head coordinates of different target positions can even be randomly distributed across the TPM without causing any calibration difficulties. This property may be important *in vivo* since, in the parietal lobes, functionally different types of cortical columns seem to be mixed together into a nontopographic cortical array (Lynch, 1980; Mountcastle, 1957, 1978).

The TPM needs to contain loci corresponding to a large number of different egocentric positions, whereas only six pairs of agonist-antagonist muscles move the two eyes (Section 1.5). In order to map head coordinates into muscle coordinates, each target position in the TPM sends sampling signals to motor representations of all the agonist-antagonist muscle positions at the head-muscle interface (HMI). A massive convergence of pathways must therefore occur from the TPM onto each muscle representation in the HMI.

One way to provide space for so many converging pathways is to represent each muscle within a large region of cells, to let each target position in the TPM project to a small subset of these cells, and to distribute the eye position signal in parallel across the entire region using many axon collaterals. In this type of anatomical realization, a potentially confusing mixture of cellular response profiles would present itself to a physiologist's electrodes. Signals due to both lights and eye positions would change rapidly from cell to cell due to target position inputs computed in head coordinates. These signals would intermix with signals due to eye positions that change slowly from cell to cell. The next paragraph explains why these influences would appear and disappear through time in a complex way, depending upon where and whether lights flash on and off and are differentially attended through time. These properties may be one reason why Motter and Mountcastle (1981, p.7) have written that "no consistent set of rules has evolved for naming the classes of neurons with different properties that can be identified in the parietal cortex in waking monkeys" and have classified as "unidentified cells" 31% of all the neurons that they studied. Perhaps, use of the new 24 channel microelectrode (Kuperstein and Eichenbaum, 1985) in parietal cortex will show how neurons can be part of collective neural group properties.

B. *Present Eye Position Signals: Corollary Discharges*

Outflow signals that move and help to hold the eye muscles in position are assumed to be the source of eye position signals (Section 1.9). This assumption is supported by data of Guthrie, Porter, and Sparks (1983), who showed that vector compensation still occured in the Mays and Sparks paradigm after all inflow signals from the eye muscles were surgically eliminated. Since these outflow signals are computed in agonist-antagonist coordinates, they can be directly relayed to the HMI. We identify the sources of these outflow signals with the tonic cells in the peripontine reticular formation (Keller, 1981) or in the vestibular nucleus (Fuchs and Kimm, 1975; Keller and Kamath, 1975; Miles, 1974).

C. *Simultaneous Calibration of the Head-to-Muscle Transform and of the Vector Difference between Target Position and Eye Position*

The HMI transforms target positions from head coordinates into motor coordinates in order to compute vector differences of target positions and present positions in motor coordinates. We will show how the HMI accomplishes both tasks using the same network equations.

First consider the mechanism which learns the transformation of target position from head coordinates into motor coordinates. Suppose that a cell population within the TPM encodes the target position by being activated before the saccade begins. Let the activity of this population be stored in STM until after the saccade is over. One might legitimately ask how any saccade whatsoever can be generated before the transformation within the HMI is learned. If the visually reactive Retinotopic Command Network (RCN) that we described in Chapter 3 did not exist, this concern would be a valid one. As it is, we consider a developmental stage before the HMI is calibrated when saccades can be unconditionally generated and corrected by visual error signals within the visually reactive RCN.

The active population within the TPM sends sampling signals over its conditionable pathways to the HMI. The HMI also receives corollary discharge signals that encode eye position as time goes on. These corollary discharge signals provide the eye position data that the conditionable pathways will learn. Not all eye positions are, however, the correct ones to learn. For example, before the saccade occurs, the corollary discharge signals encode initial eye position. The correct eye position to learn is not the initial eye position. Rather, it is the intended eye position.

This simple observation leads to our first major conclusion about HMI design. The conditionable pathways from the TPM target position to the HMI can learn only *after* a saccade is over. This property raises an important question. If the TPM target position is stored in STM throughout the saccade, then it can emit sampling signals along its conditionable pathways throughout the saccade. How can these sampling signals be prevented from encoding all the eye positions that are attained before and during the saccade? How can these sampling signals be caused to encode only the eye position that is attained after the saccade? We conclude that a gating signal exists which is capable of modulating the learning that occurs within the LTM traces of active conditionable pathways. Learning is prevented except when this gating signal is on. The gating signal turns on only after a saccade is over. A similar gating signal was needed to prevent the learning of intermodality circular reactions (Section 1.3).

If these formal constraints can be achieved, then a target position stored within the TPM can learn the eye position that is attained by the subsequent saccade. How does the HMI know whether this final eye position is the "expected", or intended, eye position, namely the eye position which corresponds to the target position that is coded within the TPM? The answer is, quite simply, that the HMI does not possess this information. The HMI transformation succeeds in learning the expected eye position only because the visually reactive RCN can learn to generate correct saccades. Thus, as a result of the visual error correction that takes place within the visually reactive *retinotopic* system, the HMI can learn accurate transformations of target positions into *motor* coordinates.

From the above discussion, one can begin to understand how a vector difference can be computed by the HMI. Learning an eye position within the HMI occurs only after a saccade is over. Before a saccade begins, an active target position that is stored at the TPM can read-out the motor coordinates which it learned on previous occasions. These are the motor coordinates of the *target* position, not of the eye's *present* position before the saccade begins.

Thus before the saccade begins, information about target position and present position are simultaneously available within the HMI. There is no danger that the conditionable pathways will forget their learned target position by relearning the present eye position, because learning occurs only after a saccade is over, not before it begins. This fact guarantees the stability of memory before the saccade begins, but it does not yet explain how the HMI can compute a vector difference of target position and present position before a saccade begins. How this occurs can be better seen by considering the form of the learning process that occurs after a saccade is over.

A corollary discharge reads eye position into the HMI in the form of a pattern of excitatory inputs. At times when learning can occur, the conditionable pathways from the TPM continue to learn until their signals can match the corollary discharge signals. Then learning stops. Thus the conditionable pathways from the TPM to the HMI are *inhibitory* pathways (Figure 4.4). These inhibitory pathways carry the "adaptive inhibitory efference copy" of the HMI (Section 4.2). When the excitatory corollary discharges equal the inhibitory conditionable TPM→HMI signals, learning stops.

Before a saccade occurs, the active target position within the TPM reads its motor coordinates into the HMI as a pattern of inhibitory signals. The corollary discharge reads its present position into the HMI as a pattern of excitatory signals. The sum of these inhibitory and excitatory signal patterns represents a vector difference of target position and present position in motor coordinates.

D. *Visually-Mediated Gating of Vector Outputs*

Since the eyes always assume some position, corollary discharges are tonically received by the HMI. Since these eye position signals are excitatory, the HMI is always active, even if no target position is read into the HMI from the TPM. Indeed, when the TPM is inactive, no inhibitory signals whatsoever are sent to the HMI. Given that the HMI is always active when the TPM is inactive, we are led to ask: what prevents the HMI from persistently generating output motor commands, and thereby eliciting series of saccades, in the absence of either visually reactive or intentional saccadic commands? Clearly, something is missing from the HMI design.

To fill this gap, we assume that the output from the HMI is multiplicatively gated to zero except when some TPM population is actively reading-out a target position to the HMI. Thus, whereas the HMI is always activated by corollary discharges, it can only generate output signals at times when a vector difference between a target position and a present position is being computed at the HMI.

The TPM can only read-out target positions at times when visual or other input sources can activate target position populations within the TPM. Thus visual signals play two distinct roles in the VCN: a specific role and a nonspecific role. Their specific role is to provide information concerning which target positions to activate within the TPM. Their nonspecific role is to enable outputs from the HMI to be released. In Sections 4.9–4.11, we will explain some paradoxical data using the simple fact that visual inputs subserve both specific and nonspecific functions within the VCN.

The reader can now appreciate what a forbidding task it would be for a neurophysiologist to characterize the function of a network like the HMI without first having a good theory of how it works. Visual signals and positional signals get mixed together to compute target positions within the TPM, only to be recoded as positional signals in motor coordinates within the HMI. Thus positional signals are encoded in two different ways within the HMI by the inhibitory TPM inputs. Superimposed on these inhibitory positional signals are excitatory positional signals due to corollary discharges. Modulating this mixture of excitatory and inhibitory positional signals are two types of nonspecific gating signals. Visual inputs influence one of these gating signals, but not the other. Thus visual signals influence the network in two different ways and positional signals influence the network in three different ways. All of these interactions occur rapidly in time, albeit at different phases of the saccadic cycle. Superimposed upon these rapid signalling events are signals which can change slowly due to learning. Although the learning takes place in motor coordinates, it is modulated by a gating signal that is computed in head coordinates. The HMI is a neurophysiologist's nightmare, despite the intuitive simplicity of its functional design.

Another summary of HMI dynamics can be given which hints at its functional role as part of a larger processing scheme. Two different types of gating signals are needed to regulate HMI dynamics. One type of gating signal is turned on before a saccade begins, and is used to regulate saccadic performance. The other type of gating signal is turned on after a saccade ends, and is used to regulate saccadic learning. When their properties are described in this way, these properties suggest the conclusion that these two types of gating signals are controlled by complementary movement and postural subsystems that help to regulate the saccadic rhythm (Chapters 9 and 11).

4.7. Modulators of Head-to-Muscle Coordinate Learning

The hypothesis that a gating signal regulates learning within the HMI leads to several experimental predictions. Such a gating signal is also called a Now Print signal in the neural modelling literature (Grossberg, 1982a). The cells which control this Now Print signal may either be transiently activated after a saccade ends (rebound cells) or may be turned on except during saccades (pause cells). Cells are known to exist that fire after a visually evoked saccade terminates, such as the refixation neurons found by Motter and Mountcastle (1981). Pause cells are also well-known saccade system components (Keller, 1981; Robinson, 1975; Schlag-Rey and Schlag, 1983). In order for pause cells to work well as sources of Now Print signals, the saccade must begin shortly after the HMI is activated by the TPM. Otherwise, the TPM target position would be able to sample the initial eye position, as well as the terminal eye position, for a significant amount of time. A critical parameter in ruling out a pause cell as a possible generator of a Now Print signal is the relative amount of time after the saccade ends as compared to before the saccade begins that the TPM command and the pause cell are simultaneously active. This ratio must be large in order for a pause cell to be an effective Now Print signal source.

A stronger test of whether a particular refixation neuron or pause cell is controlling a Now Print signal to the HMI can also be made. Suppose that such a cell could be excited on a series of saccadic trials by an electrode before each saccade occurs from a fixed target position. Then the head-to-muscle transform should gradually encode the initial eye position. Consequently, over successive learning trials, saccades in response to the fixed target position should become progressively smaller.

Gating signals of the type that are needed within the HMI have been reported in invertebrate sensory-motor learning circuits by Hawkins, Abrams, Carew, and Kandel (1983) and Walters and Bryne (1983). In these studies, the gating signal is mediated by a presynaptic Ca^{++} current that modulates the chemical transmitter system in the conditionable pathway. When a candidate HMI circuit is isolated, the possibility that a Ca^{++} current carries the Now Print signal can be tested using the same methods that have been developed in the invertebrate preparations.

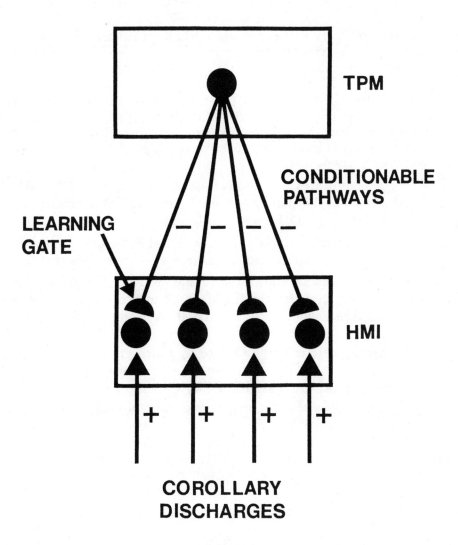

Figure 4.4. Recoding of a target position into muscle coordinates at a head-muscle interface, or HMI: The conditioned pathways learn an "adaptive inhibitory efference copy" from the corollary discharges that they are allowed to sample when the learning gate is active. When the efference copy equals the sampled corollary discharges, learning ceases.

4.8. Mathematical Design of the Head-Muscle Interface

The HMI circuit is a modified version of a motor expectancy learning circuit that was proposed by Grossberg (1972a, Figure 6). Denote by I_j the excitatory corollary discharge signal that represents the eye position corresponding to the jth muscle. Denote by $-S_i$ the ith inhibitory sampling signal that is released by the ith target position within the TPM. Let z_{ij} denote the LTM trace that exists at the synapse of the inhibitory pathway from the ith TPM target position to the jth HMI muscle representation. As in the design of the AG stage in Chapter 3, each LTM trace is assumed to control the rate of transmitter production in its synapse. Each LTM trace z_{ij} is assumed to possess the following properties (Grossberg, 1964, 1968, 1982a):

1. Trace z_{ij} computes a time-average of the product of the ith sampling signal S_i with the jth potential x_j of the HMI whenever x_j is suprathreshold $(x_j > 0)$. Otherwise, no learning occurs.

2. Trace z_{ij} multiplicatively gates the signal S_i before it can influence x_j. The net inhibitory signal that influences x_j due to S_i is thus $-S_i z_{ij}$.

3. Potential x_j reacts additively to the sum of all conditionable inhibitory signals $-S_i z_{ij}$ from the TPM and the jth excitatory corollary discharge I_j at times when it is sensitized by a gating signal from the TPM.

4. The learning rate is gated to zero by a presynaptic gating, or Now Print, signal P that is switched on after a saccade terminates.

Hypotheses (1)–(4) are instantiated by the following differential equations for the time rates of change $\frac{d}{dt}x_j$ and $\frac{d}{dt}z_{ij}$ of each potential x_j and LTM trace z_{ij}, respectively:

$$\frac{d}{dt}x_j = -Ax_j + G(\sum_{i=1}^{n} S_i)(-\sum_{i=1}^{n} S_i z_{ij} + I_j) \qquad (4.1)$$

and

$$\frac{d}{dt}z_{ij} = P\{-Bz_{ij} + S_i[x_j]^+\}, \qquad (4.2)$$

where

$$[x_j]^+ = \begin{cases} x_j & \text{if } x_j > 0 \\ 0 & \text{if } x_j < 0 \end{cases} \qquad (4.3)$$

and the gating function $G(\sum_{i=1}^{n} S_i)$ is an increasing function of $\sum_{i=1}^{n} S_i$ that vanishes when all $S_i = 0$. The suprathreshold activity pattern

$$V = ([x_1]^+, [x_2]^+, [x_3]^+, [x_4]^+, [x_5]^+, [x_6]^+) \qquad (4.4)$$

represents the instantaneous vector difference between target position and eye position in muscle coordinates for a single eye. We now summarize how equations (4.1)–(4.4) carry out the operations that were outlined in Section 4.6.

Suppose that, due to attentional processing within the TPM, at most one target position sampling signal $S_i > 0$ at any time. Without loss of generality, we can suppose that the gating function

$$G(\sum_{i=1}^{n} S_i) = \begin{cases} 1 & \text{if } \sum_{i=1}^{n} S_i > 0 \\ 0 & \text{if } \sum_{i=1}^{n} S_i = 0. \end{cases} \tag{4.5}$$

At times when no TPM target position is active, equation (4.1) reduces to the equation

$$\frac{d}{dt}x_j = -Ax_j, \tag{4.6}$$

which implies that the potential x_j rapidly decays to its passive equilibrium value, zero. In particular, no sustained output signals can be generated from the HMI at these times.

By contrast, consider times when some target position, say the ith one, is active within the TPM. At times when $S_i > 0$, equation (4.1) reduces to the equation

$$\frac{d}{dt}x_j = -Ax_j - S_iz_{ij} + I_j. \tag{4.7}$$

The LTM trace is assumed to change slowly relative to the fluctuation rate of the STM trace x_j. Hence we can assume that x_j is always in an approximate equilibrium relative to the slow time scale of z_{ij}. At equilibrium, $\frac{d}{dt}x_j = 0$. Then (4.7) implies that x_j approximately satisfies the equation

$$x_j = \frac{1}{A}(I_j - S_iz_{ij}). \tag{4.8}$$

The forgetting rate B of z_{ij} in (4.2) is also assumed to be slow relative to the learning rate $S_i[x_j]^+$. Consequently, the rate of change of z_{ij} approximately satisfies the equation

$$\frac{d}{dt}z_{ij} = PS_i[x_j]^+. \tag{4.9}$$

Equations (4.8) and (4.9) together imply that

$$\frac{d}{dt}z_{ij} = \frac{PS_i}{A}[I_j - S_iz_{ij}]^+. \tag{4.10}$$

By equation (4.10), the LTM trace changes only at times when the gating signal P, the sampling signal S_i, and the position difference term $[I_j - S_iz_{ij}]^+$ are *all* positive. Moreover, z_{ij} can increase due only to these factors. All decreases of z_{ij} are due to the very slow forgetting term

$-BPz_{ij}$ in (4.2), which can be completely ignored on the time scale of a learning trial.

Suppose that, at the onset of learning, z_{ij} is small, possibly even zero. Also suppose that, when S_i is activated across learning trials, S_i maintains a temporally stable value due to the competitive feedback interactions that store signals in STM within the TPM (Section 2.6). Finally suppose that the gating signal P becomes positive only after a saccade is over. At such times, I_j encodes the corollary discharge (present eye position) corresponding to the jth extraocular muscle, $j = 1, 2, \ldots, 6$. Due to learning within the visually reactive RCN (Chapter 3), at times when $S_i > 0$ the present eye position $(I_1, I_2, \ldots, I_6)$ gradually converges to the eye position $(I_{i1}, I_{i2}, \ldots, I_{i6})$ corresponding to the target position that activated S_i.

By (4.10), z_{ij} changes only when $S_i > 0$ and $P > 0$. When $S_i > 0$ and $P > 0$, (4.10) implies that $S_i z_{ij}$ approaches I_j as learning proceeds. Since each I_j converges to I_{ij} on learning trials when $S_i > 0$, $S_i z_{ij}$ converges to I_{ij} on these trials. The slow forgetting rate B prevents $S_i z_{ij}$ from getting stuck at I_j values that may occur before I_j converges to I_{ij}.

This argument shows that the gated signal $S_i z_{ij}$ approaches I_{ij} for *all* $j = 1, 2, \ldots, 6$. Thus activating the target position corresponding to S_i reads-out the signal pattern $(S_i z_{i1}, S_i z_{i2}, \ldots, S_i z_{i6})$ into the HMI. Due to learning, this signal pattern approaches the target position $(I_{i1}, I_{i2}, \ldots, I_{i6})$. In all, the head coordinates of S_i have learned to read their target position, expressed in agonist-antagonist muscle coordinates, into the HMI.

After learning occurs, suppose that $S_i > 0$ at a time when the eye is at the present eye position $(I_1, I_2, \ldots, I_6)$. By (4.8),

$$x_j = \frac{1}{A}(I_j - I_{ij}) \tag{4.11}$$

at these times. Equation (4.11) computes the vector difference of the present eye position and the target position, expressed in muscle coordinates. The HMI output signals are

$$V = ([x_1]^+, [x_2]^+, \ldots, [x_6]^+). \tag{4.12}$$

In pattern V, if an agonist muscle representation has a positive value, its antagonist muscle representation has a negative value, and conversely. Thus at most three of the six entries in V are positive at any time. These entries completely determine which vector difference is being computed.

4.9. Muscle Linearization and Retinotopic Recoding

As it stands, the HMI circuit clarifies some issues and raises others. The HMI design shows how target positions can be recoded into motor coordinates so that vector differences which automatically compensate for present position can be computed (Section 1.7). The HMI design also shows how the visually reactive system prevents an infinite regress from occurring: although learning within the HMI can only associate *final* eye position in motor coordinates with a TPM target position, this eye position approaches the *target* eye position due to learning within the visually reactive system.

Two major problems still need to be solved in order for the HMI to work well: linearization of the muscle response to outflow signals, and transformation of the HMI output patterns V in (4.12) from muscle coordinates into retinotopic coordinates.

A. *Linearization of Muscle Response*

The need to linearize the muscle response to outflow signals can be seen by considering equation (4.11). Each potential x_j computes the difference of present eye position I_j and target position I_{ij} in muscle coordinates. Both I_j and I_{ij} are derived from outflow signals to the muscle plant. Unless the muscle plant contracts as a linear function of these outflow signals, neither I_j nor I_{ij} provides a reliable index of where the eye is actually pointing at any time. Thus a circuit is needed which can linearize the muscle plant's response to outflow signals, despite the fact that the muscle plant is nonlinear (Section 1.10).

This argument can be made more vividly by noting that the output V of the HMI is based upon a vector *difference* of target position and present position. *Infinitely* many choices of these positions can generate the *same* vector difference. The function of each fixed vector difference is to encode a determinate distance and direction that the eye must move to foveate a light. If the many individual target positions and present positions that lead to a fixed vector difference do not accurately reflect where the eye actually is or intends to go, then the vector difference itself cannot encode how the eye must move to foveate a light. A single vector difference could then be generated by combinations of target positions and present positions that do not represent the same distance and direction of motion between the actual present eye position and the actual position of a light on the retina.

These considerations strongly suggest that the muscle response is linearized by a separate learning circuit. In Chapter 3, we considered many possible ways whereby the saccadic control system could, in principle, compensate for muscle plant nonlinearity. The design of the HMI suggests a particular scheme. Given that a separate circuit linearizes the muscle response, the simulation described in Figure 3.12B indicates that a retinotopic sampling map may be sufficient to control the LTM traces which are tuned by second light error signals at the AG stage.

This conclusion does not imply that adaptive compensation for initial eye position is no longer needed. Indeed, such compensation occurs within the circuit that linearizes the muscle response (Chapter 5). However, this circuit delivers its conditioned signals to a processing stage that occurs

after, rather than before, the saccade generator (SG). Only a retinotopic
sampling map is needed, for purposes of correcting individual saccades, to
deliver conditionable signals before the SG stage. Despite this fact, there
are other reasons why converging conditionable pathways from more than
one sampling map are needed at a stage prior to the SG stage, as we will
see in Chapter 9.

B. *Retinotopic Recoding*

The HMI transforms the multimodal target position map of the TPM
into a much simpler unimodal motor map. However, muscle coordinates
are the wrong coordinates from which to generate saccadic commands.
Such commands need to be generated in retinotopic coordinates, so that
they can benefit from second light visual error signals (Chapter 3). We
are hereby led to appreciate more fully the simple but subtle deviousness
of sensory-motor systems. Visual signals in retinotopic coordinates are
recoded as target positions in head coordinates, then recoded as target
positions in muscle coordinates, so that they can be recoded as vector
differences in muscle coordinates, only to be recoded into retinotopic coordinates once again. The circle from vision to motor coordinates and
back to vision is hereby closed.

How can a vector difference in muscle coordinates be recoded into
retinotopic coordinates? Are these two types of information dimensionally compatible? Another subtlety is explicated by the answer: although
a target position in muscle coordinates is dimensionally incompatible with
retinotopic coordinates, a vector difference in muscle coordinates is dimensionally compatible with retinotopic coordinates. This is true because of
the way in which a vector difference is computed. In order to compute
a target position, initial eye position is added onto the retinal position
of the light. In order to compute a vector difference, initial eye position
is subtracted from target position. The addition-then-subtraction of initial eye position from retinal position shows that the vector difference is
retinotopically consistent. Of course, this description ignores all the coordinate transformations and time delays that make these transformations
functionally meaningful. Just adding and subtracting initial eye position
seems meaningless, even absurd, outside of this functional context. However, this description shows that the vector differences that are computed
in muscle coordinates within the HMI can, in principle, be mapped back
into retinotopic coordinates. We suggest how this is done in Chapter 11.

We can now explain why we have often used the term "retinotopic"
coordinates instead of "retinal" coordinates. We use the term "retinal"
coordinates only to describe the frame in which lights on the retina are
registered. The more general term "retinotopic" coordinates is used to
describe any coordinate system, including vector differences, that can be
mapped in a one-to-one way on retinal coordinates.

Before considering our solutions to the muscle linearization and retinotopic recoding problems, we describe some saccadic data that are clarified
by properties of HMI dynamics.

4.10. Saccade Staircases and Automatic Compensation for Present Position

Schiller and Stryker (1972) have shown that a sustained electrode input to the monkey superior colliculus (SC) causes a staircase, or succession, of saccades of equal amplitude. In particular, Schiller and Stryker (1972) showed differences in evoked saccades due to electrical stimulation of superior colliculus and abducens oculomotor nucleus in the monkey. In the abducens nucleus, saccade amplitude was proportional to stimulation duration. In the deeper layers of the superior colliculus, stimulation longer than about 25 ms evoked a saccade whose amplitude was determined by collicular location. When stimulation duration exceeded 150 ms, two saccades were evoked with an intervening fixation. With prolonged stimulation a staircase of identical saccades was produced. The current threshold for generating such a staircase decreases by a factor of 20–100 as the electrode moves from the superficial layers to the deep layers of the SC. We will therefore focus on how such a staircase can be elicited from the deep layers of the SC.

Hikosaka and Wurtz (1983) have also generated saccade staircases from the SC. They accomplished this by injecting bicuculline, a GABA antagonist, into the SC. This manipulation, which decays over a time course of minutes, was made to directly test their hypothesis "that SN [substantia nigra] cells exert tonic inhibition on SC cells and that the pause in SN cell discharge before saccadic eye movements allowed the burst of activity in the SC cells. If this hypothesis were correct, application of GABA agonists and antagonists in the SC should clearly affect the initiation of saccades" (p.368), and this is what Hikosaka and Wurtz confirmed.

The existence of staircases *per se* will be explained in Section 7.6, after we have analysed how inputs to the saccade generator (SG) are normally updated after each saccade. In this section, we will comment upon two issues that are related to saccade staircases: Since saccade staircases can *sometimes occur* in response to a sustained input to the SG, then what prevents them from *always* occurring in response to any sustained command to the SG? Since each saccade in a saccade staircase starts out at a different initial position of the eyes, and since the same electrode input amplitude causes all of these saccades, why doesn't the size of successive saccades change due to the nonlinearity of the muscle plant, as it may in some species?

The main issue raised by the first question derives its interest from a comparison of the Mays and Sparks (1980) data with the Schiller and Stryker (1972) data. In both experiments, an electrode input to the SC was used. In the Mays and Sparks (1980) paradigm, our theory claims that the saccadic control system compensated for the movement caused by the electrode input by updating the present eye position input to the HMI, and computing the vector difference of the updated present eye position with the target position of the light. The vector difference then generated the command whereby the second saccade foveated the light.

Given that eye position is updated at the HMI after a saccade, and that present position signals are excitatory, why doesn't *every* saccade cause its own saccade staircase by updating present position at the HMI and thereby generating another saccade? Thus the Mays and Sparks (1980) and Schiller and Stryker (1972) experiments, which seem to be unrelated when described in lay language, raise serious design issues when their implications are considered on the mechanistic level.

In our theory, this question is answered as follows. The TPM cannot activate a target position solely in response to eye position signals. A combination of visual signals and eye position signals is needed. The HMI, in turn, can generate output signals only at times when the TPM is actively reading a target position into the HMI. Thus, whereas eye position inputs to the HMI are updated by electrode-induced saccades in the Schiller and Stryker paradigm, these signals cannot elicit outputs from the HMI.

By contrast, an attended light input can activate a target position within the TPM. When the saccade caused by this light is over, the updated present position input to the HMI typically equals the target position input to the HMI. The target position and present position then cancel each other by vector subtraction. Thus although the HMI is capable of generating an output in this case, no saccade staircase is generated because the output equals zero.

These conclusions depend critically upon the idea that visually-dependent TPM activation controls the output gate of the HMI. Other authors have also realized that some sort of output gating is needed to control automatic compensation for present position. These authors have not, however, chosen the gating source that we require. For example, in his important review of arm movement control, Hyvärinen (1982, p.1115) wrote: "Joint neurons in area 5 discharge more vigorously during active than passive movements...and arm-projection and hand-manipulation neurons probably receive sensory signals from joints, muscles, and skin during active movements. It appears likely that the sensory activity in these neurons is 'gated' by inputs related to the preparation of the motor act...in the form of corollary discharge from motor structures". Hyvärinen thus suggested that the corollary discharges, not visually modulated target position commands, are the source of the gating signals. If this were so in the HMI, saccade staircases would relentlessly occur in the dark due to the tonic nature of the corollary discharges. We venture to say that a similar catastrophe would occur if corollary discharges gated the HMI that automatically compensates for present position in the arm control system.

The requirements imposed by HMI design also provide a simple answer to the question: Why are all the saccades in the saccade staircase equal in size, despite the nonlinear nature of the muscle plant? Our answer derives from the hypothesis that the muscle plant response is linearized by a separate adaptive circuit, so that the corollary discharges to the HMI have behavioral meaning. Equal electrode inputs generate equal movements from this linearized plant. In Chapter 5, we will state a prediction capable of testing this explanation.

We also note the report of Hikosaka and Wurtz (1983) that saccade oscillations can occur in their paradigm. In every case, a visual fixation point existed in their experiments. These oscillations may be due to saccades elicited by the fixation point that alternate with the drug-induced saccades. Such an oscillation could occur when a visually elicited activation is strong enough to competitively inhibit the drug-induced activation. Alternatively, the mechanism whereby saccades return to the head-in-center position may be at work. These alternatives can experimentally be differentiated by studying monkeys in the dark or in front of a homogeneous fixation screen.

4.11. Corrective Saccades in the Dark: An Outflow Interpretation

Shebilske (1977) has collected data which he used to argue for the existence of inflow signals from the eye muscles to the saccadic command system. He analysed the saccades of human subjects in response to briefly flashed lights that were turned off before the end of the saccades. Shebilske discovered that on trials wherein the first saccade to the light was incorrect, a second corrective saccade was directed towards the target with high probability. Since the light was no longer on, Shebilske argued that an internal representation of the position of the target in space was stored in STM. Shebilske (1977, p.46) also assumed that "outflow encodes the internal eye position." This assumption led him to conclude that the present eye position signals which are used to generate a corrective saccade must be inflow signals. Otherwise, since intended position and outflow are the same, there would be no basis for computing the discrepancy between present eye position and intended eye position.

An alternative explanation that uses outflow signals to provide present eye position information can be given for these data using properties of the HMI. Let the TPM store a target position in STM which reads-out a movement command to the HMI. Suppose that the many processing steps leading from the TPM through the HMI towards the cells that establish the new position of the eyes are susceptible to occasional encoding errors due to internal system noise. Also suppose that the signals from these outflow cells to eye muscles are almost always correctly interpreted. In other words, whereas Shebilske (1977, p.46) claims that "outflow encodes the intended eye position," we suggest that outflow does not always encode the intended eye position.

Suppose that after the first saccade occurs, the incorrect outflow signal, which has been obeyed by the muscles, is also used to generate a corollary discharge to the HMI. Since the muscles obeyed this outflow signal, it provides a veridical estimate of eye position after the saccade terminates. When the vector difference of target position and corollary discharge is computed at the HMI, a new command is generated which is capable of eliciting a corrective saccade in the dark.

Shebilske (1977, pp.45–46) reviews two test conditions to confirm his inflow hypothesis. Both test conditions are compatible with the above outflow interpretation.

The main point of this discussion is to suggest that the Shebilske (1977) data are compatible with the same mechanism that we have used to explain the Mays and Sparks (1980) data. Recently, Guthrie, Porter, and Sparks (1983) have shown that vector compensation occurs in the Mays and Sparks paradigm after surgical elimination of all inflow signals from the eye muscles. In the light of our conceptual bridge between the two experimental paradigms, these recent data provide further support for an outflow interpretation of Shebilske's results. Evidence for outflow but not inflow has also been found using loaded contact lens (Skavenski, Haddad, and Steinman, 1972). They performed experiments in which they either fixed inflow signals or fixed outflow signals and tested for perceived monocular visual direction. In the first experiment, a suction contact lens was put on an eye and one of three loads was attached to the lens. The subject fixated a target straight ahead with a load on. In order to maintain this fixation, the subject had to increase the amount of outflow. Measurements of perceived direction were made by having the subject move a test target to the perceived straight ahead. The mean shift of perceived direction increased monotonically with increasing loads on the contact lens. Since loading the eye does not affect inflow, it was concluded that perceived direction is computed using outflow.

In the second experiment, a red target was exposed to the left eye while the loaded right eye was exposed to brief flashes of a white target. The subject was asked to match the direction of the white target to the red target. Here it was assumed that because the two eyes are yoked, the left eye maintained a constant outflow for both eyes, since it was exposed to a constant target. The right eye rotated passively under load, thereby varying inflow. There was no change in the mean perceived direction of the red target when the amount of passive rotation was subtracted from the measurements to account for shifts in the retinal locus. Again it was concluded that inflow does not contribute to perceived visual direction.

CHAPTER 5
ADAPTIVE LINEARIZATION OF
THE MUSCLE PLANT

5.1. Fast Corrective Saccades vs. Slow Muscle Linearization

The use of outflow signals to determine present position at the HMI, and our outflow interpretation of the Shebilske (1977) data about corrective saccades (Section 4.11), do not deny that inflow signals play an important role in saccadic dynamics. In fact, our analysis stressed the need to linearize muscle plant responses to the outflow signals that determine present position at the HMI. In order to linearize muscle responses to outflow signals, information about the muscle plant's characteristics must somehow be used. Inflow signals supply this type of information. The process whereby inflow information is used is a slowly varying adaptive process. The corrective saccades studied by Shebilske (1977) occur on a much faster time scale than the adjustment of this slow recalibration process. Thus there is no contradiction in simultaneously advocating an outflow interpretation of the Shebilske (1977) data and an inflow interpretation of muscle linearization.

We will use the role of inflow in adaptive muscle linearization to explain several types of data, such as the data of Steinbach and Smith (1981) on the pointing behavior of patients after surgery on their extraocular muscles to correct strabismus (Section 5.4), and the data of Ron and Robinson (1973) and Vilis, Snow, and Hore (1983) concerning the role of the cerebellum in preventing dysmetria (Section 5.3).

5.2. Muscle Linearization Network

We hypothesize that a *Muscle Linearization Network* (MLN) exists wherein an inflow signal helps to linearize the size of a muscle contraction in response to outflow signals (Figure 5.1). This hypothesis does not imply that the muscle plant becomes more linear, but only that the muscle response to outflow signals becomes more linear, so that outflow signals can be used as a good estimator of present eye position in the HMI.

The MLN shares several basic design properties with the retinotopic command network (RCN) of Chapter 3. This comparison, as well as later ones in the text, will clarify our contention that distinct sensory-motor systems share common design features, including common brain regions. For example, in both the MLN and the RCN, the source of movement signals branches into two parallel pathways. One pathway generates an unconditioned movement signal. The other pathway generates a conditioned movement signal. This latter pathway passes through the AG stage, or cerebellum. The size, or gain, of the conditioned signal is determined by error signals to the AG stage. The unconditioned and conditioned movement signals then converge at a stage subsequent to the source of the unconditioned movement signal.

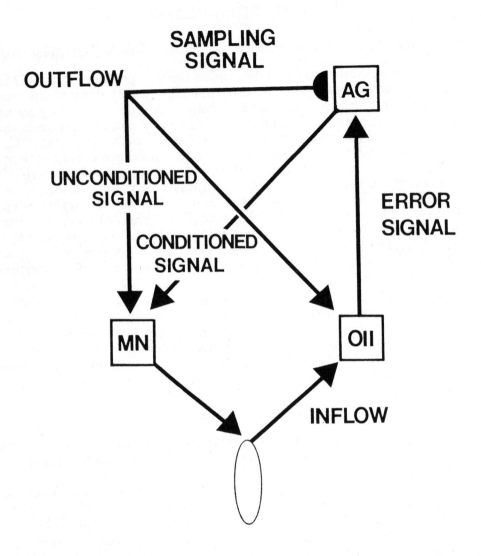

Figure 5.1. Some main features of the muscle linearization network, or MLN: The outflow-inflow interface (OII) registers matches and mismatches between outflow signals and inflow signals. Mismatches generate error signals to the adaptive gain (AG) stage. These error signals change the gain of the conditioned movement signal to the motoneurons (MN). Such an MLN adaptively linearizes the responses of a nonlinear muscle plant to outflow signals. The outflow signals can therefore also be used as a source of accurate corollary discharges of present eye position.

In the MLN, the unconditioned movement signal is clearly an outflow signal. The error signal is determined by a matching process that compares outflow signals with inflow signals, such that perfect matches generate no error signals and large mismatches generate large error signals. These error signals are delivered to the AG stage, where they alter the gain of the corresponding conditioned pathway. This conditioned pathway also arises from the source of outflow signals. The unconditioned and conditioned movement signals then converge at a stage subsequent to the source of outflow movement signals.

A number of informative technical problems must be solved in order for the MLN to work well. We will suggest solutions to these problems in stages. First, we will specify the MLN macrocircuit in greater detail. A possible macrocircuit is depicted in Figure 5.2. Fuchs and Becker (1981) noted the uncertainties of connectivity among brain stem saccade-related cells. The fact that modifications of the macrocircuit can achieve similar functional properties, and that modifications may exist across species, should be kept in mind throughout the subsequent discussion.

Figure 5.2 builds upon the conclusion (Keller, 1974, 1981; Luschei and Fuchs, 1972; Robinson, 1975) that medium lead burst (MLB) cells, which are the target cells of the saccade generator (SG), activate both tonic (T) cells and burst-tonic motoneurons (MN). The T cells, in turn, also excite the MN cells. The MN cells innervate the eye muscles which move and hold the eyes in place. The firing rate of T cells changes smoothly with eye position, whereas the firing rate of MN cells exhibits a burst during a saccade that returns to a position-dependent steady discharge level between saccades. Chapter 7 describes and models these cell types in greater detail.

We assume that the T cells are the source of the unconditioned outflow pathway to the MN cells. Given the other design constraints upon the MLN circuit, this hypothesis implies that the T cells also give rise to three other types of pathways. One pathway has already been mentioned: the pathway that provides corollary discharges to the HMI (Chapter 4). The other two pathways are used to control the conditioned movement signals that linearize the muscle response. One pathway sends excitatory signals to a network called the *outflow-inflow interface* (OII). The OII carries out the matching of outflow signals with inflow signals that generates error signals to the adaptive gain (AG) stage, or cerebellum. A non-zero error signal is generated only if a mismatch between outflow and inflow occurs. The fourth type of pathway from the T cells also reaches the cerebellum. This is the conditioned movement pathway that samples the error signals from the OII to the AG stage. This conditioned pathway thereupon projects to a stage subsequent to the T cells but prior to the muscles. We identify this target of conditioned movement signals as the MN cells.

In summary, the total saccade-related signal from the T cells to the MN cells is assumed to derive from a direct unconditioned pathway and an indirect conditioned pathway through the cerebellum. The size of the

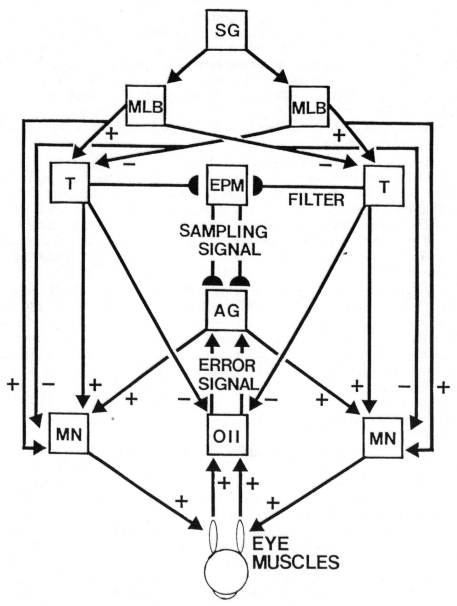

Figure 5.2. Some finer details of the muscle linearization network, or MLN: As in Figure 5.1, the OII generates error signals to the AG stage which alter the gain of the conditioned pathway to the MN. The sampling signals of these conditioned pathways are generated by an eye position map (EPM) which recodes outputs from tonic (T) cells of the saccade generator (SG). The medium lead bursters (MLB) of the SG excite their T cells and MN cells while they inhibit antagonist T cells and MN cells. The T cells also excite the corresponding MN cells and generate outflow signals to the OII, where they are matched against inflow signals.

conditioned signal is modified until a match between direct tonic cell outflow and muscle inflow is achieved. The conditioned pathway supplements
the direct pathway signal until the muscle response to the direct pathway
signal is linear. This property enables the output from the total tonic cell
population to provide accurate corollary discharges to the HMI despite the
existence of nonlinearities of muscle response in the absence of cerebellar
compensation. It should be noted, however, that this sort of adaptive OII
calibration does not guarantee accurate foveation. It merely guarantees a
linear muscle response to whatever signals happen to activate the T cells.

5.3. Cerebellar Direct Response Cells

Before considering more technical questions about MLN design, we
summarize two types of data that are clarified by the existence of a circuit
like the MLN.

The existence of an indirect conditioned cerebellar pathway suggests
an important role for oculomotor nuclei that occur between tonic cells
and eye muscles. A cellular interface is needed at a stage subsequent to
the tonic cells but prior to the muscles at which the total outflow signal,
both unconditioned and conditioned, to the muscles can be computed.
Figure 5.2 thus predicts the existence of a pathway from the AG stage, or
cerebellum, to the MN cells of the oculomotor nuclei.

Ron and Robinson (1973) have reported the existence of saccade-
related *direct response cells* in the dentate nucleus of the cerebellum. Direct electrical activation of these cells can elicit saccades with the remarkably short latency of 5–9 msec. These reaction times are consistent with
the existence of a direct pathway from the direct response cells to the
MN cells of the oculomotor nuclei. Our theory suggests that a subset of
the direct response cells may be part of the conditioned movement pathway that linearizes muscle responses. If so, selective transection of this
pathway should destroy the linearity of muscle responses.

Partial support for this hypothesis follows from the experiments of
Vilis, Snow, and Hore (1983). These authors have shown that lesions of
the medial cerebellar nuclei cause different degrees of dysmetria in different
eye muscles. Such lesions do not, however, distinguish between cerebellar
pathways to the oculomotor nuclei and to other saccade-controlling pathways, such as the SG. For example, in addition to direct response cells,
Ron and Robinson (1973) have also reported the existence of cerebellar
cells that elicit saccades with a much longer latency (12–16 msec.). These
latter signals have properties compatible with their action at the SG. They
may thus be part of the conditionable pathway of the RCN (Chapter 3).
Hepp, Henn, Jaeger, and Waespe (1981) have described saccade-related
burst-tonic mossy fibers in the cerebellar vermis having properties compatible with an SG action.

Thus, although many properties of these cerebellar pathways remain
to be worked out, our theory provides a robust explanation of why certain
cerebellar pathways should activate saccades at or before the SG, while

other cerebellar pathways should activate saccades at a much later processing stage, notably the MN cells. In fact, our theory suggests that a distinct cerebellar pathway, which helps to hold the eyes in a stable postural position between saccades, also projects to the MN cells (Chapter 8).

5.4. Adaptation to Strabismus Surgery

Steinbach and Smith (1981) have reported data that suggest a role for inflow signals in the eye movement control system. By contrast, the data of workers like Guthrie, Porter, and Sparks (1983) and Skavenski, Haddad, and Steinman (1972) have supported a role for outflow control and against inflow control. We now suggest how properties of the MLN can explain the Steinbach and Smith (1981) data without contradicting the data about outflow control.

Steinbach and Smith (1981) studied the arm-pointing behavior of patients who had been operated upon to correct strabismus. In such an operation, some eye muscles are detached from the eyeball and cut. Then the muscles are reattached to the eyeball to determine a new direction in which the eye will point at rest. After such an operation, a patient's eyes are bandaged for 7–48 hours. During this recovery period, a patient experiences no visual cues.

The arm-pointing behavior of patients was tested immediately after their bandages were removed. They were asked to point at test lights with one of their arms. The patients were not able to see their arms during this task. Despite the absence of visual signals of any kind, including visual error signals, during the bandaged interval, the arm-pointing behavior demonstrated a considerable amount of adaptation to the operation. The only obvious change due to the operation was in the eye muscles near their point of attachment, and not in the outflow pathways to them. These data thus suggest a role for inflow signals in controlling the adaptation process whereby conditioned outflow compensates for the operation.

This suggestion is further supported by Steinbach and Smith's observations of subjects who had experienced two successive strabismus operations. The Golgi tendon organs corresponding to the operated eye's medial rectus and lateral rectus muscles were thereby presumed to be destroyed. Adaptation to the eye's new position in its orbit was not observed in the pointing behavior of these patients. These data suggest that inflow signals, possibly mediated by the Golgi tendon organs, play an important role in this type of adaptation.

A possible explanation of these data in terms of MLN properties is the following. Suppose that a surgical lesion in an eye muscle alters the inflow signal that the muscle generates. Then mismatches between outflow signals and inflow signals can occur at the OII even when the patient's eyes are bandaged, since these outflow-inflow comparisons do not require visual signals. These mismatches generate error signals to the AG stage that slowly change the conditioned gain of the outflow signals. Two properties of this conditioned change cannot be explained until we more precisely characterize the OII microcircuit; namely, why the adaptive change tends to compensate for the surgical lesion if the proprioceptors are spared, yet why no adaptation occurs if the proprioceptors are removed, even though such removal would seem to produce the biggest outflow-inflow mismatches. These issues thus probe finer aspects of how matches and mismatches are computed within the OII. For the moment, let us simply assume these properties of adaptation in order to complete our argument.

Even if we assume these properties, further argument is needed, because these properties do not in themselves explain how adaptation of an eye movement command can influence movement commands to the arms. To answer this question, we must ask how computations within the eye-head system generate movement commands to the hand-arm system. Our analysis of how circular reactions are learned (Section 1.3) suggests that such commands are mediated via head coordinate maps. In particular, the target position map, or TPM, of the eye-head movement system generates a command to the TPM of the hand-arm movement system.

This conclusion raises the possibility that the positional signals used to compute target positions in the TPM are inflow signals. The data of Guthrie, Porter, and Sparks (1983) seem to contradict this possibility, since vector compensation can occur normally in the absence of any inflow signals. If, however, outflow, rather than inflow, is used to compute target positions in the TPM, then how do changes in eye muscle inflow alter arm-pointing behavior at all?

We suggest that when the patient first sees the target light, no effect of the inflow change is experienced at the TPM. Instead, the subject's eyes saccade to foveate the target. This saccade benefits from the inflow-mediated changes in the total movement signal during the time that the eyes were bandaged. The saccade is therefore erroneous, but less erroneous than it would have been without the benefit of OII-driven gain changes. After this eye movement is over, the target light is again registered on the retina, at a new non-foveal position. This new retinal position can instate a new target position within the TPM. This second target position does reflect the inflow-mediated gain change. In fact, any further eye movements that the subject makes in an effort to foveate the target light can activate target positions at the TPM that reflect the inflow-mediated gain change. In the Steinbach and Smith (1981) experiment, subjects made from six to ten pointing responses. All but the first of these TPM target positions are suggested by the theory to activate pointing behavior which reflects adaptation to the surgical lesion.

One can test whether only this adaptive mechanism is recalibrated due to strabismus surgery by analysing pointing behavior that occurs before a patient moves his eyes. Then no major differences should exist between the arm-pointing behavior of patients who have had one strabismus operation and those who have had two strabismus operations.

Before describing OII design in greater detail, we pause to summarize some of the different concepts of "error correction" that have thus far arisen.

5.5. Error Correction with and without Adaptive Gain Changes

Data such as those of Steinbach and Smith (1981), Shebilske (1977), and Vilis, Snow, and Hore (1983) show that the term "error correction" must be used with care. Corrective saccades in the dark (Section 4.11) can use the HMI to "correct a saccadic error" without necessarily altering the parameters that control saccades. This is not the same type of "error correction" as occurs when second lights generate error signals that adaptively change the parameters of saccadic commands within the AG stage (Chapter 3). Indeed, in the Shebilske paradigm, there is no second light to act as an error signal, even though a corrective saccade can occur. Moreover, the HMI is part of the Vector Command Network, or VCN, whereas the second light error signals are elaborated as part of the Retinotopic Command Network, or RCN.

Conversely, a nonfoveating saccade can occur in which the light source is kept on and the outflow signal accurately encodes the vector command from the HMI. On such a trial, no corrective saccades of the Shebilske type will be generated if the target position and the final eye position agree at the HMI. However, adaptive learning could still occur because the second light is not foveated. Moreover, the nonfoveated second light can generate a second saccade. Such a second saccade, although tending to move the light towards the fovea, is not "corrective" in the Shebilske sense. Finally, inflow-mediated gain control of the outflow signal via the OII, albeit an adaptive change, is not the same adaptive change that causes accurate foveating saccades. The OII exists, moreover, in a different system: the Muscle Linearization Network, or MLN. One must clearly distinguish between VCN-mediated corrective saccades, RCN-mediated adaptive saccadic learning, RCN-mediated foveating second saccades, and MLN-mediated adaptive muscle compensation in order to avoid conceptual and terminological confusions.

5.6. Matching within the Outflow-Inflow Interface

The matching mechanism that we suggest for the OII helps to simultaneously solve several functional problems:

1. It can compensate for differences in the absolute size scales of outflow signals and inflow signals by computing the *relative* sizes of the signals corresponding to agonist-antagonist muscle pairs. Thus the computational unit within the OII is a spatial pattern, or normalized motor synergy (Section 1.10), rather than the amplitude of a single outflow or inflow signal.

2. It can match the inflow synergy against the outflow synergy. A perfect match occurs if the inflow synergy is a linear function of the outflow synergy. Poor matches occur if the inflow synergy exhibits nonlinear distortions. The error signal emitted from the OII increases as the match deteriorates.

3. Despite this last property, if the OII receives no inflow signals, then the muscle plant is not further linearized.

We will first summarize formal circuits that imply these properties before considering physical mechanisms that can generate their formal relationships. Several different, but closely related, formal circuits can achieve the desired properties. We summarize two of them to articulate the issues that need further neural data to be completely resolved. Two types of formal designs will be described, those in which the agonist inflow signal is an increasing linear function of the amount of agonist *contraction*, and those in which the agonist inflow signal is an increasing linear function of the agonist muscle *length*. Since amount of muscle contraction varies inversely with muscle length, these circuits embody testably different properties.

Figure 5.3 summarizes the main formal properties of an OII design whose inflow signals increase with muscle contraction. Figure 5.4 summarizes an OII model whose inflow signals increase with muscle length. Suppose that, within a prescribed time interval, the tonic cell outflow signal to an agonist muscle equals α and to the corresponding antagonist muscle equals β. Suppose that the muscle contractions caused by these outflow signals are $C(\alpha)$ and $C(\beta)$, respectively, and that the inflow signals are proportional to the amount of contraction; viz., $kC(\alpha)$ and $kC(\beta)$, where k is a positive constant.

The absolute sizes of these outflow signals and inflow signals might vary on very different size scales. We therefore assume that these size scales are normalized before their resultant spatial patterns are compared. Such a normalization scheme defines a "big" agonist outflow signal as one that is large relative to its antagonist contraction. Thus we assume that the outflow signal pattern (α, β) is transformed into the spatial pattern

$$\left(\frac{\alpha}{\alpha + \beta}, \frac{\beta}{\alpha + \beta}\right) \tag{5.1}$$

and that the inflow signal pattern

$$\left(kC(\alpha), kC(\beta)\right) \tag{5.2}$$

is transformed into the spatial pattern

$$\left(\frac{C(\alpha)}{C(\alpha) + C(\beta)}, \frac{C(\beta)}{C(\alpha) + C(\beta)}\right), \tag{5.3}$$

except if $k = 0$. If $k = 0$, equation (5.3) is replaced by $(0,0)$. Then the two spatial patterns are matched as follows.

The inflow spatial pattern (5.1) generates topographic excitatory signals and the outflow spatial pattern generates topographic inhibitory signals to the comparator region. Error signals are generated only if one of

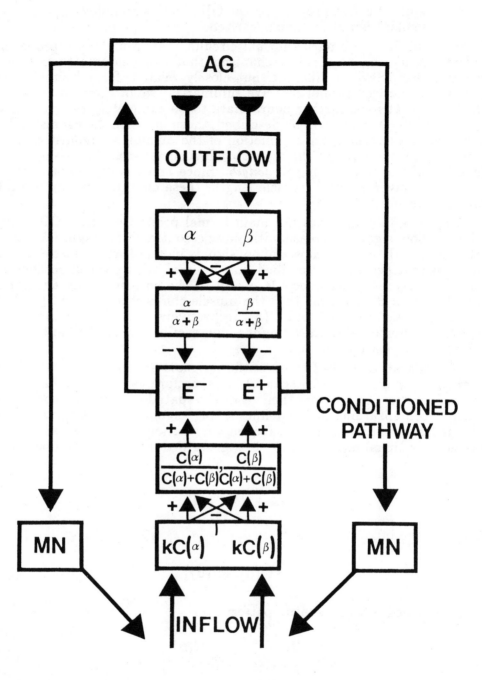

Figure 5.3. Microstructure of an outflow-inflow interface (OII) whose inflow signals vary monotonically with the amount of muscle contraction: See text for details.

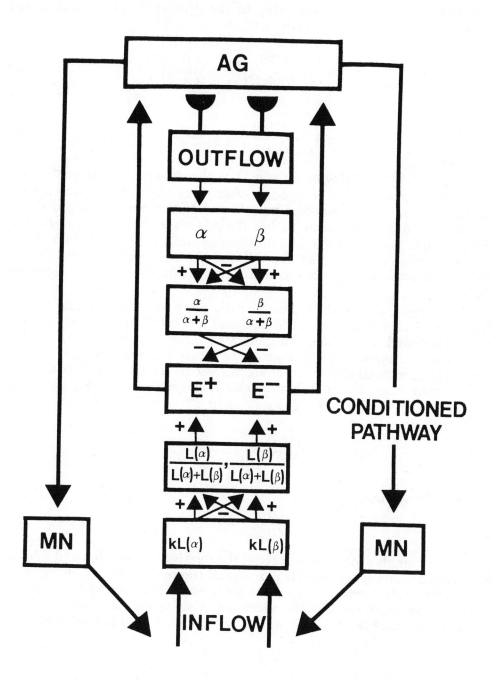

Figure 5.4. Microstructure of an outflow-inflow interface (OII) whose inflow signals vary monotonically with muscle length: See text for details.

the net potentials corresponding to the agonist inputs or antagonist inputs is positive. In other words, let

$$E^+ = \left[\frac{C(\beta)}{C(\alpha) + C(\beta)} - \frac{\beta}{\alpha + \beta}\right]^+ \qquad (5.4)$$

and

$$E^- = \left[\frac{C(\alpha)}{C(\alpha) + C(\beta)} - \frac{\alpha}{\alpha + \beta}\right]^+ \qquad (5.5)$$

where $[\xi]^+ = \max(\xi, 0)$ and E^+ (E^-) is the agonist (antagonist) error signal. We suppose that the agonist error signal E^+ acts to increase the conditioned gain of the agonist muscle and to decrease the conditioned gain of the antagonist muscle within the AG stage. The antagonist error signal E^- has the opposite effect on these muscles at the AG stage. Thus the error signals generated by the OII and the error signals generated by second light error signals obey similar laws within the AG stage (Section 3.13).

To understand how these formal rules work, note that if the agonist muscle contracts less than its outflow signal command, then its conditioned gain is increased due to the OII-generated error signals in (5.4). Subsequent outflow signals therefore generate larger contractions and smaller error signals, until finally no error signals occur. To test whether no error signals occur when the muscle response is linearized, consider equations (5.4) and (5.5). Both error signals E^+ and E^- equal zero if

$$\frac{C(\alpha)}{C(\alpha) + C(\beta)} = \frac{\alpha}{\alpha + \beta}. \qquad (5.6)$$

Equation (5.6) implies

$$\frac{C(\alpha)}{C(\beta)} = \frac{\alpha}{\beta}. \qquad (5.7)$$

Thus error signals are not generated if the relative contraction and dilation of an agonist-antagonist muscle pair equals the relative size of the agonist-antagonist outflow signal. This is the basic linearity property that we seek. In particular, suppose that the agonist and antagonist outflow signals to the tonic cells mutually inhibit each other in a push-pull fashion, such that

$$\alpha + \beta = \gamma \qquad (5.8)$$

where γ is constant. Also suppose that the amount of contraction of the agonist is balanced by the amount of dilation of the antagonist, such that

$$C(\alpha) + C(\beta) = \delta. \qquad (5.9)$$

Then (5.7) implies

$$C(\alpha) = p\alpha, \qquad (5.10)$$

where the proportionality constant $p = \gamma^{-1}\delta$.

Suppose, by contrast, that the agonist muscle contracts nonlinearly in response to the outflow signals; for example, suppose that the agonist muscle contracts too little. Then by (5.4) and (5.5),

$$E^+ > 0 = E^-, \tag{5.11}$$

so that the agonist conditioned gain will be increased and the antagonist conditioned gain will be decreased due to conditioning. The inequalities (5.11) are due to the fact that the match of *agonist* signals in (5.5) gives rise to the *antagonist* error signal, and the match of *antagonist* signals in (5.4) gives rise to the *agonist* error signal. This model predicts that the agonist-antagonist symmetry axis is reversed somewhere between the OII, which is a target for the outflow and inflow signals from the tonic cells and muscles, respectively, and the cerebellum, which receives OII-activated error signals via climbing fibers. The model of Figure 5.4, in which length-based inflow signals are used, also predicts a reversal of symmetry axis. This reversal occurs, however, within the OII in the matching of outflow and inflow signals.

5.7. An Explanation of the Steinbach and Smith Data

Equations (5.1)–(5.5) provide an explanation of why an absence of inflow signals prevents adaptation to strabismus surgery. If all inflow signals are prevented, then, since the inflow constant $k = 0$ in equation (5.2), equations (5.4) and (5.5) reduce to

$$E^+ = [-\frac{\beta}{\alpha + \beta}]^+ = 0 \tag{5.12}$$

and

$$E^- = [-\frac{\alpha}{\alpha + \beta}]^+ = 0, \tag{5.13}$$

so that no error signals at the AG stage are generated. Another way to state this conclusion is in terms of inflow signals to the cerebellum. In equations (5.4) and (5.5), inflow signals provide the excitatory drive for generating error signals to the cerebellum. This model predicts that cutting all inflow pathways will eliminate a major source of inflow which reaches the cerebellum via climbing fibers. Cutting all of these inflow pathways should also prevent the eye movement system from linearizing muscle responses after nonlinearities are induced by other experimental manipulations. Cutting the inflow pathways need not disrupt the linearity of muscle response in the absence of other experimental manipulations, because the inflow signals give rise to error signals, not to the conditioned movement signals that maintain a linear muscle response.

We can now show how the effects of strabismus surgery are compensated for by this OII model. Suppose that an agonist muscle is cut and shortened before being reattached to the eyeball. Suppose that such an operation has two simultaneous effects: It causes the eye to point more in the direction of the agonist muscle, and it weakens the inflow signal from this muscle. Due to the weakening of the agonist inflow signal, equations (5.4) and (5.5) imply that

$$E^+ = 0 < E^-. \tag{5.14}$$

Consequently, the gain of the antagonist muscle will increase, thereby tending to shift the eye back towards its original position. One might therefore ask why strabismus surgery does not always fail? The theory suggests two reasons: The backward shift merely tends to relinearize the muscle responses. Second light error signals assume the major load of recalibrating the conditioned gains which will ensure accurate foveation despite the surgical change in eye position.

5.8. A Role for Golgi Tendon Organs in Muscle Linearization

Steinbach and Smith (1981, p.1408) concluded from their data "that in some not yet understood way the tendon end organs are important elements in a scheme for eye position proprioception...This is a difficult hypothesis because all established facts about tendon organ function indicate a role in phasic responses to stretch and never any suggestion of a role in supplying positional information." The models in Figure 5.3 and 5.4 indicate two different ways in which Golgi tendon organs might contribute to muscle linearization. Both of these models are based upon observations that Golgi tendon organs respond to increases in muscle tension. Tendon organs exhibit a high threshold when activated by passive stretch, but are exquisitely sensitive to active muscle contraction (Granit, 1962; Houck and Henneman, 1967; Kandel and Schwartz, 1981). Thus during active contraction of an agonist eye muscle, its Golgi tendon organs can emit an output signal that increases with the amount of muscle contraction. Since the antagonist muscle is passively stretched during an active agonist contraction, its Golgi tendon organ may respond much less, or not at all. If the antagonist tendon organ does respond, however, its signal would be expected to increase, rather than decrease, due to the progressive contraction of the agonist muscle. Data concerning the properties of Golgi tendon organs during saccadic eye movements seem not to be available, so our discussion of this matter will consider several mechanistic possibilities that are compatible with functional requirements.

One possibility is that, as an agonist muscle contracts, the increase of MN input to the agonist muscle coexists with a progressive decrease in MN input to the antagonist muscle. Such a decrease could cause a progressive reduction of tension in the antagonist muscle. The increase in $C(\alpha)$ and the decrease in $C(\beta)$ that was assumed in equation (5.3) could hereby be achieved. Van Gisbergen, Robinson, and Gielen (1981), by contrast, have shown that the MN input to the antagonist muscles of monkeys are totally shut off during saccades. Thus a different source of progressively decreasing antagonist inputs $C(\beta)$ is needed to establish the ratio scale in equation (5.3).

One possibility is that the Golgi tendon organs of the agonist muscle provide the input for both $C(\alpha)$ and $C(\beta)$ using a push-pull mechanism. Figure 5.5 depicts such a mechanism. Figure 5.5 is based upon the hypothesis that there exist agonist and antagonist tonic cell populations which receive push-pull inflow inputs from the contracting muscle. These tonic cells, in turn, input to the mechanism that computes the ratio scale. Thus, suppose that during an agonist contraction, the agonist inflow signal is $kC(\alpha)$ and the antagonist inflow signals is approximately 0. Let the baseline activity of both the agonist and the antagonist tonic cell populations equal M. Then their activities after inflow input are

$$\big(M + kC(\alpha), M - kC(\alpha)\big). \tag{5.15}$$

Since M is larger than the maximal inflow signal, both terms in (5.15) are nonnegative. Next, the activities (5.15) generate a spatial pattern

$$\left(\frac{1}{2}(1 + \frac{kC(\alpha)}{M}), \frac{1}{2}(1 - \frac{kC(\alpha)}{M})\right). \tag{5.16}$$

Each activity in (5.16) is computed by dividing the corresponding activity in (5.15) by the sum of both activities in (5.15). Equation (5.16) is now used instead of (5.3) to compute the error signals E^+ and E^- in (5.4) and (5.5). Thus

$$E^+ = \left[\frac{1}{2}(1 - \frac{kC(\alpha)}{M}) - \frac{\beta}{\alpha + \beta}\right]^+ \tag{5.17}$$

and

$$E^- = \left[\frac{1}{2}(1 + \frac{kC(\alpha)}{M}) - \frac{\alpha}{\alpha + \beta}\right]^+. \tag{5.18}$$

To test whether no error signal is emitted when the muscle response is linearized, we set E^+ and E^- equal to zero, as in Section 5.6. No error signal is emitted if

$$C(\alpha) = \frac{M}{k}\left(\frac{\alpha - \beta}{\alpha + \beta}\right). \tag{5.19}$$

If, moreover, agonist and antagonist outflow signals to the tonic cells are mutually inhibitory, as in (5.8), then

$$C(\alpha) = q\alpha - r \tag{5.20}$$

where $q = 2M(k\gamma)^{-1}$ and $r = M(k)^{-1}$. Thus this model also generates error signals until the amount of muscle contraction is a linear function of the outflow signals. All of our other conclusions about muscle linearization and about the Steinbach and Smith (1981) data also hold, with the

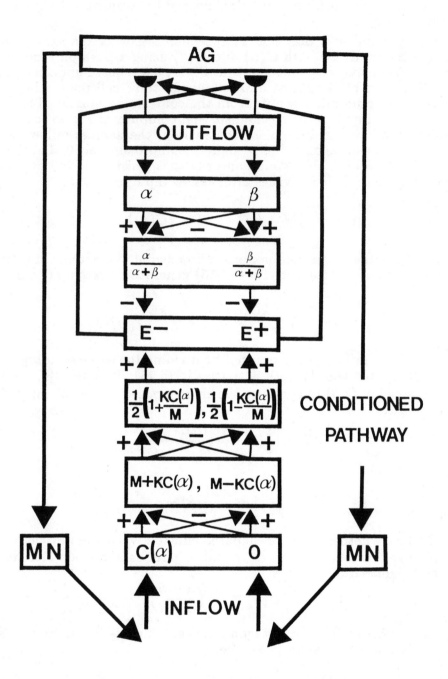

Figure 5.5. Microstructure of an outflow-inflow interface (OII) whose inflow signals are derived only from the muscles that are actively contracting: See text for details.

exception of one refinement. If all inflow signals are cut in Figure 5.5, then the tonic cells continue to register basal activities (M, M), and the normalized pattern $(\frac{1}{2}, \frac{1}{2})$ continues to input to (E^-, E^+). Thus error signals $E^+ = [\frac{1}{2} - \frac{\beta}{\alpha+\beta}]^+$ and $E^- = [\frac{1}{2} - \frac{\alpha}{\alpha+\beta}]^+$ can reach the AG stage. These error signals will not influence muscle linearization, however, if there are approximately as many eye movements in an agonist direction as there are in the corresponding antagonist direction, because both error signals are measured relative to the value $\frac{1}{2}$.

For completeness, we note that an alternative model, based upon length-dependent inflow signals (Figure 5.4), is also consistent with the Steinbach and Smith (1981) data. The length-dependent inflow signals would be derived from the muscle spindles (Granit, 1962; Kandel and Schwartz, 1981), rather than from the Golgi tendon organs. A single strabismus operation could alter the match between inflow length information and outflow commands. It remains to say how destruction of all inflow signals from the Golgi tendon organs could prevent adaptation. In a spindle-based model, these data seem to require the assumption that inflow from the Golgi tendon organs is also used. Such inflow would not, however, be used to compute the state of muscle contraction. It would act to nonspecifically gate the error signals to the cerebellum. Only during active muscle contractions would these error gates be activated, thereby enabling muscle linearization to occur.

5.9. Dynamic Linearization: Adaptive Sampling during Saccades

All of the above models of the OII share an important, and surprising, functional property. They all predict that the cerebellar learning which linearizes eye muscle responses takes place *during* saccades, and at a very fast sampling rate. In models which use Golgi tendon organ inflow, as in equation (5.15), this conclusion follows from the fact that, during posture, agonist and antagonist tensions must be equal in order to hold the eye in a fixed position. Hence, after a saccade is over, the outputs from both agonist and antagonist Golgi tendon organs should be equal too. Their ratio cannot, therefore, be used to compute deviations from muscle linearity. In a spindle-based model, as in Figure 5.4, the Golgi tendon organ output that gates cerebellar error signals would be expected to be much larger during a saccade, when the agonist muscle is actively contracting, than after. Hence error signals would be much more effective during a saccade in this model too.

The idea that adaptive sampling takes place during a saccade makes sense from an intuitive vantage point. The forces on the eye muscles during a saccade are very different from the forces that act between saccades. Hence conditioned gains that were learned during posture might be the wrong gains to ensure muscle linearity during movement. Furthermore, if one waits until a movement is over to learn these gains, then the accumulated nonlinearity due to an entire saccade would have to be compensated for at the terminal saccadic position. By contrast, if the learning circuit is fast enough to deliver sampling and error signals several times during a saccade, say within 15 or 20 msec., then conditioned gains could be learned for components of each saccadic movement in which not too much nonlinearity has accumulated. The saccade would hereby be broken down into movement "frames," each of whose nonlinear distortions could separately be dealt with as a function of eye position within that frame.

If the model is confirmed in which Golgi tendon organs supply inflow to the OII, it will provide a new functional role for these organs as sensors of dynamic muscle contraction, as well as for the rapid conduction velocity of their afferent fibers.

Two more mechanisms need to be specified to complete our discussion of OII design.

5.10. An Agonist-Antagonist Ratio Scale

This section suggests a simple mechanism whereby an input pattern (I_1, I_2) can be transformed into a spatial pattern

$$\left(\frac{I_1}{I_1 + I_2}, \frac{I_2}{I_1 + I_2}\right). \tag{5.21}$$

The transformations (5.1), (5.3), and (5.16) within the OII are all special cases of this problem. The desired transformation can be accomplished by a feedforward on-center off-surround network whose cells obey membrane equations (Section 2.6). In the special case of an agonist-antagonist interaction, an on-center off-surround anatomy is a push-pull anatomy.

Let $x_1(t)$ be the potential of the agonist population and $x_2(t)$ be the potential of the antagonist population. A simple version of the networks used in Section 2.6 is sufficient. Suppose that

$$\frac{d}{dt}x_1 = -Ax_1 + (B - x_1)I_1 - x_1I_2 \tag{5.22}$$

and

$$\frac{d}{dt}x_2 = -Ax_2 + (B - x_2)I_2 - x_2I_1. \tag{5.23}$$

Define the total input $I = I_1 + I_2$. Then (5.22) and (5.23) can be rewritten as

$$\frac{d}{dt}x_1 = -Ax_1 + BI_1 - x_1I \tag{5.24}$$

and

$$\frac{d}{dt}x_2 = -Ax_2 + BI_2 - x_2I. \tag{5.25}$$

If the potentials x_1 and x_2 equilibrate quickly to changes in the inputs I_1 and I_2, then $\frac{d}{dt}x_1 \cong 0$ and $\frac{d}{dt}x_2 \cong 0$ at all times. Thus

$$x_1 \cong \frac{BI_1}{A + I} \tag{5.26}$$

and

$$x_2 \cong \frac{BI_2}{A + I}.$$ (5.27)

If the total input I exceeds constant A by a sufficient amount, then

$$x_1 \cong \frac{BI_1}{I_1 + I_2}$$ (5.28)

and

$$x_2 \cong \frac{BI_2}{I_1 + I_2}.$$ (5.29)

The desired transformation can thus be defined by

$$(I_1, I_2) \rightarrow (x_1, x_2).$$ (5.30)

5.11. Sampling from a Spatial Map of Outflow Position

We assume that the tonic (T) cells in Figure 5.2 are the source of outflow signals to the MN cells as well as the source of sampling signals to the AG stage. The T cells cannot, however, project directly to the AG stage, for the same reason that the HMI cannot project directly to the AG stage. Sufficiently different spatial patterns of activity must give rise to different sampling pathways with their own LTM traces. Only in this way can different outflow patterns learn different conditioned gains to compensate for different degrees of muscle nonlinearity at different eye muscle positions.

The T cell and HMI examples hereby focus our attention upon a functional problem that is of general importance: How can activity patterns across a fixed set of cells be parsed by a spatial map, such that sufficiently different patterns activate different cell populations within the spatial map? The next chapter addresses this issue.

Within the MLN, sufficiently distinct tonic cell outflow patterns activate different cellular locations within such a spatial map. We therefore call the map an *eye position* map (EPM). Each spatial locus in the EPM sends a separate sampling pathway to the cerebellum. Each such pathway adaptively encodes all gain changes that are caused by OII-induced error signals while the sampling pathway is active. These gain changes, in turn, differentially alter the cerebellar feedback signals to the MN cells of the oculomotor nuclei. Chapter 3 explains how a single sampling pathway can simultaneously encode gain changes that differentially influence all the eye muscles and thereby control all the eye muscles in a synergetic, or coarticulated, fashion.

CHAPTER 6
SPATIAL MAPS OF MOTOR PATTERNS

6.1. The General Problem: Transforming Pattern Intensities into Map Positions

The problem of this chapter is to analyse how different activity patterns over a fixed set of cells can be transformed into different spatial foci of activity at the next processing stage. We call a network which encodes information by activating cells in different locations a *spatial map*. Our problem is thus to transform different activity patterns over a fixed set of cells into a spatial map. In the case of the HMI, the activity patterns represent difference vectors. Hence the spatial map is consistent with retinotopic coordinates (Section 4.8). We therefore call such as spatial map a retinotopic map, or RM. As we noted in Section 5.11, the spatial map that recodes tonic cell outflow patterns is called an eye position map, or EPM. Such an EPM is consistent with head coordinates, rather than retinotopic coordinates.

Although an RM and an EPM encode different types of information, they can arise from the same mechanisms. The formal problem to be solved is the same, no matter what interpretation is given to the activity patterns that must be spatially parsed.

Several types of mechanisms are consistent with these functional requirements. The available neural data do not unambiguously force the choice of one mechanism above all others. Evolutionary variations could, moreover, choose different solutions across species. We therefore analyse several possible spatial mapping models, much as we described several possible models of saccadic error correction in Section 3.18. Each of these models leads to testable differences that future experiments can attempt to measure, and the collection of all the models provides a deeper conceptual insight than any one model could provide.

To fix ideas, we will henceforth discuss the special cases of mapping HMI vectors into an RM, or of T cell outflow patterns into an EPM. The same considerations hold for transforming any set of muscle-coded activity patterns into a spatial map.

6.2. Antagonistic Positional Gradients, Contrast Enhancement, and Coincidence Detectors

The first model executes a transformation that requires no learning. It exploits the organization of muscles into agonist-antagonist pairs. A similar construction exists for sensory fields that possess natural left-to-right and/or bottom-to-top symmetry axes. A similar map seems, for example, to exist in the auditory system of the owl (Konishi, 1984).

The model's inputs are grouped into agonist and antagonist pairs. Both inputs need to be positive, except in the extremal cases where one input is maximally active and the other is shut off. In the MLN, both agonist and antagonist tonic cells can directly give rise to positive inputs. By contrast, only one output from each agonist-antagonist pair of the HMI can be positive. Hence such outputs need to activate tonically active cells in a push-pull fashion, as in equation (5.15), before these tonic cells can generate inputs to the model.

Denote the input pair by (I_1, I_2). The model first maps each input pattern into a one-dimensional spatial map in such a way that different map positions correspond to different input ratios I_1/I_2. To see how this happens, denote the population with input activity I_i by v_i, $i = 1, 2$. Let each population v_i send pathways to a field F_1 of cells. Since there are many cells in F_1, we approximate the field of cells by a continuous one-dimensional medium. Let S be the spatial variable of this medium, and let P_{iS} denote the strength of the pathway from v_i to position S in F_1. Suppose for definiteness that

$$P_{1S} = -Pe^{-\mu(\nu-S)^2} \qquad (6.1)$$

and

$$P_{2S} = Pe^{-\mu(\omega-S)^2}. \qquad (6.2)$$

In other words, each cell population v_i sends a broad spatial gradient of connections to F_1 (Figure 6.1). Each spatial gradient connects to F_1 according to a simple random growth law. By equation (6.1), the best connection of v_1 is to position $S = \nu$. Population v_1 contacts other positions S within F_1 with a strength that decreases as a Gaussian function of their distance $|\nu - S|$ from position v. By equation (6.2), the best connection of v_2 is to position $S = \omega$. Population v_2 contacts other positions S within F_1 with a strength that decreases as a Gaussian function of their distance $|\omega - S|$ from position ω. Suppose that $\nu < \omega$. The connections from v_1 to F_1 are assumed to be inhibitory. The connections from v_2 to F_2 are assumed to be excitatory. The total input at position S due to the activity pattern (I_1, I_2) is

$$J(S; I_1, I_2) = -I_1 P_{1S} + I_2 P_{2S}. \qquad (6.3)$$

We denote by $S(I_1/I_2)$ the position S which receives the *maximal* input in response to input pattern (I_1, I_2). As the input pattern (I_1, I_2) changes, the position $S(I_1/I_2)$ changes too, and depends only on the ratio I_1/I_2. Thus the antagonistic interaction of a pair of Gaussian positional gradients can convert spatial patterns into spatial maps. Before proving this fact, we summarize the subsequent two stages of the model.

The input pattern to the field F_1 is contrast-enhanced and normalized by on-center off-surround interactions within F_1 (Section 2.6). Thus each activity pattern (I_1, I_2) activates a sharply tuned population of cells within F_1 at and near position $S(I_1/I_2)$. This contrast-enhancement operation converts F_1 into a one-dimensional spatial map of the agonist-antagonist

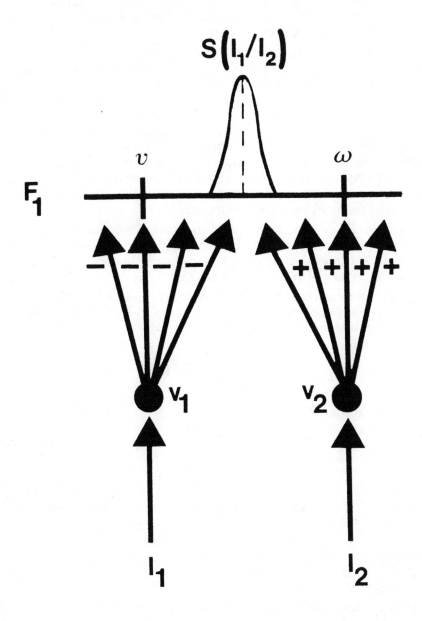

Figure 6.1. Mapping an agonist-antagonist pair (v_1, v_2) of cell populations into a spatial map F_1: In response to the input pattern (I_1, I_2), the maximally activated position is $S(I_1/I_2)$, which depends only upon the ratio of I_1 to I_2. Population v_1 gives rise to a broadly distributed inhibitory spatial gradient. Population v_2 gives rise to a broadly distributed excitatory gradient.

input patterns (I_1, I_2). [A similar organization helps to explain the peak shift and behavioral contrast that can occur during discrimination learning experiments (Grossberg, 1981).]

We now consider how to generate a spatial map of more than one agonist-antagonist activity pattern. In cases where just two agonist-antagonist patterns are needed, this can be done by letting each location in F_1 activate parallel strips of cells at the next stage F_2 (Figure 6.2). Assume that the other agonist-antagonist pair also activates parallel strips of cells in F_2, but that the strips of the different agonist-antagonist pairs are not parallel. The ideal case is one in which the two types of strips are mutually perpendicular. Finally, suppose that the cells within F_2 are coincidence detectors that respond only if they are simultaneously activated by a pair of strips. Such coincidence detectors are easily designed due to the fact that the inputs from F_1 to F_2 are normalized.

Such a field F_2 computes a two-dimensional spatial map of the two pairs of agonist-antagonist input patterns. This procedure can be iterated to generate an n-dimensional spatial map, but it becomes physiologically implausible for values of n much larger than 3.

It remains to determine the position $S(I_1/I_2)$ at which the input pattern $J(S; I_1, I_2)$ of equation (6.3) is maximal. To locate this position, we determine the solutions of the equation

$$\frac{\partial}{\partial S} J(S; I_1, I_2) = 0. \tag{6.4}$$

Equation (6.4) implies that

$$\frac{(S - \omega)}{(S - \nu)} e^{[(S-\nu)^2 - (S-\omega)^2]} = \frac{I_1}{I_2}. \tag{6.5}$$

Both I_1/I_2 and the exponential term are nonnegative. Hence (6.5) has a solution only if the ratio $(S - \omega)(S - \nu)^{-1}$ is also nonnegative. This is true only if $S \le \nu$ or $S \ge \omega$. Since $\nu < \omega$ and the connections from v_1 to the cells around position $S = \nu$ are inhibitory, it is clear that some nonnegative inputs $J(S; I_1, I_2)$ are found in the region $S \ge \omega$, which we consider henceforth.

Introducing the new variable $y = S - \nu$, we rewrite (6.5) in the form

$$\frac{(y - \lambda)}{y} e^{\mu[y^2 - (\lambda - y)^2]} = \frac{I_1}{I_2}, \tag{6.6}$$

where $\lambda = \omega - \nu$. Equation (6.6), in turn, implies that

$$f(y) = \frac{e^{\mu \lambda^2} I_1}{I_2} \tag{6.7}$$

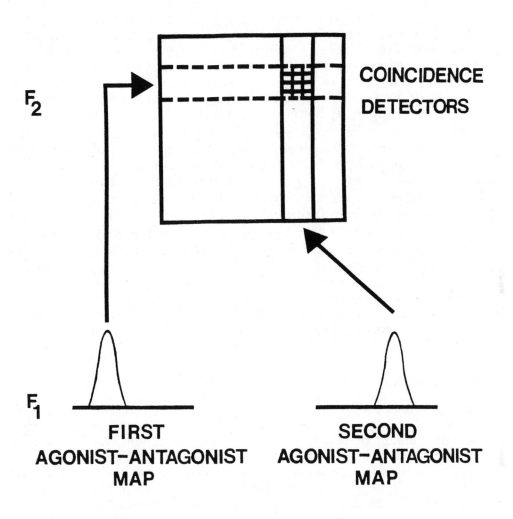

Figure 6.2. Coincidence detectors at level F_2 selectively respond to pairs of spatial positions at F_1 which are activated by different agonist-antagonist cell populations.

where

$$f(y) = \frac{(y - \lambda)}{y} e^{2\mu\lambda y}. \tag{6.8}$$

Since $y - \nu = S \geq \omega$, it follows that $y \geq \lambda$. As y increases from λ to ∞, $f(y)$ increases from 0 to ∞. Thus given *any* nonnegative choice of the ratio I_1/I_2, there exists a value $y(I_1/I_2)$ of y between λ and ∞ that satisfies (6.7). Moreover, as the ratio I_1/I_2 increases, the value of $y(I_1/I_2)$ also increases. In terms of the positional variable $S = y + \nu$, this means that the position $S(I_1/I_2)$ at which $J(S; I_1, I_2)$ is maximal increases from ω to ∞ as the ratio I_1/I_2 increases from 0 to ∞.

Of course, it makes no sense to talk about an infinite field of cells. Thus it is necessary to consider how the maximal range of input ratios I_1/I_2 can be coded by a finite interval of cells. Inspection of (6.7) and (6.8) shows that a choice of parameters such that λ is small and $\mu\lambda$ is sufficiently large facilitates this goal. Then the function $(y - \lambda)y^{-1}$ in (6.8) rapidly jumps from 0 towards its maximum value 1 as y increases above λ. Function $e^{2\mu\lambda y}$ in (6.8) grows quickly as a function of y, thereby being able to match a larger range of ratios I_1/I_2 in (6.7). Finally the coefficient $\mu\lambda^2$ in (6.7) can be relatively small even though $\mu\lambda$ is relatively large, because λ is small. Thus the main constraint is that the amount of shift $\lambda = \omega - \nu$ of the antagonistic positional gradients should be small relative to other parameters of the problem. Increasing the spatial decay rate μ of these spatial gradients enables a wider range of input ratios I_1/I_2 to be encoded within a fixed interval.

6.3. Position-Threshold-Slope Shift Maps

The previous model illustrated the importance of using antagonistic quantities to convert activities into positions. The next model describes a different version of this general idea. In this model, the antagonism is not derived from the interaction of an agonist-antagonist pair. The antagonism arises from a *single* motor activity. Using such a model, the HMI does not have to preprocess its outputs by putting them through a tonic push-pull process. To fix ideas, we consider how such a model would convert the vector differences $V = ([x_1]^+, [x_2]^+, \ldots, [x_6]^+)$ of the HMI into activated positions within the RM.

Using this model, each suprathreshold activity $[x_j]^+$ at the HMI generates a signal $[x_j]^+ P_j(r, \theta)$ to a position (r, θ) at the first stage F_1 of processing, which is depicted for convenience as a surface in polar coordinates (r, θ). The path strengths $P_j(r, \theta)$ define positional gradients from each HMI population v_j to F_1. The total input from the HMI to position (r, θ) of F_1 is the sum

$$S(r, \theta) = \sum_{j=1}^{6} [x_j]^+ P_j(r, \theta) \tag{6.9}$$

of these signals (Figure 6.3). Then an output signal

$$T(r,\theta) = \Big[S(r,\theta) - \Gamma(r,\theta)\Big]^+ \tag{6.10}$$

is emitted to the second stage F_2 of processing, which is the RM. Recall that the notation $[\xi]^+$ stands for $\max(\xi, 0)$.

By (6.9), the input $S(r,\theta)$ to F_1 is the sum of output signals $[x_j]^+$ weighted by the path strengths $P_i(r,\theta)$. In other words, the HMI vector $V = ([x_1]^+, [x_2]^+, \ldots, [x_6]^+)$ is *filtered* by the path strength vector $P(r,\theta) = (P_1(r,\theta), P_2(r,\theta), \ldots, P_6(r,\theta))$ at position (r,θ). For simplicity, we have assumed that F_1 equilibrates rapidly to this input, and that the equilibrium activity at each position (r,θ) equals its input $S(r,\theta)$. Then $S(r,\theta)$ gives rise to the output signal $T(r,\theta)$ in (6.10). The map $S(r,\theta) \to T(r,\theta)$ from F_1 to the RM is topographic, whereas the map $V \to S(r,\theta)$ from the HMI to F_1 is built up from the convergent filtering action of six positional gradients.

Equation (6.10) says that a signal is emitted to the RM only if $S(r,\theta) > \Gamma(r,\theta)$. Thus $\Gamma(r,\theta)$ is the *signal threshold* of the (r,θ) pathway. The signal $T(r,\theta)$ grows linearly as a function of suprathreshold values of $S(r,\theta)$, as in the classical Hartline-Ratliff equation (Ratliff, 1965) and other models of neural pattern discrimination (Grossberg, 1970, 1976a).

Both the positional gradients $P_j(r,\theta)$ and the signal thresholds $\Gamma(r,\theta)$ depend upon the position (r,θ) within F_1. A larger choice of $P_j(r,\theta)$ says that an input $[x_j]^+ P_j(r,\theta)$ to (r,θ) grows with a steeper slope as a function of $[x_j]^+$. A larger choice of $\Gamma(r,\theta)$ says that a larger total input $S(r,\theta)$ to (r,θ) is needed to fire a signal to the RM. Both $P_j(r,\theta)$ and $\Gamma(r,\theta)$ are assumed to increase with r. Thus cells at F_1 with larger radial positions r are more sensitive to their inputs and have higher output thresholds than cells with smaller radial positions r. This covariation of cell position, signal threshold, and signal slope causes a shift to occur in the spatial locus of maximal total activity at the RM as an HMI signal $[x_j]^+$ increases. Low intensity inputs cause maximal activity to occur at the low threshold end of the RM, whereas high intensity inputs cause maximal activity to occur at the high threshold end of the RM. Due to the role of correlations in cell position, threshold, and slope in generating this shift in activity locus, we call this mechanism a *Position-Threshold-Slope* (PTS) *Shift*. Populations of cells in which threshold and slope covary across cells have been found, for example, in the abducens and oculomotor nuclei (Luschei and Fuchs, 1972; Robinson, 1970; Schiller, 1970).

The input pattern to the RM that is caused by a PTS shift is contrast-enhanced and normalized before it is stored in STM as an RM activity peak. This is accomplished by endowing the RM with a suitably designed recurrent on-center off-surround shunting network (Section 2.6). A simple

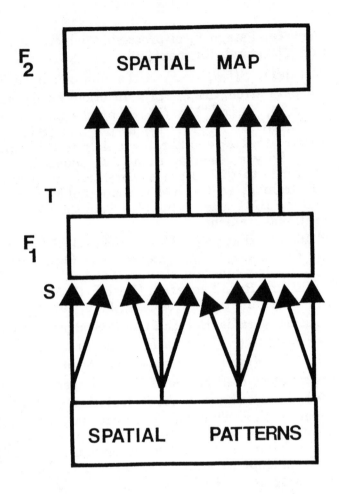

Figure 6.3. A position-threshold-slope (PTS) shift: Spatial patterns of activity within an HMI, or other source of spatial patterns, give rise to broadly distributed outputs that converge upon the network level F_1. Level F_1 maps topographically to level F_2. Due to the parameters of the broad spatial interactions and the topographic mapping, different spatial patterns activate different positions at F_2. The inputs S and outputs T are defined by equations (6.9) and (6.10).

rule that approximates the dynamics of such a network is

$$x(r, \theta) = \left[\frac{T(r, \theta)}{\max_{(R, \phi)} T(R, \phi)} \right]^n, \tag{6.11}$$

where $n > 1$. By (6.11), all nonmaximal $T(r, \theta)$ generate a small $x(r, \theta)$ if n is chosen sufficiently large, whereas the maximal $T(r, \theta)$ generates an $x(r, \theta) = 1$ no matter how large n is chosen.

A 3-dimensional (one dimension for every agonist-antagonist pair) PTS shift can be designed so that every realizable HMI pattern V generates a different activity peak within the RM. Moreover, continuous variations in one or more activities within V cause continuous changes in the RM position. This PTS shift mechanism works well formally and uses known types of parametric correlations within neuronal populations. The most demanding constraint concerns the spatial juxtaposition of the six populations that respond to the six signals $[x_j]^+$ in V, $j = 1, 2, \ldots, 6$. Each population corresponds to a different muscle of one eye. In order for the PTS shift mechanism to work well, all six populations must be topographically placed in such a way that any three contiguous eye muscles are represented by three contiguous populations. The simplest way to accomplish this is to arrange the populations as a sector map (Figure 2.2).

Figures 6.4 and 6.5 summarize a computer simulation of how the RM changes position as a function of V. We now describe the parameters used in this simulation. This description is rather technical, and can be skipped if the reader wishes to go to the next issue.

In any realizable monocular pattern V within the HMI, at most three consecutive components can be positive at any time. This is true because, if three contiguous muscles contract to saccade the eye, then their three antagonist muscles must relax. By "consecutive" components, we mean "consecutive modulo 6," so that positive components (x_5, x_6, x_1) and (x_6, x_1, x_2) are considered consecutive. If we consider the set of all realizable patterns V, then we can group them in terms of patterns which correspond to saccades in the same direction. When we do so, a convenient representation of the positive pattern components becomes apparent.

For example, consider the direction and length of the saccade encoded by a prescribed pattern V. Suppose that pattern V^* encodes a saccade in the same direction, but of greater length. Then the same muscles that contract in response to V also contract in response to V^*, but each contracting muscle must contract more in response to V^*. In other words, each of the positive components in V^* is larger than its corresponding component in V. This argument constrains the possible combinations of positive entries that can realize patterns V.

We can represent patterns V whose saccades have increasing length but the same direction as triples of points on a succession of nonintersecting, expanding, closed curves. The distance of a point from the origin represents the size of a positive x_i in V. The direction of the point with

POSITION—THRESHOLD—SLOPE MAP

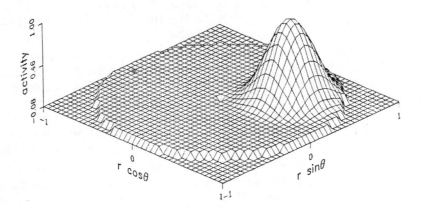

MUSCLE REPRESENTATION

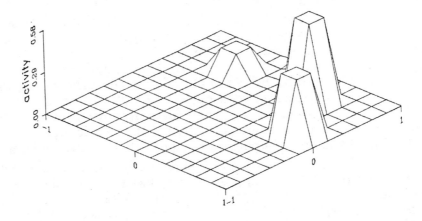

Figure 6.4. Computer simulations of a transformation from an HMI into a retinotopic map (RM) using a PTS shift. See text for details.

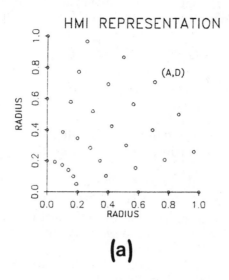

(a)

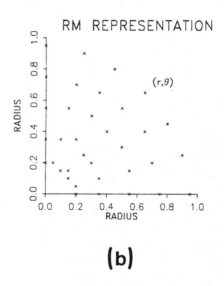

(b)

Figure 6.5. Computer simulation of a transformation from an HMI in (a) to an RM in (b). The parameters (A, D) and (r, θ) which define the coordinates of the transformation are defined in equations (6.12)–(6.14). Due to the radial symmetry of the map, a similar transformation holds in all four quadrants. The similarity of the polar grid in (r, θ) coordinates to that in (A, D) coordinates says that the map is approximately linear.

respect to the horizontal axis represents the direction in which its corresponding muscle contracts. This observation can be expressed more formally as follows. We represent each HMI output in the form

$$[x_i]^+ = Af(|\,D - D_i\,|), \tag{6.12}$$

$i = 1, 2, \ldots, 6$. In (6.12), the parameters D_i and the function $f(w)$ are fixed. They embody the constraints on saccadic length and direction that we have just summarized. The variables A and D change as a function of V. Variable A encodes amplitude information and variable D encodes directional information. Thus the representation (6.12) expresses the six-dimensional vector V as a two-dimensional vector (A, D) in polar coordinates. This is possible due to the manner in which the parameters D_i and the function $f(w)$ absorb the extra degrees of freedom.

Parameter D_i represents the ith direction of contraction, $i = 1, 2, \ldots,$ 6. Each pattern V defines a value A that increases with the length of the saccade. Function $f(w)$ modulates the amplitude of A in a manner that depends upon which direction is under consideration. In particular, function $f(w)$ has the following properties:

i) $f(w) > 0$ if $-\pi/2 < w < \pi/2$;

ii) $f(w) = 0$ if $-\pi \leq w \leq -\pi/2$ or if $\pi/2 \leq w \leq \pi$;

iii) $f(w)$ increases if $-\pi/2 < w < 0$;

iv) $f(w)$ decreases if $0 < w < \pi/2$;

v) $f(w)$ is 2π-periodic.

Using function $f(w)$, each pattern V defines a value D that represents the direction of the saccade. For example, if $D = D_3$, then the saccade moves in a direction close to that represented by the third muscle. This follows from properties (iii) and (iv), since then $x_3 = Af(0)$, whereas $x_2 = Af(|\,D_3 - D_2\,|) < Af(0)$ and $x_4 = Af(|\,D_3 - D_4\,|) < Af(0)$. Moreover at most three contiguous x_i's are positive. This is because it is assumed that $|\,D_3 - D_5\,| > \pi/2, |\,D_3 - D_6\,| > \pi/2, |\,D_3 - D_1\,| > \pi/2$, and so on. Thus by property (ii), if $D = D_3$ then $x_1 = x_5 = x_6 = 0$. A similar analysis holds for any choice of D such that $-\pi \leq D \leq \pi$.

The PTS shift hypothesis implies that both the path strength $P_i(r, \theta)$ and the threshold $\Gamma(r, \theta)$ are increasing functions of r. The gradient nature of the HMI→RM map suggests, in addition, that $P_i(r, \theta)$ decreases as θ deviates from the direction represented by D_i. In our simulations, the thresholds $\Gamma(r, \theta)$ were chosen independent of θ for simplicity, but an increase of $\Gamma(r, \theta)$ as θ deviates from D_i is also physically plausible.

We numerically analysed several choices of the functions $f(w)$, $P_i(r, \theta)$, and $\Gamma(r, \theta)$ and the parameters D_i in order to understand the PTS shift map. Our results indicated that a certain amount of regularity in these functions as i, r, and θ vary generates a more uniformly distributed mapping function; that is, a mapping function whose chosen position within the RM does not change very slowly as a function of certain changes in V and very quickly as a function of other changes in V. Map uniformity is not, however, an end in itself, since all that is needed is an (approximately) one-to-one map.

The essentially linear map described in Figures 6.4 and 6.5 was generated using the following functions. First the $[x_i]^+$ in (6.12) were expressed in terms of the functions $D_i = \frac{(i-1)\pi}{3}$, $i = 1, 2, \ldots, 6$, and $f(w) = [\cos w]^+$. Then the PTS shift was defined using the positional gradients

$$P_i(r, \theta) = r\Big[\cos(\theta - D_i)\Big]^+,$$
(6.13)

in (6.9), and the signal thresholds

$$\Gamma(r, \theta) = \gamma r^2$$
(6.14)

in (6.10), where $\gamma = .8$.

6.4. Self-Organizing Spatial Maps

The design of a 3-dimensional PTS shift map requires careful preprocessing of the HMI output vector, say via a sector map. An alternative solution to the spatial mapping problem does not need to impose this topographic constraint. In this solution, each input $[x_j]^+$ is again used to generate a PTS shift, but only within its own population. Distinct populations do not have to be embedded within a sector map. The output signals from these independent PTS shifts are the inputs to an adaptive coding model. This model for developmental map formation has also been used to explain several other types of data (Grossberg, 1976a, 1976b, 1982a). Thus, in this solution, a carefully, but plausibly, prewired network topography is replaced by a less carefully prewired network that can develop its own topography. Consequently, this self-organizing model can handle input vectors of any dimension.

The adaptive filter executes the same types of computations that were used to calibrate the TPM→HMI transform. Once again, the component signals $[x_j]^+$ in a vector input pattern such as V are the starting point of the computation. The signals $[x_j]^+$ cannot themselves be used as the inputs to the adaptive filter from the HMI to the RM because V encodes information about saccade direction *and* length. Why this is so is explained in later paragraphs. Instead, the intensities $[x_j]^+$ are first converted into spatial maps using one-dimensional PTS shifts. Then the total activity of all the active PTS shifts is normalized, or conserved, by long-range shunting lateral inhibition. Finally, the normalized positional activities S_j corresponding to each $[x_j]^+$ are used as the inputs to the adaptive filter. The adaptive filter interacts with the RM to establish a spatial map of patterns V within the HMI (Figure 6.6). We now describe this self-organizing spatial map in greater detail.

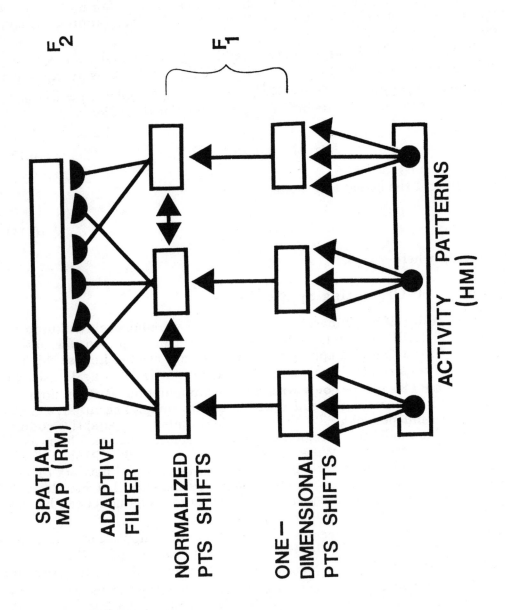

Figure 6.6. A self-organizing spatial map: Activity patterns within an HMI, or other source of spatial patterns, map into 1-dimensional PTS shifts, whose activities are normalized within F_1. Then F_1 generates output signals to F_2 via an adaptive filter. See text for details.

In a one-dimensional PTS shift, each intensity $[x_j]^+$ gives rise to an input that is uniformly distributed (in a statistical sense) across a population of cells. The signal thresholds and suprathreshold sensitivities (slopes) of the cells within each population are nonuniformly distributed within the population. Cells with lower thresholds tend to be found at one end of the population, cells with higher thresholds are found at the other end of the population, and cells with intermediate thresholds are found in between the two ends. Cells with higher thresholds are more sensitive to suprathreshold inputs. In other words, if the threshold of the cell's signal function is higher, then the slope of the signal function is steeper in the suprathreshold range. Thus the equation

$$T_j(r) = \left[[x_j]^+ - \Gamma_j(r)\right]^+ P_j(r) \qquad (6.15)$$

defines the output from the jth muscle coordinate of the HMI to the radial position r of the jth PTS shift population. Since $\Gamma_j(r) \geq 0$, (6.15) can be simplified to read

$$T_j(r) = \left[x_j - \Gamma_j(r)\right]^+ P_j(r), \qquad (6.16)$$

which shows that the jth output can be computed directly from the HMI potential x_j. In (6.16), both the threshold $\Gamma_j(r)$ and the path strength $P_j(r)$ are assumed to increase with r. The largest signal $T_j(r)$, across all values of r, defines the PTS position activated by x_j.

Denote by F_1 the stage that receives the output signals (6.16) from *all* the HMI potentials x_j. Thus F_1 contains all the separate PTS shifts. We assume that F_1 normalizes its response to this total input and stored it in STM. Denote the normalized STM activities of F_1 by S_i. Keep in mind that $i \neq j$ because a whole population of cells corresponds to each HMI potential x_j. These normalized activities S_i are the inputs to the adaptive coding model.

Each output signal S_i from F_1 generates an input signal $S_i C_{ik} z_{ik}$ to each population v_k of the spatial map. Parameter C_{ik} is the strength of the path that carries S_i to v_k, and z_{ik} is the LTM trace of this path. For simplicity, suppose that all $C_{ik} = 1$. This choice implies that the spatial gradients from the HMI to the RM are nonspecifically distributed to all RM populations. Then the signal due to S_i at v_k is $S_i z_{ik}$. All of these signals are added to generate the total input

$$T_k = \sum S_i z_{ik} \qquad (6.17)$$

that is received by v_k.

Suppose that the RM responds to these inputs by satisfying the following properties:

1. It enhances the potentials x_k in the RM that correspond to the largest inputs T_k and suppresses the activities of all other potentials.

2. It conserves, or normalizes, the total activity of the enhanced potentials.

3. It stores the normalized and enhanced activities x_k in STM until the RM is attentionally reset by auxiliary signals.

Letting x_k be the activity of v_k, these rules can be approximated by the computation

$$x_k = \begin{cases} 1 & \text{if } T_k > \max\{\epsilon, T_m : m \neq k\} \\ 0 & \text{otherwise,} \end{cases} \qquad (6.18)$$

which is a variant of (6.11).

6.5. Activity-Dependent Map Formation

Then the enhanced activities x_k, and only these activities, change the weights of the LTM traces z_{ik}. This adaptive coding postulate assumes that code learning is dependent upon post-synaptic activation. Singer (1983) has reported compatible data in the visual cortex. Due to (6.18), this postulate implies that learning occurs at the LTM trace z_{ik} only if $x_k = 1$; that is, only if v_k is activated. The role of the learning rule is to guarantee that the pattern $z_k \equiv (z_{1k}, z_{2k}, z_{3k}, \ldots)$ of LTM traces abutting v_k becomes parallel, or proportional, to a time average of all the signal patterns $S \equiv (S_1, S_2, S_3, \ldots)$ that are active at F_1 when v_k is active in the RM. If v_k is active only when a single signal pattern S is active, then z_k becomes proportional to only this signal pattern. The simplest possibility is thus that z_{ik} approaches S_i as learning proceeds. If a larger set of signal patterns is active when v_k is active, then the tuning curve of v_k will become coarser, other things being equal.

The simplest learning law that embodies these properties is

$$\frac{d}{dt}z_{ik} = (-Bz_{ik} + S_i)[x_k]^+. \qquad (6.19)$$

Equation (6.19) is conceptually the same learning law as equation (4.2) within the HMI. Term S_i in (6.19) plays the role of S_i in (4.2), and term $[x_k]^+$ in (6.19) plays the role of both P and $[x_j]^+$ in (4.2).

When a series of vector patterns V sends signals from the HMI to the RM through time, the interaction of fast contrast enhancement and normalization in the RM with slow LTM adaptation parses the patterns V in such a way that different patterns across the HMI activate topographically distinct regions of the RM. Many refinements of this mechanism can be implemented. For example, the prewired gradients C_{ik} in (6.18) can be chosen so that strong agonist activations in the HMI tend to activate a given region of the RM, whereas strong antagonist activations in the HMI tend to activate a complementary region of the RM. For present purposes, the most important property of this model is that it is temporally stable. That is, because a small number of populations in F_1 is mapped into a large number of populations in the RM, once a topographic parsing by the RM of patterns across the HMI is established, this spatial map will endure through time unless the system suffers some type of internal damage.

We will now indicate in greater detail how the rules (6.17)–(6.19) work together to control spatial map formation within an RM or EPM, and along the way explain why the output from the HMI or tonic cells must be fed into PTS shifts before the normalized PTS shift response generates inputs to the adaptive coding model.

Since, by (6.18), $x_k = 0$ or 1, (6.19) can be rewritten as

$$\frac{d}{dt}z_{ik} = (-Bz_{ik} + S_i)x_k. \tag{6.20}$$

For notational simplicity, also let $B = 1$. By (6.20), $x_k = 0$ implies that $\frac{d}{dt}z_{ik} = 0$. Consequently, no learning occurs in z_{ik} unless v_k is activated. If $x_k = 1$, then (6.20) implies

$$\frac{d}{dt}z_{ik} = -z_{ik} + S_i. \tag{6.21}$$

By (6.21), z_{ik} approaches S_i whenever v_k is active. In other words, the LTM pattern z_k approaches the signal pattern S as learning proceeds. This property holds for any S that is active when v_k is active. Thus, integrating equation (6.21) shows that $z_k(t)$ is a time average of all the signal patterns S that were active when v_k was active before time t.

The definition in (6.17) of the total input T_k to v_k shows why training each z_k to become parallel to a different signal pattern $S^{(k)} = (S_1^{(k)}, S_2^{(k)}, S_3^{(k)}, \ldots)$ enables each $S^{(k)}$ to selectively activate its v_k. Under these circumstances, in response to any signal pattern S, $T_k = \sum_i S_i S_i^{(k)}$ and $T_m = \sum_i S_i S_i^{(m)}$ for all $m \neq k$. If we choose $S = S^{(k)}$, then $T_k = \sum_i [S_i^{(k)}]^2$ whereas $T_m = \sum_i S_i^{(k)} S_i^{(m)}$ for all $m \neq k$. Other things being equal, $T_k > T_m$, $m \neq k$, because $S^{(k)}$ is parallel to itself in T_k but $S^{(k)}$ is not parallel to any of the other signal patterns $S^{(m)}$ in T_m, $m \neq k$. Whenever $T_k > T_m$, $m \neq k$, it follows by (6.18) that $x_k = 1$ and all $x_m = 0$, $m \neq k$. In other words, $S^{(k)}$ is coded by v_k.

In order to guarantee that $T_k > T_m$ whenever $z_k = S^{(k)}$ and $z_k \neq S^{(m)}$, $m \neq k$, one problem still needs to be overcome. The total signal $\sum_i S_i$ needs to be constant (conserved, normalized) across all signal patterns S. Otherwise, the encoding mechanism can fail as follows. Let $z_k = S^{(k)}$ and $z_m = S^{(m)}$, $m \neq k$, but suppose that each signal $S_i^{(m)}$ in $S^{(m)}$ is larger than the corresponding signal $S_i^{(k)}$ in $S^{(k)}$. Then $\sum_i S_i^{(m)} > \sum_i S_i^{(k)}$, so the total signal is not normalized. In this situation, T_m can be larger than

T_k even if $S = S^{(k)}$ because, although z_k is parallel to S, each LTM trace in z_m is larger than the corresponding LTM trace in z_k. The total activity across F_1 was normalized to deal with this problem.

6.6. Coding of Movement Length and Direction

In many coding problems, normalizing the input pattern itself causes no difficulty. If, however, we directly normalized the signals $[x_j]^+$ from the HMI and fed these normalized signals into the adaptive filter, then a serious problem would have been caused. The patterns V at the HMI represent saccade direction *and* length. Normalizing these patterns would collapse all saccadic commands with the same direction into a single normalized command S. Length differences of these saccades could not be distinguished by this mechanism.

This problem is solved by letting each $[x_j]^+$ input to a 1-dimensional PTS shift. This transformation maps HMI intensities into PTS positions in an approximately one-to-one fashion. Normalizing the positive *intensities* of the activated PTS *positions* does not alter the one-to-one property of the map. No loss of saccadic length or direction information occurs if normalization acts on output signals from PTS shifts. Then the normalized PTS shift pattern S can be fed as input signals to the adaptive coding model to generate a spatial parsing of HMI patterns across the RM.

6.7. Normalization of Total PTS Shift Map

It remains to say how the total output from all the PTS shifts can be normalized. The physiologically simplest schemes feed the PTS intensities as inputs into an on-center off-surround network whose cells obey membrane equations (shunting interactions) and whose off-surrounds are broadly distributed across the network. A network with particularly nice properties undergoes both feedforward and feedback on-center off-surround interactions. The inputs and the feedback signals activate the same populations of interneurons, which distribute both types of signals to the rest of the network. The feedback signals are chosen to be linear functions of population activity. The choice of linear feedback signals may cause confusion unless further commentary is provided.

Section 2.6 noted that linear feedback signals can create an amplification instability in networks whose function is to *phasically* store activity patterns in STM. In networks that react to *tonically* active input sources, such as the HMI or tonic cells, the amplification instability becomes the functionally useful property of temporally maintaining a stable baseline of activity or tone. A simple network that instantiates this concept is

$$\frac{d}{dt}S_i = -CS_i + (D - S_i)(I_i + S_i) - S_i \sum_{r \neq i}(I_r + S_r), \tag{6.22}$$

(Grossberg, 1973, 1978b), where the I_i are the inputs to F_1 due to the PTS shifts and the S_i are the normalized activations caused by these inputs within F_1. For simplicity, suppose that the total input $\sum_i I_i$ to (6.22) is small compared to the total number of sites D in each population, and let $D > C$. Then, in response to *any* PTS shift pattern $(I_1, I_2, I_3, \ldots)$, the total activity $\sum_{i=1} S_i$ of (6.22) approximates the constant value $D - C$ and S_i becomes proportional to I_i. When a new PTS shift pattern is input to the network, the total activity remains normalized as the normalized activities of S_i adjust themselves to become proportional to the new inputs I_i.

These several spatial mapping models—which have used antagonistic positional gradients, contrast enhancement, normalization, coincidence detectors, PTS shifts, and adaptive coding mechanisms—define a domain of testable possibilities which future experiments need to address. Of particular interest is the question of whether an RM and an EPM are both designed using the same mechanisms, or whether the different preprocessing requirements of HMI outputs and T cell outputs have induced evolutionary specializations of their spatial mapping mechanisms.

CHAPTER 7
SACCADE GENERATOR AND SACCADE RESET

7.1. Saccade Generator

In Section 2.5, we described learning requirements that suggest the need for a saccade generator (SG). An SG must be capable of shutting off its own output signal, thereby terminating a saccadic movement, while its input signal remains on. In this chapter, we will describe some implications of the existence of an SG. Robinson and his colleagues (Keller, 1981; Raybourn and Keller, 1977; Robinson, 1981) have contributed substantially to this problem. We will discuss how general properties of the SG impose new design constraints on networks that input to the SG. A detailed SG design must be also developed, however, in order to clearly state the properties of these input sources and how they may interact with SG cells.

7.2. Converting an Intensity Code into a Duration Code

In order for the SG output to shut off before its input shuts off, some measure of output size must accumulate and act as an inhibitory signal that counteracts the input. The net SG output must, moreover, change as a systematic function of SG input, not only to generate saccades in response to unconditioned inputs, but also to alter a saccade as the conditioned input corresponding to a fixed unconditioned input changes due to learning. In our discussions of both unconditioned inputs (Chapter 2) and conditioned inputs (Chapter 3), larger SG inputs are required to generate larger saccadic movements.

At first glance, it would appear that two qualitatively different types of circuits could, in principle, accomplish this goal (Grossberg, 1970, Section 3). In one circuit, a feedforward inhibitory interneuron v_1 accumulates the activity that counteracts the input at v_2 (Figure 7.1a). In the other circuit, a feedback inhibitory interneuron v_2 accumulates the activity that counteracts the input at v_1 (Figure 7.1b). These two designs lead to significantly different predictions about the input circuits that activate the SG. A feedforward inhibitory interneuron cannot, however, effectively carry out the required task. This is because the range of output sizes that a feedforward inhibitory interneuron can accomodate is insufficient for SG purposes. Either smaller inputs could not be shut off at all, which is unacceptable, or the total range of output sizes would be much too restricted. To mathematically prove these assertions herein would take us too far from our charted course. They are implied by Theorem 1 in Grossberg (1970, p.297). We therefore consider the simplest version of a feedback inhibitory interneuron (Figure 7.1b).

In such a circuit, some measure of output size accumulates and feeds back as an inhibitory signal that counteracts the input. Since the functional role of the SG output is to move the eye to its target position, the simplest accumulating measure of output size is the outflow signal itself.

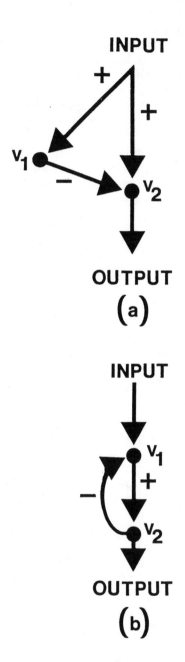

Figure 7.1. (a) A feedforward inhibitory interneuron v_1 inhibits the excitatory effect of the input at v_2; (b) When v_2 is excited by v_1, it feeds inhibitory signals back to v_1, thereby tending to inhibit the excitatory effect of the input upon v_1.

This argument suggests an agonist interaction like that depicted in Figure 7.2. In Figure 7.2, an input to burst (B) cells generates signals to the tonic (T) cells. The T cells integrate this input through time. This integrated T cell activity generates outflow signals to the motoneurons (MN), thereby causing them to move. In addition, the T cells generate an inhibitory feedback signal to the B cells and an excitatory feedforward signal to the MN cells. As this inhibitory signal builds up due to the integrative action of the T cells, it progressively weakens the excitatory effect of the input on the B cells. When the inhibitory T cell feedback completely cancels the input, the B cells shut off (hence their name), thereby terminating SG input to the T cells and allowing the saccade to end.

To see how this kind of network can work, consider the simple model

$$\frac{d}{dt}x = -Ax + I - By \tag{7.1}$$

and

$$\frac{d}{dt}y = f(x) \tag{7.2}$$

where $x(t)$ is the activity of the model B cells, $y(t)$ is the activity of the model T cells, and I is the input size. Suppose that $f(x)$ is a nonnegative increasing function such that $f(0) = 0$. Also suppose that $f(x)$ has a finite maximum, say 1, and that most inputs I which perturb $x(t)$ are large enough to drive $f(x)$ close to its maximum. Then when I turns on, $x(t)$ is activated and starts to grow. Function $f(x)$ rapidly grows to 1. By (7.2), $y(t)$ integrates the value 1 through time, hence grows (approximately) linearly with t. Thus $y(t) \cong t$. The net input $I - By$ to the B cells in (7.1) therefore satisfies

$$I - BY \cong I - Bt. \tag{7.3}$$

Thus the net input becomes zero at (approximately) time

$$t_I = \frac{I}{B}. \tag{7.4}$$

Thereafter the decay rate $-A$ of $x(t)$ and the negativity of $I - By$ drive $x(t)$ to zero.

The critical property of this circuit is that $y(t)$ integrates the (approximate) input 1 for a time interval of (approximately) I/B in duration, before $x(t)$ shuts off its input to $y(t)$. Thus the tonic outflow signal increases at an (approximately) constant rate for a duration that increases (approximately) linearly with the input intensity I. These linear properties break down at the small input sizes I such that $f(x)$ does not equal 1, and at the transitional times when $x(t)$ is increasing from equilibrium and decreasing back to equilibrium. Despite these caveats, it is clear that

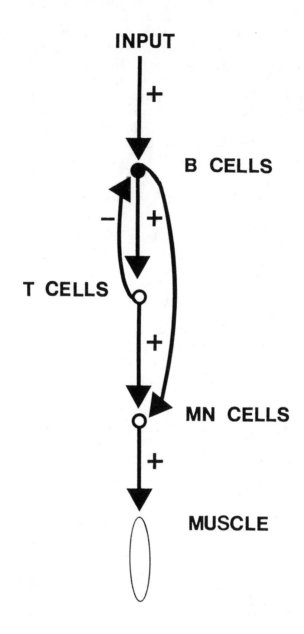

Figure 7.2. A simple saccade generator (SG) circuit: The input excites burst cells (B) which, in turn, excite tonic cells (T) and motoneurons (MN). The T cells inhibit the B cells. In such a circuit, the duration of B cell activity increases with the intensity of the input. (Filled circles are phasically active cells. Open circles are tonically active cells.)

such a system can generate movement signals that expand and contract in a regular way as the input increases and decreases over an unlimited range. In other words, such a system can convert an *intensity* code (I) into a code for temporal *duration* (t_I). Using such a code, the duration of a saccade should covary with the duration of burst cell activity. This is also true in the data (Luschei and Fuchs, 1972).

7.3. Summation of Retinotopic and Initial Eye Position Signals to the Saccade Generator

We can now draw several important conclusions about the inputs to the SG. By Chapter 5, T cell outputs generate the outflow signals that determine the position of the eyes in the head. Thus, after an accurate saccade terminates, the T cell feedback to the SG encodes the target position of the eyes. Since this T cell feedback signal cancels the total input to the SG, the total input to the SG also encodes the target position of the eyes.

We concluded in Chapters 3 and 4, by contrast, that the movement commands to the SG are computed in retinotopic coordinates. Retinotopic commands from the visually reactive movement system are derived from a retinotopic map (RM) that is activated by retinal lights (Chapter 3). Retinotopic commands from the intentional and predictive movement systems are derived from an RM that is activated by difference vectors (Chapter 6). We are hereby led to articulate the following important design problem: How can retinotopic commands be converted into target position commands before activating the SG?

The following conclusion now seems inevitable: at the SG, an RM adds its movement signal to a signal from an eye position map (EPM). In order for the sum of RM and EPM signals to encode the target position of the eye, the EPM signal must encode the initial position of the eye before the saccade begins.

7.4. The Eye Position Update Network

The primary functional role of the EPM map is to form part of a network that updates initial eye position signals to the SG after each saccade terminates. We call this network the *Eye Position Update Network* (EPUN). The existence of an EPUN is implied by the fact that T cell feedback shuts off the SG: After a correct saccade terminates, the T cell feedback cancels the total SG input. In order to prepare for the next saccade, the RM command that encoded the previous saccade command must be shut off, so that a new RM command can replace it. By the time that the new RM command is instated, a new EPM command must also be activated, so that the total RM + EPM command can encode the new target position. The new EPM command encodes, as always, the initial eye position. However, this new *initial* eye position is the *target* eye position of the previous saccade.

This summary suggests that the following sequence of events occurs between two successive saccades:

$$RM_1 + EPM_1 \rightarrow EPM_1 \rightarrow EPM_2 \rightarrow RM_2 + EPM_2. \qquad (7.5)$$

In (7.5), $RM_1 + EPM_1$ stands for the total SG input that caused the first saccade. After the saccade is over, the RM_1 input shuts off. This event does not cause a new saccade to occur because the T cell feedback, having cancelled the total input $RM_1 + EPM_1$, can also cancel the EPM_1 input alone. Then the eye position input is updated by the new initial position input EPM_2. The input EPM_2 approximately matches the T cell feedback, hence does not cause a new saccade. Finally, a new RM_2 input is activated. If the T cell feedback cancels the EPM_2 signal, then the RM_2 input generates a burst within the SG whose size depends upon the RM_2 command alone.

Some variation on the timing of the reset events in (7.5) is also consistent with functional requirements. For example, both RM_1 and EPM_1 may be simultaneously reset. It is not, however, permissible for EPM_1 to be reset before RM_1 is reset. Then the new total command $RM_1 + EPM_2$, which approximately equals $2RM_1 + EPM_1$, could elicit a spurious saccade in response to the increment RM_1.

7.5. Two Types of Initial Position Compensation: Eye Position Update and Muscle Linearization

This discussion suggests that both the RM and the EPM activate conditionable pathways through the adaptive gain (AG) stage that contribute to the total SG input. We already know that the RM must activate such a conditionable pathway (Chapter 3). The conclusion that the EPM also controls a conditionable pathway follows from the possibility that the size scale of the EPM signals is initially either much too large or much too small to balance the T cell feedback that is registered before and after saccades. Unless this calibration problem is solved, the conditionable RM pathway would have to compensate both for initial position errors of the unbalanced EPM and T cell inputs and for saccadic foveation errors. By contrast, if both the RM and the EPM control conditionable pathways, then they can cooperate to correct initial position errors and saccadic foveation errors.

One of the major lessons of Chapter 3 was to show how multiple sampling maps can cooperate to generate the total adaptive gain needed to correct saccadic foveation errors. Since both the RM and the EPM can activate conditionable pathways, they could, in principle, share the adaptive load to correct saccadic foveation errors, as in equations (3.34) and (3.35). Under normal circumstances, the MLN obviates much of the need for such cooperation by directly linearizing the response of the muscle plant, thereby enabling the RM to absorb most of the adaptive load needed to correct saccadic errors, as in equations (3.25) and (3.26).

The analysis in Chapter 5 suggests experimental tests of whether the EPM controls a conditionable pathway. Suppose, for example, that certain pathways from cerebellar direct response cells to MN cells carry the conditioned signals that linearize muscle responses (Section 5.3). If these pathways of the MLN were cut, then dysmetria should be caused due to the subsequent nonlinear muscle responses. As a result, the corollary discharges to the HMI would inaccurately encode the actual positions of the eyes. Any movement commands based upon HMI vectors would consequently lead to saccadic errors for two reasons: The vectors themselves would be incorrectly calibrated, and the total input to the SG would not compensate for muscle nonlinearity. By contrast, visually reactive saccades due to retinal lights would lead to saccadic errors for only one reason: They would not be erroneous due to incorrectly calibrated vectors. They would be erroneous only due to the nonlinearity of the muscle plant.

If such visually reactive saccades could be evoked sufficiently often, the adaptive cooperation of RM and EPM signals at the SG should substantially correct the dysmetria. By contrast, adaptation to vector-based RM commands might show less correction, because the corollary discharges from which the vectors are computed would continue to be miscalibrated. Ablating the frontal eye fields can cause only visually reactive saccades to occur, whereas ablating the superior colliculus can cause only intentional and predictive saccades to occur (Schiller, Sandell, and Maunsell, 1984). Such lesions, in concert with lesions of the pathway from cerebellar direct response cells to MN cells, may therefore be useful to test whether the EPM input to the SG is conditionable.

Another test of EPUN properties can be made by using paradigms in which saccade staircases are generated.

7.6. Saccade Staircases

The EPUN helps to explain saccade staircases of the type found by Schiller and Stryker (1972). In their experiments, a sustained electrode input to the deep layers of the superior colliculus caused a series of saccades of equal size. The EPUN design explains the existence of saccade staircases as follows.

The electrode input initially adds an RM input to the total SG input. A saccade is hereby generated. This RM input does not turn off, because the electrode does not turn off. On the other hand, after the saccade is over, the EPM input is updated, as in (7.5). The EPM input hereby increases by an amount corresponding to the length of the saccade. This new EPM input cancels the new level of T cell feedback. Hence the extra RM input due to the sustained electrode input can cause a second saccade. This argument can clearly be iterated to conclude that a saccade staircase will occur.

An intriguing feature of this explanation emerges when we ask why all the saccades in the saccade staircase are of approximately equal size. In Section 4.9 we noted that one factor is the *absence* of initial eye position compensation from the HMI. We have just noted that the staircase *per se* is due to the *presence* of initial eye position compensation from the EPUN. Further argument is needed to explain the equal sizes of the saccades. Equal increments in total input to the SG do not imply equal saccade sizes if the muscle plant is nonlinear. However, the muscle plant is functionally linear due to the action of the MLN. A series of equal saccades is the result

This explanation shows that appropriate properties of three adaptive circuits (VCN, EPUN, and MLN) are needed to reconcile the properties of saccadic staircases with the greater body of saccadic data. Suitable manipulations in any of these circuits should therefore yield predictable changes in the properties of saccadic staircases. For example, cutting the cerebellar direct response pathways that are assumed to linearize muscle response in the MLN is predicted to elicit saccades of unequal sizes in a saccade staircase. Preventing the reset of the neurons that are assumed to update the EPM in the EPUN is predicted to cause just one saccade to be generated. This latter property can be used to discover what brain region houses this EPM.

Our explanation of saccadic staircases implies that during normal adult saccades, the RM input is shut off after the saccade is over. Any mechanism that prevents this reset event can elicit saccadic staircases. Perhaps saccadic staircases in infants (Salapatek *et al.*, 1980) are due to the fact that (cortical) mechanisms have not yet developed their ability to reset stored retinotopic commands after a nonfoveated target is shut off. Since the sizes of the saccades in these staircases are approximately equal, the more primitive MLN has presumably already developed by this developmental stage.

7.7. Circuit Design of the Eye Position Update Network

The EPUN is built up by using many of the same design principles as the RCN (Chapter 3), VCN (Chapter 4), and the MLN (Chapter 5). This fact illustrates that, once a network module has been synthesized by the evolutionary process, it may be specialized in many ways by hooking it up to different input and output pathways. The EPUN network is designed as follows.

As in the MLN, T cell activity is mapped into an EPM which sends sampling signals to the AG stage (Figure 7.3). Instead of using the OII-generated error signals of the MLN at the AG stage, the EPUN uses the second light error signals of the RCN and VCN. As in the RCN and VCN, the conditionable pathways from the AG stage project to the SG.

Both retinal lights and HMI vectors are encoded within an RM before a saccade begins and are stored in STM there until after the saccade is over. In this way second light error signals can correct foveation errors due to the RM command (Chapter 2). The hypothesis that RM + EPM signals cooperate at the SG leads to the suggestion that the EPM is activated using similar temporal rules: The T cell input to the EPM is encoded and stored in STM before a saccade begins, and is not reset until after the saccade is over. The EPM thus represents *initial* eye position right after the saccade ends, and the total RM + EPM input represents target position.

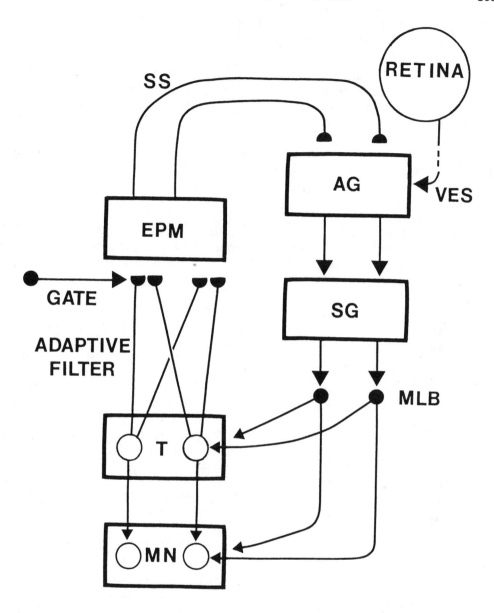

Figure 7.3. An eye position update network (EPUN): This network updates the present eye position signal to the saccade generator (SG) after a saccade is over. Due to this network, the retinotopically coded saccadic commands computed by the retinotopic command network (RCN) can activate the SG by the correct amount to foveate a target light. Abbreviations: T = tonic cells, MN = motoneurons, EPM = eye position map, AG = adaptive gain stage, VES = visual error signals, MLB = medium lead bursters.

Thus any second light error signal that the saccade might generate can correct the cooperating conditionable pathways of this composite target position command.

The discrete sampling of T cell signals by the EPM is controlled by some type of gating action, because the T cells are tonically active and are thus always on. Several functional variations on this gating concept are readily imagined, and await future data to select among them. For example, a pause cell, or cell that is on except during a saccade (Section 7.8), could provide an excitatory gating action either at the synaptic knobs of T cell pathways to the EPM (Figure 7.3) or at the axon hillocks of these pathways. In the former case, the gating action could also modulate the plasticity of the adaptive filter which maps T cell outputs into EPM positions (Chapter 6). Alternatively, a burst cell, or cell that is on only during a saccade, could provide an inhibitory gating action at synaptic knobs or axon hillocks. Neural data which may provide interpretations of EPUN cells are reserved until Chapter 11, where we will also make several predictions about movement and postural subsystems.

7.8. A Saccade Generator Circuit

In this section, we describe a more complex SG model than the simple feedback inhibitory circuit of Figure 7.2. This circuit utilizes cell types such as pause cells, two types of burst cells, tonic cells, and motoneurons that will play a role in our later discussions. Data concerning such cell types were described by Luschei and Fuchs (1972). The circuit illustrates how agonist and antagonist movement signals can work together in a push-pull fashion. In particular, antagonist bursts can occur near the end of a saccade and isometric coactivation of medium lead bursters can occur when a saccade moves in a direction perpendicular to the preferred axis of the bursters (van Gisbergen, Robinson, and Gielen, 1981). The circuit also has the property that its accuracy can vary with the network's level of arousal, notably that saccadic undershoots can occur in a fatigued or insufficiently aroused state, as in the data of Bahill and Stark (1979). In our SG circuit, the last three properties are all explained by the same mechanism.

Figure 7.4 depicts how such a model SG circuit controls a left-right pair of mutually antagonistic muscles. To describe this circuit's properties, we consider how cells that contract the right muscle interact with each other and with the other cells of the network. A total RM + EPM input is received by the long-lead burster (LLB) population v_2. Population v_2 sends excitatory signals to the medium-lead burster (MLB) population v_6. Population v_6 also receives powerful inhibitory signals from the pauser (P) population v_3. The LLB cells cannot supraliminally activate the MLB cells until the P cells shut off. The inputs to the LLB cells can build up gradually through time and over spatially dispersed populations that can receive inputs from several sources of RM and EPM inputs. When the total LLB input reaches a critical size, the LLB population can directly inhibit the P cells v_3, and thereby indirectly disinhibit the MLB cells v_6.

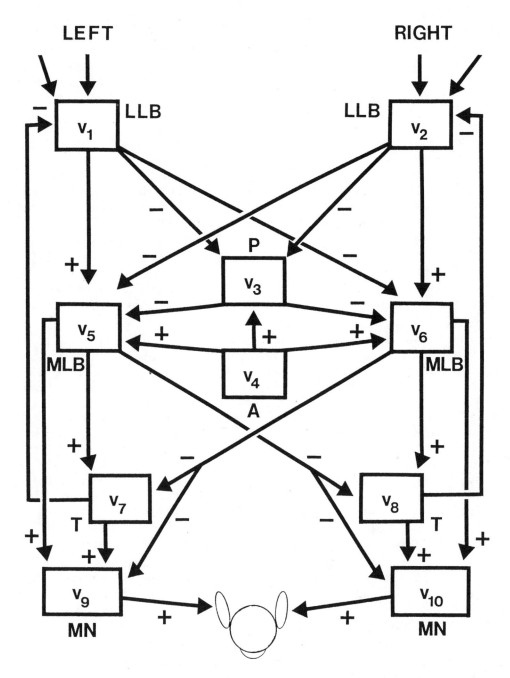

Figure 7.4. A saccade generator (SG) circuit: The text describes how the circuit works. Abbreviations: LLB = long lead burster, MLB = medium lead burster, T = tonic cell, MN = motoneuron, P = pauser, A = arousal.

The gradual and spatially dispersed build-up of input to the LLB cells is hereby translated into a rapid and focussed onset of activity at the MLB cells.

The MLB cells activate their tonic (T) cells v_8 and their motoneuron (MN) cells v_{10}, also called burst-tonic cells. The T cells v_8 integrate their inputs, and relay this integrated activity to the MN cells v_{10}. Thus the MN cells receive integrated MLB input from the T cells, as well as direct MLB inputs. The MN cells, in turn, contract the right muscle. The direct MLB inputs enable their MN cells to generate a large initial signal to the eye muscles. This initial burst can overcome muscle inertia and any changes in total muscle input that may occur during the transition from posture to movement (Chapter 8). The T cell input, on the other hand, helps the eye to attain its final position and to maintain this position after the saccade is over. The T cells also generate the inhibitory feedback signals to the LLB cells which terminate the saccade, as in Figure 7.2.

Due to inhibitory feedback from the T cells, recording from the LLB cells will not easily disclose the existence of inputs from an eye position map (EPM), as in equation (7.5). This is because the T cell feedback tends to cancel the EPM input to the LLB cells. Inhibition of the T cell input should unmask the EPM input contribution to the LLB cells in such a circuit.

Activation of the right muscle circuitry also affects the left muscle circuitry. In order to understand how this happens in the circuit of Figure 7.4, we must first explain how the arousal (A) cells v_4 work. These A cells control the generalized "excitability" of the entire circuit. In particular, population v_4 determines the tonic activation level of the P cells v_3. The A cells also generate inputs to the MLB cell populations v_5 and v_6. The balance between A cell excitation and P cell inhibition keeps the MLB cells off between saccades. When the P cells v_3 are turned off by inputs from the LLB cells v_2, the unmasked input from the A cells v_4 combines with LLB input at v_6 to provide a strong onset of MLB activation. The primary function of the A cell population is thus to bring the size of MLB activation by unconditioned LLB inputs into a reasonable range at an early developmental stage, such that later conditioned changes in LLB inputs can correct any remaining errors of saccade length and direction.

When an input to the LLB cells v_2 initiates a saccade, the v_2 cells also inhibit the MLB cells v_5 of the left muscle. This inhibitory signal to v_5 cancels the excitatory signal from the A cells v_4 after the P cells v_3 are shut off. Thus the LLB cells v_2 simultaneously inhibit the P cells v_3 and the antagonistic MLB cells v_5 using broadly distributed off-surround pathways.

This hypothesis has important experimental implications. The antagonist MLB cells v_5 are shut off at the beginning of a saccade by the agonist LLB cells v_2. However, as the saccade progresses, the inhibitory feedback from the agonist T cells v_8 gradually shuts off the LLB cells v_2. As a result, LLB inhibition of the MLB cells v_5 gets progressively smaller, until the v_5 cells receive a net excitatory input from the A cells v_4. In other words, the MLB cells v_5 experience an *antagonistic burst* towards the end of a saccade, as also occurs *in vivo* (van Gisbergen, Robinson, and Gielen, 1981).

The hypothesis that an antagonistic burst may be due to disinhibition of a tonic arousal signal has not been made in other SG models. Should it prove to be false, the A cells could be removed without destroying most of the circuit's properties. An antagonistic burst could also, for example, be due to weak coactivation of antagonist LLB cells during an agonist saccade. This hypothesis can be tested in several ways. For example, the circuit in Figure 7.4 predicts that the maximal size of this antagonistic burst in v_5 varies monotonically with the maximal size of the agonist burst in v_6, and that both maximal sizes should decrease during drowsy states that cause saccadic undershoots.

In order to achieve a push-pull effect at each antagonistic muscle pair, the MLB cells v_6 inhibit the antagonist T cells v_7 and the MN cells v_9 when they excite their own T cells v_8 and MN cells v_{10}. This type of push-pull effect has been reported at abducens MN cells by van Gisbergen, Robinson, and Gielen (1981). These authors also reported that burst neuron discharge rate closely followed the difference between target position and eye position signals during a saccade, thereby providing strong evidence for their hypothesis that T cell inhibition shuts off the saccade-generating burst.

7.9. Computer Simulations of a Saccade Generator Model

Figure 7.5 describes computer simulations of a model circuit of the type depicted in Figure 7.4. For completeness, we also summarize the differential equations that were used in this simulation. In order to simplify the model and to minimize the number of free parameters, we chose parameters equal to 1 and linear signal functions wherever possible.

Long Lead Bursters

$$\frac{d}{dt}x_1 = -x_1 + I_1 - x_7 + x_7(0) \tag{7.6}$$

$$\frac{d}{dt}x_2 = -x_2 + I_2 - x_8 + x_8(0) \tag{7.7}$$

Pausers

$$\frac{d}{dt}x_3 = -x_3 + x_4 - f(x_1) - f(x_2) \tag{7.8}$$

Arousal Cells

$$x_4 = \text{constant}$$

Medium Lead Bursters

$$\frac{d}{dt}x_5 = -x_5 + x_1 + x_4 - g(x_2) - g(x_3) \tag{7.9}$$

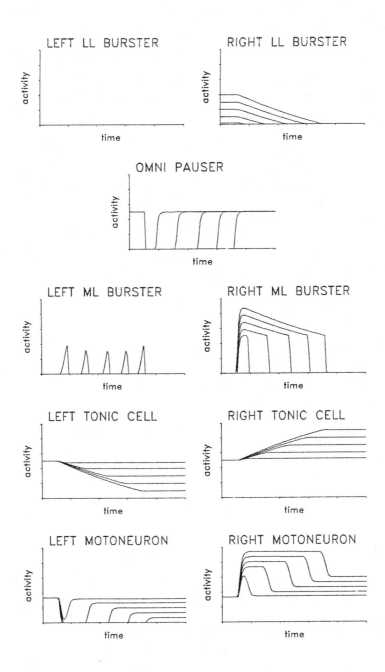

Figure 7.5. Computer simulation of a saccade generator (SG) circuit: The graphs depict the time evolution of cell activity in response to a series of constant inputs of increasing intensity to the right long lead burster population.

$$\frac{d}{dt}x_6 = -x_6 + x_2 + x_4 - g(x_1) - g(x_3) \tag{7.10}$$

Tonic Cells

$$\frac{d}{dt}x_7 = C(x_5 - x_6) \tag{7.11}$$

$$\frac{d}{dt}x_8 = C(x_6 - x_5) \tag{7.12}$$

Motoneurons

$$\frac{d}{dt}x_9 = -x_9 + x_5 - x_6 + x_7 \tag{7.13}$$

$$\frac{d}{dt}x_{10} = -x_{10} + x_6 - x_5 + x_8 \tag{7.14}$$

Initial data were chosen as follows:

$$x_1(0) = x_2(0) = x_5(0) = x_6(0) = 0 \tag{7.15}$$

$$x_3(0) = x_4(0) = x_7(0) = x_8(0) = x_9(0) = x_{10}(0) = \frac{1}{2} \tag{7.16}$$

Parameters, signal functions, and inputs were chosen as follows:

$$C = .01, \tag{7.17}$$

$$f(w) = \frac{w}{.001 + w}, \tag{7.18}$$

$$g(w) = \frac{w}{.02 + w}, \tag{7.19}$$

$$I_1 \equiv 0$$

$$I_2 = .02, .1, .2, .3, .4 \text{ on trials } 1 - 5.$$

In equation (7.6), term $x_7(0)$ is used to encode the EPM input corresponding to the target position attained by the previous saccade, which is hypothesized to equal the T cell inhibitory feedback from v_7 at the end of this saccade. Term $x_8(0)$ in equation (7.7) has a similar interpretation.

7.10. Comparison of Computer Simulations with Neural Data

Properties of model SG cells are similar to data on the response characteristics of various cell types in the deep layers of the superior colliculus, peripontine reticular formation, and oculomotor nuclei. Figure 7.6 schematizes the neural responses leading to a saccade. It highlights the main properties of the various cell types found in unit recordings by Luschei and Fuchs (1972) and Raybourn and Keller (1977).

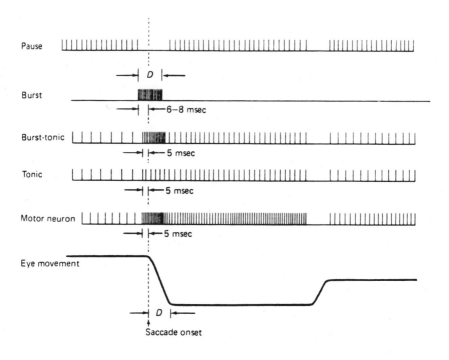

Figure 7.6. A schematic representation of the electrical activity recorded from cells in a saccade generator. Reprinted by permission of the publisher from "Oculomotor System" by P. Gouras, **Principles of Neural Science**, E.R. Kandel and J.H. Schwartz (Eds.), p.402. Copyright 1981 by Elsevier Science Publishing Co., Inc.

Agonist medium lead bursters (MLB) tend to burst to near saturating levels during saccades. The burst duration is proportional to the saccade length in the MLB's direction of action. Antagonist MLB cells burst slightly shortly before the saccade ends. Both MLB's have been found to burst equally to saccades orthogonal to the MLB's direction of action (van Gisbergen *et al.*, 1981). In the model, this occurs when a saccadic command shuts off the pausers v_3. These pausers are assumed to be omnipausers which are shut off by every saccadic command. If the saccade is perpendicular to an antagonist pair of LLB populations, then no other inputs perturb the corresponding circuit. Consequently both agonist and antagonist MLB populations are equally activated during the saccade.

The duration of pauser inactivity due to a saccadic command is proportional to saccade length. The tonic cell activity is proportional to present eye position. The motoneuron, or burst-tonic cell, activity is also proportional to eye position between saccades. In addition, motoneurons burst during saccades with a burst duration similar to that of the MLBs.

All of these properties of the experimental data appear in our model. Moreover, our simulations use the same neuron model for all cell types. The varied response characteristics seen in our simulations depend entirely on the connections, input and output signal functions, and parameter choices between the model cells. These cellular characteristics are thus emergent properties due to choices of network interactions and reaction rates. This type of model provides an alternative to control theory models whose transfer functions may not correspond to neural mechanisms. In particular, we have suggested that antagonist bursts near the end of a saccade, isometric coactivation during perpendicular saccades, and undershoot during a fatigued state may all be due to a common neural mechanism. This is not the type of explanation that is easily made by a control theory model.

CHAPTER 8
POSTURAL STABILITY AND
LENGTH-TENSION REGULATION

8.1. Separate Postural and Movement Systems

Two distinct types of adaptive circuits have thus far been invoked to ballistically move the eyes to target positions. The muscle linearization network (MLN) compensates for the nonlinearity of the oculomotor plant, whereas the retinotopic command network (RCN) and vector command network (VCN) use visual error signals to alter the direction and length of saccades. Neither of these mechanisms suffices to maintain the position of the eye during gaze. This is because both types of movement circuits are used to calibrate the proper direction and length of a saccade, but not the tensions needed to maintain gaze after a saccade is over. As Section 1.12 noted, unequal lengths of agonist and antagonist muscles must coexist with equal tensions in these muscles to maintain gaze after the saccade is over.

Figure 7.4 provides a more precise understanding of this design issue. In Figure 7.4, the medium lead burster (MLB) population v_6 that excites the motoneuron (MN) cells v_{10} of an agonist muscle also completely inhibits the MN cells v_9 of the antagonist muscle. In particular, the inhibition of the antagonist MN by the agonist MLB prevents the antagonist tonic (T) cells from reading-out their signals to the antagonist muscle during the saccade. This push-pull arrangement prevents the antagonist muscle from unnecessarily slowing down during a rapid agonist contraction. In particular, the force exerted by the antagonist muscle on the eyeball is much reduced during a saccade.

By contrast, as soon as the saccade is over, the MLB inhibition is removed from the antagonist MN cells, and the full impact of T cell output is felt at the antagonist muscle. The balance of tensions between agonist and antagonist muscles consequently changes. In order to prevent the eye from drifting away from its target position after the saccade is over, an additional circuit is needed to compensate for any imbalances that may exist in agonist-antagonist tensions. This circuit must be able to do its work without altering the muscle lengths that were attained by a saccade. Thus movements and postures must be regulated by different control systems in order to preserve the lengths achieved by movement, yet compensate for the tension changes that occur during posture.

The postural system, no less than the movement system, must be capable of learning. The intrinsic tension characteristics of the eye muscles may change through time. The degree of tension imbalance at each combination of agonist-antagonist muscle lengths may also differ, and could not be effectively counterbalanced by a prewired mechanism.

193

8.2. Tension Equalization Network

Figure 8.1 describes a network capable of learning to generate equal agonist-antagonist tensions without undermining the length characteristics of the movement system. This circuit is called a *Tension Equalization Network* (TEN). The goal of the TEN is to prevent post-saccadic drifts from occurring. It does so by using motions of visual cues with respect to the retina as error signals after a saccade is over. Visual motions with respect to the retina can also occur when the eyes are moving due to active movement commands. In order not to confuse these two types of motion, gating mechanisms are needed which enable learning to occur only when the eye is not in an active movement mode. Another type of gating must also occur within the TEN. Read-out of postural signals from the conditioned pathways of the TEN must also not be allowed except in the postural mode. If equalizing tensions were imposed upon agonist and antagonist muscles in the movement mode, then movements would be impaired. It remains to discuss whether the gating mechanism which shuts off learning except in the postural mode is the same gating mechanism which shuts off output signals except in the postural mode. This would, of course, be the most parsimonious solution.

8.3. Design of the Tension Equalization Network

The TEN shares many of the design features that are used by the MLN and the EPUN. It also shares design features with networks capable of vestibulo-ocular reflex (VOR) adaptation. As in the MLN and the EPUN, the TEN spatially encodes T cell activity patterns at an eye position map (EPM). The EPM, in turn, sends conditionable pathways to the adaptive gain (AG) stage.

The error signals which these pathways sample at the AG stage are neither the error signals from the outflow-inflow interface (OII) of the MLN, nor the second light error signals of the EPUN. The TEN needs to use error signals that can measure the amount of post-saccadic drift. At first broach, one might think that an OII-activated error signal might be suitable, because it could use inflow signals to register motions of the eye muscles with respect to outflow commands. This possibility seems less tenable when one considers the physiological mechanisms whereby inflow signals are generated. If Golgi tendon organs were used as the inflow source, the mechanism would fail totally both because the tendons are insensitive to passive stretch and because tension-regulating feedback from the TEN would confound whatever length-predictive information the tendons did deliver. Length-based inflow signals could also be altered by tension-regulating feedback from the TEN.

We suggest that visual error signals are used by the TEN. These error signals must be capable of correcting post-saccadic drifts even in the absence of moving visual targets. Hence we suppose that directionally tuned error signals are activated by motions of the whole visual field. The accessory optic system is capable of generating error signals of this type

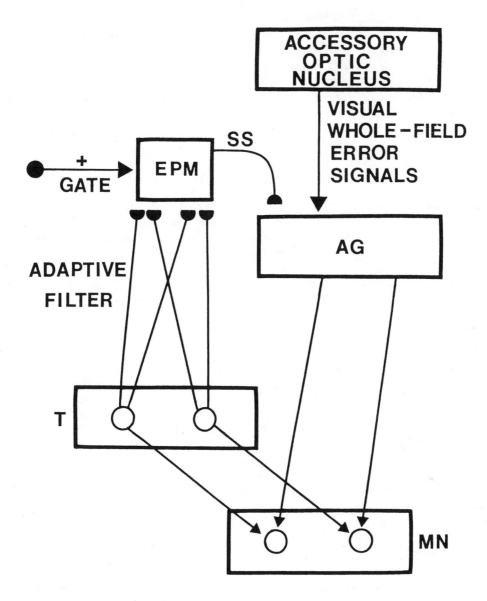

Figure 8.1. Circuit diagram of a tension equalization network (TEN): This network prevents post-saccadic drift from occurring during gaze. It adaptively balances agonist-antagonist tensions even though the agonist-antagonist muscle lengths are unequal. As in the muscle linearization network (MLN) of Figure 5.2., an eye position map (EPM) is the source of sampling signals to the adaptive gain (AG) stage. As in the circuit for vestibulo-ocular reflex (VOR) adaptation of Figure 8.3, whole-field visual error signals are used, rather than second light error signals. Abbreviations: T = tonic cells, MN = motoneurons.

(Simpson, Soodak, and Hess, 1979). Directionally-tuned whole-field visual error signals can, for example, be generated by a network whose cells fire only if they receive convergent inputs from a sufficiently large number of cells tuned to a similar direction. We assume that a whole-field visual motion in a direction opposite to a prescribed muscle's direction of contraction causes the strength of the conditioned pathway to the AG strip of that muscle to increase and the strength of the conditioned pathway to the AG strip of the antagonist muscle to decrease (Figure 8.2).

As in the MLN, the AG stage sends pathways directly to the MN cells. The pathway

$$T \text{ cell} \rightarrow EPM \rightarrow AG \rightarrow MN \qquad (8.1)$$

can influence muscle tensions without altering the tonic cell outputs that determine muscle length. In order for the TEN to work well, the conditioned pathways to these MN cells must be active only in the postural mode, and learning must be possible only in the postural mode. Both of these requirements can be achieved by a single gating signal that nonspecifically inhibits the TEN somewhere between the T cells and the AG stage in Figure 8.1. The cells which give rise to such an inhibitory gating action must be active only during a saccade. Burst cells could therefore be the sources of this inhibitory gating signal.

The TEN accomplishes its function in the following way. During a saccade, its conditioned pathways to the MN cells are inactivated by gating signals. After the burst cells shut off, these conditioned pathways are disinhibited, as the T cells register the outflow signal pattern corresponding to where the eyes should be. If the eyes then begin to drift in their orbits, these outflow signals do not change. Hence they provide a stable source of sampling signals to the AG stage. Each distinguishable T cell outflow pattern can control a different conditionable pathway (Figure 8.2) to the AG stage. Each such pathway can learn to control conditioned gains of all relevant muscles at the AG stage. These gains change as a result of learning in a way that tends to prevent future drifts when the eye ends up in the same, or a similar, outflow position. In short, the TEN is indifferent to how the eye got to where it is at the end of a saccade. Wherever that might be, the TEN uses its outflow-activated sampling pathways to hold it there.

It is important to realize that the TEN is designed to accomplish this goal without interfering with the functioning of other adaptive circuits. For example, the RM and EPM sampling maps of the EPUN have already determined an outflow pattern across the T cells before the TEN is allowed to turn on after a saccade terminates. The MLN has also achieved an approximately linear muscle plant response via the MN cells before the TEN is allowed to turn on. By the time the TEN turns on, the T cell pattern that activates its EPM has already been determined, and the positions of the eyes in the head have also been determined. It remains only for the TEN to resist passive eye movements after the active movement signals shut off, and to do so via the MN cells so as not to disturb the other computations that got the eyes to wherever they might be. Thus,

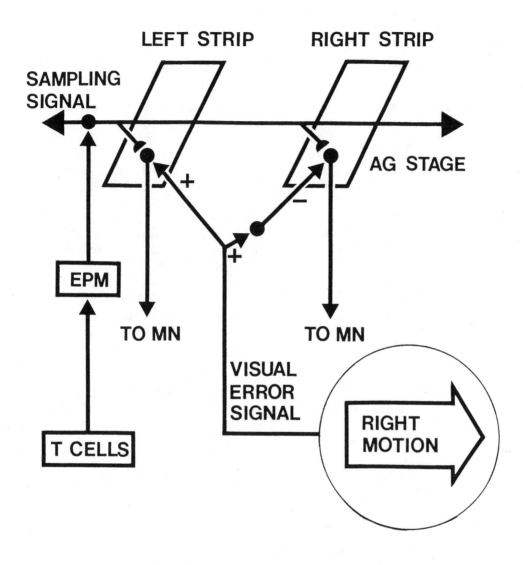

Figure 8.2. Influence of whole-field visual error signals on the adaptive gain (AG) stage: A whole-field motion to the right on the visual field causes the conditioned gain in the left motor strip to increase and in the right motor strip to decrease. Alternatively, competition between the agonist-antagonist strips could cause the net gain of the right motor strip to decrease, as in Figure 3.6b.

at times when the TEN is turned on, the signals from the MN cells to the eye muscles explicitly encode the tension requirements that hold the eyes in place, but implicitly encode both length and tension information that prevent the eyes from moving from wherever they were intended to be.

8.4. Adaptive Step Gain and Pulse Gain: Correcting Post-Saccadic Drift

Several laboratories, notably the laboratory of D.A. Robinson, have reported data that are compatible with the existence of separate cerebellar movement and gain subsystems, notably with properties of the TEN circuit as a model of gain control during gaze. The cerebellar direct response cells that Ron and Robinson (1973) discovered may be included in TEN circuits as well as in MLN circuits. In addition to the cerebellar direct response cells, which elicit saccades with the remarkably short latency of 5–9 msec., Ron and Robinson (1973) have reported the existence of cerebellar cells that elicit saccades with a much longer latency (12–26 msec.). These latter signals have properties compatible with their action as conditioned movement signals to the SG. Hepp, Henn, Jaeger, and Waespe (1981) have also reported saccade-related burst-tonic mossy fibers in the vermis having properties compatible with an SG action.

Optican and Robinson (1980) have reported cerebellar data that more directly support the existence of separate movement and gaze cerebellar pathways. They studied the effect of discrete cerebellar lesions upon the movement (pulse) and gaze (step) components of saccadic movements. Lesions of the vermis, paravermis (lobes IV–IX) and the fastigial nuclei abolished adaptive control of the pulse component, but not of the step component. Lesions of the flocculus abolished adaptive control of the step component.

Optican and Robinson (1980) also operated on the medial and lateral recti of one eye. They showed that saccade lengths and post-saccadic drift in the weakened eye were corrected only when the eye was exposed to visual experience. This fact is compatible with the use of visual error signals to recalibrate both saccade length and post-saccadic drift. Our theory suggests, however, that different visual cues are used to calibrate the pulse and step gains; namely, localized second light error signals and whole-field visual motions, respectively. This prediction may be testable by ablating the accessory optic nucleus instead of the flocculus, and testing whether the pulse gain recovers from an eye muscle operation, whereas the step gain does not. Optican and Robinson (1980) also commented (p.1071): "The fact that the time constant of the postsaccadic drift was about 40 ms presents a puzzle. This is much shorter than the dominant time constant of the orbital mechanics, which has a mean value in rhesus monkeys of about 200 ms." This property is explained in our theory by the fact that the muscle gain during post-saccadic drift is modulated by active signals from the TEN, not only by passive muscle properties. Thus cutting the pathways subserving the gain control signals can cause saccadic overshoots or undershoots to occur even if the muscles are undamaged. This fact is consistent with the observation of Optican and Robinson (1980) that cerebellectomy caused both saccadic overshoots and post-saccadic drifts.

8.5. Relationship to the Vestibulo-Ocular Reflex

We have suggested that directionally-sensitive whole-field visual motions generate the error signals of the TEN, and that the accessory optic nucleus may be a source of these error signals to the cerebellum. It has been suggested that the accessory optic nucleus also generates the whole-field error signals that are used to adaptively calibrate the VOR (Simpson, Soodak, and Hess, 1979). Figure 8.3 summarizes a VOR model which maximizes the functional homology with the TEN circuit. As in the TEN, a whole-field visual error signal in the VOR circuit acts to change conditioned gains in order to prevent slippage of visual cues across the retina. Within the TEN, the EPM that samples these error signals is activated by T cells. Within the VOR circuit, the EPM that samples these error signals is activated by the vestibular canals (Ito, 1984). In both the TEN and VOR circuits, different head positions can control different synergies of conditioned gains capable of preventing motions of the eyes relative to the visual world. Also in both circuits, a whole-field visual drift towards the right strengthens the eye motion to the left. In the TEN, the strengthened eye motion to the left prevents post-saccadic drift to the right during posture. In the VOR circuit, the strengthened eye motion to the left prevents relative motion of the visual field to the right during a head movement.

The functional homology between the TEN and the VOR circuits calls attention to the possibility that sampling signals within the VOR circuit may be gated at some stage between the vestibular canals and the cerebellum. In the TEN, this gate is opened only in the postural mode. Such a posture-dependent gating action would also be useful in the VOR circuit. This can be seen by noting that a saccade may accompany a head movement. The head movement can activate the VOR sampling pathways as the saccade may generate visual whole-field motions. Saccades thus generate whole-field error signals at times when the VOR circuit is already correctly calibrated. A posture-dependent gating action can prevent saccade-generated whole-field motions from erroneously altering the VOR gains. In species where the VOR circuit can compensate for head movements during saccades, this gating action is likely to occur at the synaptic knobs of the sampling signal pathway within the AG stage. That is, a posture-dependent nonspecific gating input is likely to occur at the parallel fiber-Purkinje cell synapse of the cerebellum. At such a locus, the posture-dependent gate can prevent learning from occurring except in the postural state, but could nonetheless allow read-out of the conditioned gains to occur even during saccades.

These comparisons between the TEN and the VOR circuits suggest that both circuits may sample error signals that are registered within the same part of the cerebellum. The cerebellar lesion experiments of Optican and Robinson (1980) are compatible with the hypothesis that the flocculus may be the cerebellar region where these whole-field error signals

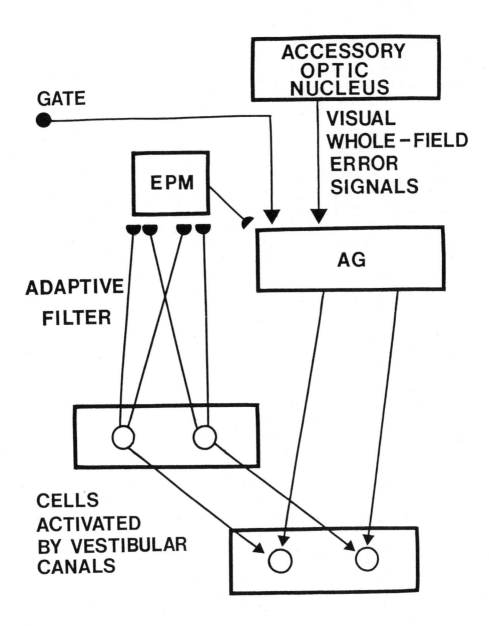

Figure 8.3. Circuit diagram for vestibulo-ocular reflex adaptation: This circuit is intended to suggest possible homologs with the circuit of Figure 8.1 that adaptively prevents post-saccadic drift.

are sampled by both circuits. This hypothesis is further strengthened by the results of Ito *et al.* (1974), who showed that lesions of the flocculus also impair VOR adaptation.

8.6. Cerebellar Functional Heterogeneity

Our analyses of circuits such as the RCN, VCN, MLN, EPUN, and TEN suggest that at least three different types of error signals are registered within the cerebellum: second light visual error signals, OII-activated error signals, and visual whole-field error signals. These results thus provide an evolutionary rationale for subdividing the cerebellum into regions which are functionally specialized to receive different types of error signals. Our analyses also suggest how all of these error signals can take advantage of a common delivery system by climbing fibers feeding into a fractured somatotopy, a hemifield competition, or both (Chapter 3). Several different learning circuits can sample error signals to each of these functionally distinct regions, much as both the TEN and VOR circuits have been hypothesized to sample the flocculus. Each of these different learning circuits maps RMs or EPMs onto the cerebellar topography. Hence multiple copies of several different type of sampling maps need to be superimposed upon maps of several different types of error signals, just to move the eyes and hold them in place (Figure 8.4).

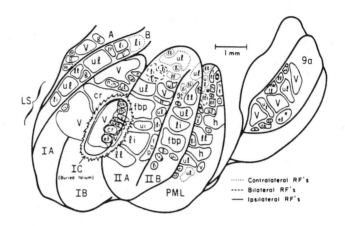

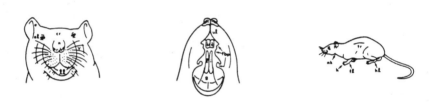

Figure 8.4. Multiple somatotopic representations in cerebellar cortex: Tactile mossy fiber projections to the granule cell layer of the cerebellar cortex are arranged in a patch-organized mosaic as shown. Letters within each patch indicate the body region that projects to that patch. Abbreviations: LS = lobulus simplex, IA and IB = the two surface folia of crus I, IC = the buried folium of crus I revealed in the "cutaway" of the overlying crus I and II, IIA and IIB = the two folia of crus II, PML = paramedian lobule, 9a = uvular folium IXa. From Bower *et al.*, *Brain and Behavioral Evolution*, **18**, 1981, 1–18. Reprinted with permission.

CHAPTER 9
SACCADIC RHYTHM AND
PREDICTIVE MOVEMENT SEQUENCES

9.1. Rhythmic Choices among Multiple Movement Sources

Chapter 8 provided a simple example of a functional rhythm in a sensory-motor system. During such a rhythm, movement and postural subsystems turn on and off intermittently through time, thereby supplementing and complementing each other's computational competences. The demands upon the postural subsystem are always the same: Hold the eyes in place no matter how they got there. The choice of movement subsystems is more varied. A visually reactive saccade may occur. Or a saccade that is triggered by an intermodality signal, such as a sound, may occur. Or a saccade may be volitionally produced, as in the rear view mirror problem (Section 1.13). Or a preplanned sequence of predictive movements may occur, as in a dance. As one ascends the evolutionary ladder from visually reactive to predictive movements, sensory cues play an increasingly limited role.

The remarkable capability of humans to override the influence of sensory cues has been experimentally analysed (Murphy, Haddad, and Steinman, 1974; Steinman, 1965). Such studies led Steinman (1976, p.121) to write: "Perhaps the most striking aspect of human oculomotor performance is its independence from stimulus variables. By this I mean that a normal human adult can look about in his visual world and attend whatever region catches his fancy undisturbed by this distinction of light on his retina, or, in perceptual terms, the way the visual world looks at a particular moment."

Special purpose networks are required to achieve a nonobligatory reaction to sensory cues. For example, patients with discrete frontal lobe removals for intractable epilepsy produce reflex-like saccades to visual stimuli (Buchtel and Guitton, 1980; Goldberg and Bushnell, 1981). In normal humans making intentional saccades, a slow negative shift of scalp potentials begins approximately 650 msec. before an eye movement and is largest in amplitude over the frontal region (Kurtzberg and Vaughan, 1982). This potential does not occur before a visually reactive saccade. The ability of normal humans and higher mammals to override momentary visual stimuli shows that the relationship between saccadic decisions and learned calibrations is not a simple one. As in our discussion of the rear view mirror problem, we will suggest how an intentional saccadic command can take advantage of learned calibrations due to visually reactive saccades even though the intentional command suppresses visually reactive commands. We will suggest that an intentional command does not both inhibit and sample the same visually reactive locus. Intentional commands need a separate subsystem to calibrate some parameters of their saccades, yet also rely on the visually reactive subsystem to calibrate other saccade-related parameters. We will relate this formal property with data demonstrating the existence of separate saccade-generating subsystems in the superior colliculus and the frontal eye fields, such that each subsystem is capable of its own vector compensations (Schiller and Sandell, 1983; Schiller, True, and Conway, 1979).

The dichotomy between intentional saccades and visually reactive saccades does not imply that neurons within the intentional subsystem are insensitive to light signals. Quite the contrary must be true in order for visual signals to initiate the calibration of movement commands within this subsystem. We compare this property with the existence of visually responsive cells in the frontal eye fields, whose activities are enhanced only when the animal makes an eye movement to a stimulus in its receptive field (Goldberg and Bushnell, 1981; Wurtz and Mohler, 1976). Despite the ability of light to calibrate the intentional subsystem, this subsystem must be able to inhibit the visually reactive subsystem, say via inhibitory signals from the prefrontal eye fields to the SC (Goldberg and Bushnell, 1981; Holmes, 1938). The intentional subsystem must also be susceptible to activation by signals other than those elicited by visual cues, notably by internally generated commands capable of encoding sequential cognitive plans. The fact that lights may help to calibrate the intentional subsystem in no way implies that only lights can activate this subsystem.

In this chapter, we consider a network that is capable of encoding a predictive sequence of movements in long-term memory, and of reading-out this movement sequence at will. This model will put us in a better position to integrate the networks which process visually reactive, intermodality, intentional, and predictive movements into a single global processing scheme in Chapter 11.

9.2. Distinguishing Correct Predictive Saccades from Incorrect Individual Saccades

The basic nature of a predictive competence may be better appreciated through the following example. Consider the two light-and-movement sequences:

I. Incorrect Light-Activated Saccade
light 1—incorrect movement 1—light 2—movement 2

II. Correct Light-Activated Predictive Saccade
light 1—light 2—correct movement 1—correct movement 2

In both case (I) and case (II), two successive, nonfoveated lights strike the retina. In case (I), both lights are due to a single source that remains on continuously, whereas in case (II) each light is due to a different source that is flashed on only briefly. In case (I), we want the second nonfoveated light to be the source of an error signal which corrects the saccade caused by the first light. We also want this second light to be able to trigger a second saccade. These properties can be realized by a retinotopic command network, or RCN (Chapter 3). In case (II), by contrast, we do not want the second nonfoveated light to be a source of an error signal, because the first predictive saccade is correct. However, we still want the second nonfoveated light to trigger a second predictive saccade.

How does the saccadic system know whether the second nonfoveated light in a light sequence should or should not trigger an error signal? Cases (I) and (II) differ in terms of how lights and movements are interspersed during visually reactive and predictive saccades, respectively. An analysis of these differences leads to the conclusion that each light activates two parallel pathways that are capable of triggering saccadic motions. The first pathway is the more direct one that leads through the network analog of the superior colliculus. The second pathway is more indirect, and leads through the network analog of the frontal eye fields. The second pathway subserves the predictive capability of the saccadic model.

This bifurcation of pathways is not the bifurcation between sampling pathways and error signal pathways that was introduced in Chapter 2. Both of the pathways in the present bifurcation are sampling pathways. We therefore need to explain how both of these sampling pathways work together to achieve the desired properties of both cases (I) and (II).

9.3. The Temporal Control of Predictive Saccades

In Section 1.16, we suggested that predictive saccades are encoded as target positions in a target position map (TPM) computed in head coordinates. Several target positions can simultaneously be stored in short term memory (STM) by such an TPM. The positions so stored are assumed to have already been influenced by attentional factors. We will review data which suggest that such TPMs may lie within, or closely interact with, the posterior parietal cortex or the frontal eye fields. These data can be interpreted using our explanation of how a spatial pattern of stored lights can be read-out as a temporal sequence of predictive saccades. Thus we are considering how a *parallel* internal representation is transformed into *serial* behavior. We will show how such an TPM interacts with a head-muscle interface, or HMI (Chapter 4), to generate the correct temporal sequence of vector commands. In the light of these results, we will consider in Section 9.10 the difficulties that need to be overcome by a system in which stored retinotopic positions are directly recoded as difference vectors, rather than first being recoded in a TPM before being compared with present position to generate a difference vector.

The minimal network design capable of controlling the STM storage and sequential read-out of predictive saccades uses two successive TPMs, denoted by TPM_1 and TPM_2. The spatial map TPM_1 initially stores all the relevant target positions in STM. The map TPM_2 selects and stores only the target position which controls the current saccade, and interacts directly with the HMI to generate output vectors. We call this entire control structure a *Predictive Command Network* (PCN).

The main functional insight that is embodied by PCN design is that matches and mismatches between target positions and present positions at the HMI regulate the sequential performance and learning of predictive saccades (Grossberg, 1978a, 1980). In particular, a match at the HMI can cause the next target position command to be read into the HMI, thereby causing a mismatch between the new target position and the present position. This mismatch generates the next saccade. In other words, as the network attains its present target, it resets itself to attain its next intended target. Once the PCN circuit is nonspecifically activated by a volitional signal, this match-mediated reset scheme can automatically run off its intended saccades until the entire predictive sequence has been performed.

In order to gradually develop this insight into a precise circuit design, a functional description of network operations will first be given. Then a specific network realization, along with possible cell-type identifications, will be suggested. Several closely related network realizations can be envisaged, and more than one version may be used across different species.

9.4. Storage of Temporal Order Information

A. *Storage of Temporal Order, Target Match, and Memory Reset*

Stage TPM_1 is assumed to store in STM the temporal order information of attended target positions. The temporal order information is encoded by a spatial pattern of activation across the target positions, with more intensely activated positions tending to be performed first. Grossberg (1978a, 1978c, 1986) has derived STM codes whereby temporal order information can be laid down in a way that permits its stable long term memory (LTM) encoding as a unitized motor plan. It turns out that a suitably designed shunting competitive network can do the job (Section 2.6). A discussion of these mechanisms lies outside the scope of this chapter. A temporal order code that is based upon relative STM activity can take into account both the order of item occurrences and the motivational salience of individual items. Motivationally more salient events can be looked at at earlier times, other things being equal. Grossberg (1982b, 1982c, 1984) has described mechanisms whereby motivational salience can modulate the attention that is given to a subset of sensory cues. A discussion of these mechanisms also lies outside the scope of this chapter. For present purposes, it suffices to note that earlier occurring items will often, but not always, be stored in STM with larger activities.

B. *Read-Out and STM Storage of a Target Choice*

When a nonspecific output gate opens between TPM_1 and TPM_2, the most active target position stored within TPM_1 is read into TPM_2. This target position is chosen by a competitive interaction among the active output pathways from TPM_1 to TPM_2. Several things now happen (Figure 9.1a).

C. *HMI Mismatch, Output Gate Closure, and Target Self-Inhibition*

Consider the state of the HMI prior to the moment of target choice at TPM_2. A match may exist there due to correct execution of a prior saccade, or the HMI may be inactive. If target read-out from TPM_2 then occurs, it nonspecifically activates the HMI (Chapter 4) as it instates a new target position there in agonist-antagonist muscle coordinates. This new target mismatches the eye position corollary discharge. Thus a primary effect of target read-out is to cause a mismatch within the HMI (Figure 9.1b).

A second effect of target read-out is to prevent the read-out of other active target locations from TPM_1 until the next saccade is over. The chosen target position in TPM_2 is stored in STM until this saccade is over. During this time, it blocks further read-out there from TPM_1 and maintains the target position within the HMI.

A third effect of target read-out from TPM_1 is to prepare TPM_1 to read-out its next saccadic command after the present saccade is over. A topographically-specific inhibitory signal from the chosen target position to its source in TPM_1 accomplishes this reset event (Figure 9.1a). Although its STM source in the temporal order code of TPM_1 is inhibited, the chosen target position can remain active in STM within TPM_2 due to the internal positive feedback loops within this network.

D. *Read-Out, Reset, and STM Storage of Retinotopic Commands*

The mismatch at the HMI generates a vector difference which generates an output pattern to an RM (Chapter 4). When this happens, the eye is still at rest. This output pattern is stored in STM as a spatial location within the RM after inhibiting any command that may have previously been active within the RM.

The RM command, in turn, activates three output pathways: an unconditioned excitatory pathway to the saccade generator (SG), a prewired inhibitory pathway to the superior colliculus (SC), and a conditioned pathway to the adaptive gain (AG) stage. These signals together can generate a saccade.

While the saccadic motion is taking place, output from the HMI to the RM is prevented by offset of an output gate. The stored movement command in the RM is thus undisturbed during the saccade.

E. *LTM Printing*

After the saccade terminates, a gate opens that enables the LTM traces in the $TPM_2 \rightarrow$ HMI pathway to print the final eye position in muscle coordinates (Chapter 4).

F. *Match-Induced Reset of the TPM*

After a correct saccade takes place, a match between target position and present eye position is generated within the HMI (Figure 9.2a). Whenever a match occurs at the HMI, the stored target position in the TPM_2 is inhibited. Its target position signals to the HMI are thereby also inhibited (Figure 9.2b), a mismatch is caused at the HMI (Figure 9.2c), and the inhibitory signal from the TPM_2 to the TPM_1 output pathways is eliminated. In all, a match at the HMI induces a mismatch at the HMI by inhibiting the $TPM_2 \rightarrow$ HMI target position command.

After the TPM_2 target position is inhibited, the target positions that are active in STM at the TPM_1 stage can compete to choose the next target light and store it in TPM_2. Then the cycle can automatically

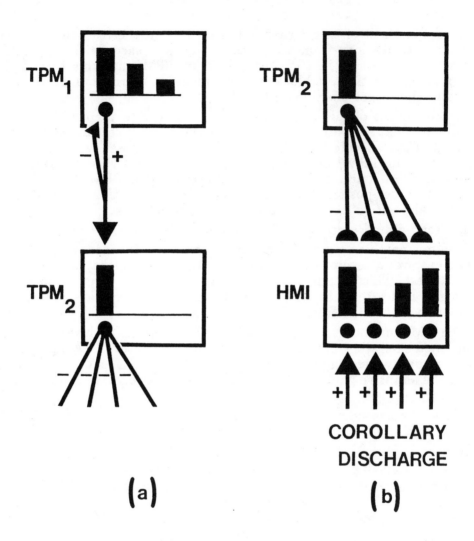

Figure 9.1. Read-out of the most active population in the first stage of the target position map (TPM$_1$): (a) When the most active target position is read-out of TPM$_1$, it self-inhibits its activity as it is stored in the second stage of the target position map (TPM$_2$); (b) Then TPM$_2$ activates its inhibitory conditioned pathways to the head-muscle interface (HMI), at which excitatory corollary discharges are also received.

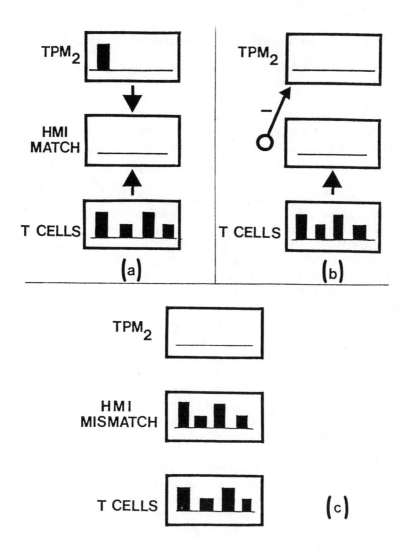

Figure 9.2. Interactions between target position map (TPM$_2$), head-muscle interface (HMI), and tonic cell (T) source of corollary discharges: (a) When target position matches present position in motor coordinates at the HMI, activity across the HMI is inhibited; (b) Inhibition of HMI activity causes the stored target position in the TPM$_2$ to be inhibited; (c) Inhibition of the TPM$_2$ also inhibits its inhibitory efference copy to the HMI. The corollary discharges can then register a mismatch at the HMI.

repeat itself until no temporal order information is stored any longer in STM within the TPM_1.

9.5. Design of a Predictive Command Network

Figures 9.3 and 9.4 together describe a formally competent microcircuit that is built up from neurally plausible components. Some cellular stages of these figures possess properties of known neuron types. The circuit thus suggests predictions about the functional roles of such cells and their interactions with other cells. Figure 9.4 provides details of HMI gating processes that could not be drawn into Figure 9.3.

The networks of TPM_1 and TPM_2 possess similar cellular architectures, even though they carry out different functional tasks. In particular, both TPM_1 and TPM_2 contain shunting on-center off-surround feedback networks (Chapter 2.6). For example, pathways 1 and 4 in TPM_1 and TPM_2, respectively, are both part of positive feedback loops in an on-center (Figure 9.3). Pathway 5 in TPM_2 illustrates a negative feedback loop in an off-surround. Despite these similarities, network TPM_1 is designed to simultaneously store a spatial pattern of temporal order information in STM. Network TPM_2, by contrast, is designed to store only one target light at a time in STM.

The subsequent discussion will show that the cells in the TPM_1 have properties similar to those of light-sensitive cells in the parietal cortex, whereas the cells in TPM_2 have properties similar to those of the light-insensitive saccade neurons in the parietal cortex (Lynch, 1980; Motter and Mountcastle, 1981). The visuomovement cells and movement cells in the frontal eye fields (Bruce and Goldberg, 1984) also have similar properties (Chapter 11). The formal properties in question were independently derived as part of a theory of of how motor commands are read-out from STM in a prescribed temporal order (Grossberg, 1978a, Section 52; 1978b). This theory predicts that similar types of cells will be found wherever this functional task is performed. The discovery of consistent parietal and frontal eye field data suggests that a convergence of theory and experiment is reflected in these network examples.

To start our discussion of the PCN microcircuit, consider a time at which a pattern of temporal order information is being stored in STM and the eye is at rest. In other words, the network has attended some lights and stored them in STM, but has not yet translated them into overt movements. At such a time, network TPM_1 is active, but network TPM_2 is inactive and no target position commands are being read by TPM_2 into the HMI. Consequently, all output gates from the HMI are closed and there exists a mismatch between corollary discharge and target position inputs to the HMI.

The activity within the TPM_1 cannot activate the TPM_2 because of the nonspecific inhibitory gating action which pathway 2 exerts on outputs from the TPM_1 (Figure 9.3). Such a gating action may *in vivo* take place at an interneuronal stage between TPM_1 and TPM_2, but we have avoided all such extra complexities to draw a simpler circuit. The cells which

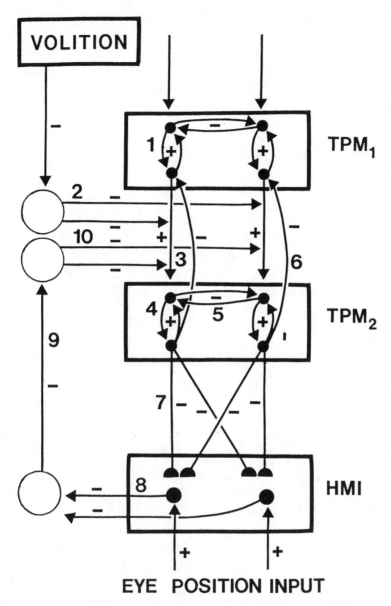

Figure 9.3. Part of the predictive command network (PCN) circuitry for storing, resetting, and sequentially reading out a series of predictive movement commands: The text describes how temporal order information that simultaneously stores several target lights in the TPM_1 can be read-out as a series of vectors from the HMI. The TPM_2 stores just one target position at a time in short term memory (STM). A match between target position and eye position at the HMI triggers read-out of the most active target position command in the TPM_1, which is then stored in the TPM_2 until its saccade is over.

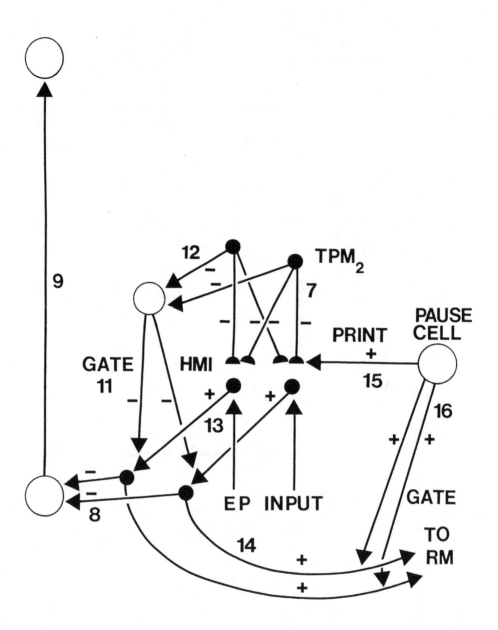

Figure 9.4. Microcircuitry of the predictive TPM$_2$ and its HMI: The text describes how light-mediated gating actions control read-out of reset signals to the TPM$_1$, read-in of target positions in motor coordinates at the HMI, and read-out of HMI vectors to the retinotopic map (RM). The RM recodes HMI vectors as focal activations within a spatial map. Abbreviation: EP = eye position.

activate the inhibitory pathway 2 are tonically active. (Tonic cells are depicted as open circles, phasic cells as closed circles.)

Pathway 10 can also gate shut the output pathways from TPM_1 to TPM_2. Pathway 10 is, however, inactive at this time. It is inhibited by pathway 9. Pathway 9 is active because pathway 8 from the HMI is inactive. Pathway 8 from the HMI is inactive because the inhibitory pathway 11 in Figure 9.4 is active. Pathway 11 is active because the TPM_2 is inactive, and thus cannot activate the inhibitory pathway 12. In all, the multisynaptic pathway $12 \rightarrow 11 \rightarrow 8 \rightarrow 9 \rightarrow 10$ is shut off whenever the TPM_2 is inactive. Thus the TPM_2 does not block its own activation by the TPM_1 at times when it is inactive. The only impediment to activation of TPM_2 by TPM_1 at such a time is the inhibitory pathway 2.

Suppose that volition acts to inhibit the nonspecific pathway 2. Volition does not need to have specific consequences of any kind in order for the PCN to respond by rapidly reading out its sequence of stored commands. We now explain how this can happen.

When pathway 2 shuts off, excitatory signals from the active TPM_1 populations can reach the TPM_2 along topographically organized pathways such as pathway 3. The largest signal causes the most rapid and vigorous activation of its receptive population. The on-center (pathway 4) off-surround (pathway 5) feedback interactions within the TPM_2 contrast enhance this input pattern until only the positive feedback loop corresponding to the largest input is active. The activity within this loop is also stored in STM by the positive feedback interaction.

This active TPM_2 population gives rise to three types of output signals. First, a topographic inhibitory feedback signal (pathway 6) from the TPM_2 to the TPM_1 inhibits its source of feedforward $TPM_1 \rightarrow TPM_2$ signals (pathway 3). The stored activity in TPM_2 hereby resets the temporal order information across TPM_1 by deleting the target position that was just stored in TPM_2. This reset event prepares TPM_1 to read-out the next-most-active population during the next saccadic cycle.

Second, activation of the TPM_2 causes the nonspecific inhibitory gating pathway 10 to turn on, thereby inhibiting further outputs from TPM_1. Thus, as one target position is being stored in TPM_2, it prevents other target positions from being read-into TPM_2. This gating action is accomplished by the multisynaptic pathway $12 \rightarrow 11 \rightarrow 8 \rightarrow 9 \rightarrow 10$. The multiple links in this pathway are needed because this pathway also controls another important property. The multisynaptic pathway $12 \rightarrow 11$ also prevents tonic read-out of eye position signals from the HMI when no target positions are registered there (Section 4.6D). Pathway $12 \rightarrow 11$ does this by gating shut all HMI outputs—including gating signals of TPM_1 outputs and inputs to the RM—whenever the TPM_2 is inactive. Pathway 8 links the HMI output gate $12 \rightarrow 11$ to the TPM_1 output gate $9 \rightarrow 10$. Pathway $12 \rightarrow 11 \rightarrow 8 \rightarrow 9 \rightarrow 10$ is thus an assemblage of two functionally distinct but synergetic subsystems.

Due to the importance of pathway $12 \rightarrow 11 \rightarrow 8 \rightarrow 9 \rightarrow 10$, we now consider in greater detail how it inhibits TPM_1 outputs. When TPM_2 gets activated, the inhibitory pathway 12 shuts off the inhibitory gating signal in pathway 11, thereby disinhibiting pathway 8. When the disinhibitory pathway 8 fires, it shuts off pathway 9, which disinhibits pathway 10, thereby shutting off outputs from the TPM_1. Pathway 8 can fire if it receives an excitatory signal from the HMI. Such a signal arises from the HMI if there is a mismatch between target position and eye position there. This property leads to a consideration of the third type of output signal that is controlled by the TPM_2.

The active population in the TPM_2 reads a target position, computed in muscle coordinates, into the HMI. This target position was learned using the mechanisms described in Chapter 4. Should this target position be different from eye position, then a mismatch will be registered in the HMI and the output pathways from the TPM_1 to the TPM_2 will be gated shut. By contrast, should this target position equal the eye position that is read into the HMI, then a match will be registered in the HMI, and the target position will cancel the eye position. Even if the inhibitory gating pathway 11 is off, no output can activate pathway 8 when a match occurs within the HMI. At such times, pathway 9 will inhibit pathway 10, thereby enabling the next target position to be read-into the TPM_2 from the TPM_1.

Thus, output along pathway 8 is contingent upon two events: activation of the TPM_2 and mismatch within the HMI. This contingency enables new inputs from the TPM_1 to reset an active TPM_2 should its target position have already been realized by prior eye movements. Were it not for this property, the sequential reset mechanism could sometimes get "stuck" before it could read-out its entire command sequence.

If the target position does not equal the eye position within the HMI, then no more signals can pass from the TPM_1 to the TPM_2, and a target position will be stored within the TPM_2, until a match can be generated within the HMI. Such a match cannot be generated by a change in target position, since the same target position will continue to be read into the HMI by the TPM_2 until a match occurs. A match can be created only if the eye moves until the eye position pattern matches the stored target position pattern.

9.6. Saccade Generation by Predictive Commands

In order for the eye to move in this way, the vector difference computed within the HMI must be able to generate a saccade, in the manner described by Chapter 4. Such a saccade can be elicited due to the second role played by the multisynaptic pathway $12 \rightarrow 11$. We have already summarized the first role of this pathway: When the TPM_2 is inactive, the tonically active gating pathway 11 inhibits the target cells at which the HMI vector is registered via pathway 13. At such times, the HMI vector encodes only eye position and would generate ceaseless saccade staircases were it not for pathway 11 (Chapter 7). By contrast, when the TPM_2 is activated, pathway 12 inhibits pathway 11. The target cells can then

TPM$_2$	HMI	12→11→8→9→10 14					
OFF	mismatch	OFF	ON	OFF	ON	OFF	OFF
ON	mismatch	ON	OFF	ON	OFF	ON	ON
ON	match	ON	OFF	OFF	ON	OFF	OFF

Table 9.1. Path activities during different target storage and matching phases of the predictive circuit in Figures 9.3 and 9.4.

register the HMI vector, which now compares target position with eye position. If a mismatch occurs, pathway 8 maintains this difference vector within the HMI by preventing STM reset of the TPM_2.

The second role of pathway $12 \rightarrow 11$ is to enable pathway 14 to carry muscle-coded vector signals to a retinotopic map (RM), where they are re-coded as an active map position and stored in STM (Chapter 6). Output signals from this RM to the saccade generator (SG) update the eye position update network (EPUN) and generate a new saccade (Chapter 7). If this saccade is correct, it causes eye position to match target position in the HMI. If the saccade is incorrect, another mismatch is caused by a vector difference in the HMI, and another corrective saccade is generated. This description thus shows how temporally discrete target position informa-tion and temporally continuous eye position information are continuously matched at the HMI.

When eye position finally comes close to matching target position within the HMI, pathway 8 becomes inactive, despite the fact that the gating pathway 11 is still inhibited. Consequently pathway 10 is inhibited via the multisynaptic pathway $8 \rightarrow 9 \rightarrow 10$, and output signals from the TPM_1 can once again reach the TPM_2. Otherwise expressed, a match at the HMI triggers a "rehearsal wave" that enables read-out of a new target position to occur from the TPM_1 (Grossberg, 1978a, 1980). The most active target position within the TPM_1 can then begin to compete with the stored target position within the TPM_2. The new target position wins this competition because the stored target position has only its pos-itive feedback pathway within TPM_2 with which to maintain its activity, whereas the new target position has both the input from TPM_1 plus its positive feedback pathway with which to become instated. As the new target position inhibits the old one within the TPM_2, it can generate a new target position input to the HMI. This new target position causes a mismatch within the HMI, which in turn causes activation of pathway 10. Pathway 10 inhibits the TPM_1 output pathways and stabilizes the STM storage of the new target position within the TPM_1.

The next saccade in the predictive sequence can then be generated by the HMI. This cycle continues until all of the stored target positions within the TPM_1 have been sequentially inhibited. After all of the saccades have been performed, the TPM_1 is inactive, the TPM_2 is left storing the last target position command in STM, and the HMI is inactive because its target position and eye position match.

Several variations on this microcircuit design can be contemplated which compute the same basic functional properties but differ in terms of testable details. One of these variations is suggested by consideration of Table 9.1. Table 9.1 summarizes how different branches of the multi-synaptic pathways $12 \rightarrow 11 \rightarrow 8 \rightarrow 9 \rightarrow 10$ and $12 \rightarrow 11 \rightarrow 8 \rightarrow 14$ are activated during different phases of the saccadic cycle. This summary suggests that these pathways are designed rather parsimoniously. Inspec-tion of Table 9.1 also shows that the pathways 8 and 10 are always on and off in-phase with each other. Consequently, pathway 8 could directly inhibit the TPM_1 output pathways, instead of acting via the multisynaptic pathway $8 \rightarrow 9 \rightarrow 10$, without altering any functional properties. We have included the tonic pathways 9 and 10 to call attention to a possible homology that may exist *in vivo* between pathway 10 and pathway 2. In Figure 9.3, both volitional signals and HMI signals play upon a general gating system whose function is to inhibit TPM_1 outputs. Pathways 2 and 10 simply mark the target cells where volitional and HMI-activated signals happen to feed into this general gating system. Thus Figure 9.3 would be "more parsimonious" than a figure in which pathway 8 directly inhibits TPM_1 outputs if such a general gating system were to exist. On the other hand, if pathway 2 inhibits not only $TPM_1 \rightarrow TPM_2$ outputs but also the TPM_2 cells, then pathways 2 and 10 could not possibly be part of the same functional system, because STM storage of activity within the TPM_2 must be able to occur while pathway 10 is active. Enabling pathway 2 to inhibit TPM_2 cells achieves a small advantage, since shutting off the volitional signal after a saccade sequence terminates would then inhibit the stored final target postion within TPM_2, and thereby completely reset the TPM_2 in preparation for the next predictive saccadic sequence. Given such an arrangement, the rationale for the multisynaptic pathway $8 \rightarrow 9 \rightarrow 10$ would collapse, and a direct inhibitory pathway 8 onto the TPM_1 output pathways might be expected to exist.

9.7. Two Types of Output Gates: Target-Driven Gates and Saccade-Driven Gates

To complete our description of PCN design, we need to consider in finer mechanistic detail several functional issues that were raised in Chapter 4. What happens if a predictive saccadic command generates a saccadic error due to inaccurate translation of a vector command into a movement, as in the Shebilske paradigm? How can a vector command be stored within the RM throughout a saccade? What prevents this stored vector command from being reset by eye positions attained during a saccade? How is learning within the HMI prevented from occurring except after a saccade terminates? We suggest that all of these functions are controlled by a single gating system. This gating system is, however, different from the *target-driven* gating system (pathway $12 \rightarrow 11$) that is modulated by storage of target positions within the TPM_2. We call the other gating system a *saccade-driven* gating system because its activity is modulated by the saccade generator (SG).

Figure 9.4 describes one possible version of the saccade-driven gating system. This version uses a pause cell input source. Such a pause cell is tonically on except during a saccade. Before and after a saccade occurs, when the pause cell population is active, it can open two gating pathways. A Now Print gate (pathway 15) enables pathway 7 from the TPM_2 to learn the eye position that was attained by the last saccade. A read-out gate (pathway 16) enables the HMI to read-out a vector command along pathway 14 to the RM, where it can be stored in STM. As soon as a saccade begins, both gates shut. Learning within the HMI therefore cannot occur during a saccade, and new vectors from the HMI cannot be read-out during a saccade. Consequently the RM command can be stored until after a saccade is over. It can thereby sample second light error signals using its conditionable pathways within the adaptive gain (AG) stage, or cerebellum (Chapter 3). After a saccade terminates, the pause cell turns on and both gates open again. It takes some time, however, for the target position within the TPM_2 to be reset, for a new vector to be computed by the HMI, for this new vector to activate the RM via pathway 14, and for the new RM input to competitively inhibit the stored RM position. During this time interval, the old RM position can sample second light error signals at the AG stage.

Reset of the RM position is accomplished in the same way that an updated target position from the TPM_1 resets the TPM_2. This type of competitive reset of the RM follows from the ability of the RM to contrast enhance and store retinotopic inputs using a shunting on-center off-surround feedback network (Chapter 6).

The conjoint action of target-driven gating and saccade-driven gating help to refine our explanation of the Shebilske (1977) data in Section 4.12. Shebilske found that incorrect saccades in response to a briefly flashed light could correct themselves in the dark. In Figure 9.4, the target-driven gate remains closed after such an incorrect saccade, because a mismatch of eye position with target position occurs within the HMI. After the incorrect saccade terminates, however, the saccade-driven gate opens, and enables the new HMI vector to instate an updated movement command in the RM. A corrective saccade ensues.

Several alternative saccade-driven gating schemes all possess the functional properties that we need, and may therefore exist *in vivo*. For example, pause cells could inhibit tonic cells that inhibit learning and vector read-out, thereby causing a disinhibitory gating reaction, rather than a direct excitatory gating reaction, in pathways 7 and 14. A saccadic burst cell population could directly inhibit learning in pathway 7 and read-out to the RM in pathway 14 (Chapter 7). To test whether one has discovered such gate-controlling cells *in vivo*, lesion experiments of several types can be carried out. For example, suppose that pathway 11 in the target-driven gating system were cut. Then outputs from the HMI could occur even in the absence of target position inputs. Saccade staircases would therefore ensue. Suppose that pathway 16 in the saccade-driven gating system were cut. Then HMI outputs could continually reset the RM during a saccade. Consequently, by the time a correct saccade was over, the RM would have received an input corresponding to the smallest vectors that it can encode. This, in itself, is not a bad property. However, if the RM were then required to relearn its conditioned AG gains, it could not do so, because it would have "forgotten" the vector which caused the saccade by the time the saccade was over.

9.8. Parietal Light-Sensitive and Saccade Neurons

The on-center cells within the TPM_1 and the TPM_2 have properties that are analogous to those of light-sensitive neurons and saccade neurons in the parietal cortex, respectively. The TPM_1 cells are light-sensitive because lights are an important information source in building up a TPM in head coordinates. If these cells in the TPM_1 store activity in STM without triggering a saccade, then their activity can persist for a long time. However, as soon as they initiate a saccade by activating the TPM_2, their activity is rapidly inhibited by negative feedback from the TPM_2 (pathway 6 in Figure 9.3). Thus these TPM_1 cells have the curious property that they shut off just when the saccade begins that their stored light might have been expected to control. Yin and Mountcastle (1977, p.1383, Figure 2A) have reported the existence of a light-sensitive cell type with similar properties in their parietal lobe data.

Supraliminal activation of TPM_2 cells, by contrast, causes these cells to generate a saccade and to persistently fire due to their STM storage until the saccade is over. These TPM_2 cells are not as sensitive to light because they are activated by TPM_1 cells, and only when the control processes which regulate pathways 2 and 10 in Figure 9.3 allow. These cell properties resemble those of the saccade neurons in the parietal cortex (Lynch, 1980; Motter and Mountcastle, 1981). In Chapter 11, we will summarize the similar properties of visuomovement cells and movement cells in the frontal eye fields (Bruce and Goldberg, 1984).

Experimental tests can be made of whether parietal light-sensitive and saccade neurons or frontal visuomovement and movement neurons are examples of TPM_1 and TPM_2 cells, respectively. Electrical stimulation of a saccade neuron should inhibit its light-sensitive source via pathway 6 in Figure 9.3. Cutting or otherwise inactivating this inhibitory feedback pathway should enable the light-sensitive neuron to remain on during the ensuing saccade. The light-sensitive cell should also respond to certain eye positions, in particular the eye positions which together with appropriate retinal positions give rise to the target position of a TPM_1 cell. The saccade neuron should remain on when an incorrect saccade occurs in the dark until after a corrective saccade of Shebilske type is made.

In addition to cells with properties of light-sensitive neurons and saccade neurons, the PCN also contains other cells with interesting characteristics. We have already noted that the target-driven and saccade-driven gating systems can be controlled by pause cells or by burst cells. In fact, several types of pause cells are included in Figure 9.4. The pause cell which controls pathway 11 will shut off just before and during a correct PCN-generated saccade and will then turn back on until the next TPM_2 command is instated. However, after an incorrect PCN-generated saccade occurs, such a pause cell will remain off until a corrective saccade of Shebilske type can be made. By contrast, the pause cells which control pathways 15 and 16 will turn off during any saccade, whether or not it is generated by the PCN and whether or not it is correct. The cells which control the "rehearsal wave" pathway 9 are also pause cells. These cells turn off only when the TPM_2 is active and a mismatch is registered within the HMI. Thus they turn off only for saccades that are generated by the PCN, and remain off during corrective saccades (Section 5.5). In addition to these differences, the onset and offset times of these different types of pause cell types are not synchronous.

Thus a neurophysiological study of a circuit such as Figure 9.4 would reveal several populations of pause cells whose local cell properties, as such, would provide an insufficient index of the cells' functional role in the network. This very difficulty also illustrates the more optimistic evolutionary theme that a small number of local cell properties can give rise to a complex repertoire of network functions.

9.9. Switching between Movement and Postural Eye Position Maps: Frontal Eye Field Control

Our analysis of the PCN has focused upon how a pattern of stored target positions can give rise to a sequence of predictive saccades. We have shown how such a stored activity pattern at the TPM_1 can sequentially activate an RM and can correct Shebilske-type errors due to mistranslation of a saccadic command between the RM and the eye muscles. This analysis calls attention to the following issues.

Before a predictive saccade takes place, the RM of the PCN and an EPM that registers initial eye position must both send their movement commands to the SG. The RM and the EPM are part of the eye position update network (EPUN) that was described in Chapter 7. *After* a predictive saccade is over, it takes some time for the next TPM_1 command to be instated within the TPM_2 and then give rise to the next RM output. In order to prevent postsaccadic drifts from occurring between these saccades, the EPM of the tension equalization network (TEN) must switch on to read-out its conditioned postural gains.

This discussion emphasizes that two different types of EPMs are turned on and off at different phases of the saccadic cycle in order to guarantee the accuracy of movements and the stability of postures. The EPM which cooperates with the RM to generate the SG input is called the *movement EPM*, or EPM_M. The EPM which controls postural gains is called the *postural EPM*, or EPM_{Pos}.

Figure 9.5 schematizes the timing of RM, EPM_M, and EPM_{Pos} onsets and offsets during a series of saccades. The durations of the EPM_M signals are not certain. They may be as long as the sillouettes drawn in Figure 9.5, or they may be more synchronous with RM durations, as illustrated by the cross-hatched area. We will develop some implications of the latter hypothesis.

Suppose that the RM and the EPM_M are synchronously switched on and off, while the EPM_{Pos} is being switched off and on. The simplest way to accomplish these properties is to suppose that the gating system which turns the RM on and off also turns the EPM_M on and off while it turns the EPM_{Pos} off and on. This gating system is a saccade-driven gating system.

It remains to suggest where the cells that carry out these EPM functions may be found. We hypothesize the the computation and storage

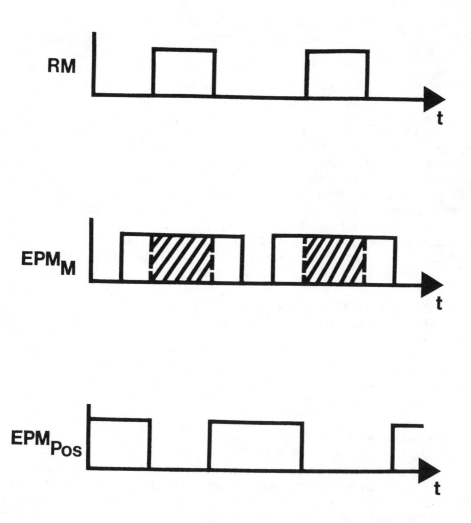

Figure 9.5. Timing of activity in the retinotopic map (RM), the movement eye position map (EPM$_M$), and the postural eye position map (EPM$_{Pos}$): The RM and EPM$_M$ activities are out-of-phase with the EPM$_{Pos}$ activities. The EPM$_M$ activities may occur only during the hatched times or during the broader time intervals that alternate with EPM$_{Pos}$ activity.

of temporal order information by the TPM_1 takes place in the frontal eye fields (FEF) as part of the frontal lobes' role in cognitive and motor planning. All of the subsequent PCN stages—TPM_2, HMI, and RM—could also, in principle, take place in the FEF, or in regions to which the FEF projects. Let us consider the hypothesis that the EPM_M and/or the EPM_{Pos} are also computed within the FEF. Is there any evidence for such an assumption? Cells within an EPM have properties analogous to those of fixation neurons, which exist in the FEF (Suzuki and Azuma, 1977). Lesions of the FEF can cause fixation deficits in monkeys (Latto and Cowey, 1971). Such a deficit could be caused, for example, by destruction of the EPM_{Pos}, since the conditioned gains needed to maintain a stable posture could not then be read into the MN cells. By contrast, both humans and monkeys can maintain visual fixation after posterior parietal lesions (Hyvärinen, 1982). Hyvärinen compares the fixity of gaze after posterior parietal damage in humans to the somatic dystonia that follows extrapyramidal cortical ablation. He concludes that "the role of the posterior parietal cortex is to interrupt fixation when an interesting visual stimulus appears in the visual periphery" (Hyvärinen, 1982, p.1112). We will discuss possible interactions between the posterior parietal cortex and the frontal eye fields in Chapter 11.

9.10. Direct Computation of Predictive Difference Vectors from Stored Retinotopic Positions?

We now consider some functional problems that would need to be solved if a neural system were to directly transform stored retinotopic positions R_1, R_2, ..., R_m into difference vectors.

A. *Getting Started*

The first problem is to get started. Consider the first light R_1 in a stored predictive sequence of retinotopically coded positions. How is R_1 encoded into a difference vector? With what stored quantity R_0 does R_1 get compared in order to compute the correct difference vector $R_1 - R_0$? To emphasize the nature of this difficulty, suppose that the last saccade was made in response to a sound, not to a light. How does the system know how to subtract R_1 from the "retinotopic" position R_0 of the sound?

These considerations suggest that a brain capable of solving this problem would encode all sources of movement commands, including auditory sources, within a *universal* retinotopic map, or URM (Figure 9.6a). Such a URM would store only the retinotopic position of the last movement command to be executed. When R_1 was read-out to be converted into a difference vector, so too would the previously stored command in R_0 in the URM (Figure 9.6b). Both retinotopic commands would be read-into a region where the difference vector $R_1 - R_0$ could be computed.

As R_1 was read-out of its RM, it would self-inhibit its RM representation to prevent perseverative performance of its movement command. It would also inhibit R_0 at the URM in order to instate itself into STM storage there. Once stored in the URM, R_1 could later be read-out along with R_2 to compute the difference vector $R_2 - R_1$ (Figure 9.6b).

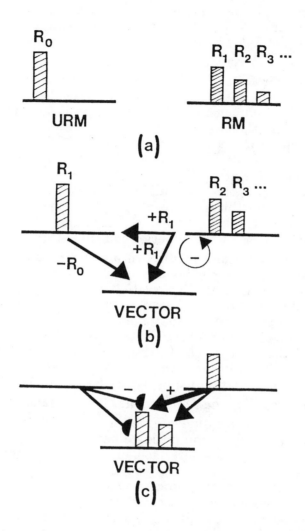

Figure 9.6. A possible circuit for direct recoding of retinotopic positions R_1, R_2, R_3, ..., into difference vectors: (a) Temporal order information is stored in short term memory at the retinotopic positions R_1, R_2, R_3, ..., of the retinotopic map (RM). A previously stored position R_0 is also active at the universal retinotopic map (URM); (b) Activation of these maps transforms R_1 and R_0 into a vector representation. R_0 is replaced in URM by R_1, as R_1 self-inhibits its activity at RM; (c) The transform from RM to the vector representation can be prewired, whereas the transform from the URM can be learned as in the head-muscle interface (HMI).

In summary, the existence of a URM and of coordinated STM reset and storage operations between the URM and all other RMs is implicit in the apparently simple idea that retinotopic commands are directly recoded into difference vectors. These constraints are relatively simple to realize compared with the following ones.

B. *Vector Sign Reversal*

Consider a pair R_1 and R_2 of retinotopic positions corresponding to horizontal eye motions. For simplicity, suppose that these positions are encoded within a 1-dimensional RM whose positions are labeled by real numbers. Consider the case in which both R_1 and R_2 lie to the right of the fovea. Suppose moreover that R_2 lies to the left of R_1. If we label the fovea with the number 0, then $R_1 > R_2 > 0$ and $R_2 - R_1 < 0$. The problem can now be stated: How can retinotopic positions with one sign (in this case positive) generate a difference vector with the correct length and opposite sign (in this case negative)? The need for such a property is strikingly illustrated by the data of Mays and Sparks concerning the quasi-visual (QV) cells of the superior colliculus (Section 4.2).

We have not succeeded in discovering any neurally plausible mechanism whereby these properties can be achieved through a mapping of an RM and a URM into another *spatial* map (Chapter 6). No plausible combination of narrow or broad excitatory or inhibitory spatial gradients seems capable of generating a spatial encoding which can simultaneously represent the length and the direction of all physically realizable difference vectors. In particular, a single difference vector can be realized by many pairs of retinotopic positions. We see no way to neurally accomplish this many-to-one transformation using signals between spatial maps.

C. *Motor Recoding and Dimensional Inconsistency*

From this perspective, one can better appreciate the type of solution that we have suggested for computing difference vectors. In Chapter 4, we introduced the head-muscle interface, or HMI, and suggested that vector differences are computed in muscle coordinates, not within a spatial map. We also showed that the same process which learns the transformation into muscle coordinates can automatically compute difference vectors. Motor coordinates are ideal for computing difference vectors because the balance of excitation and inhibition across their agonist-antagonist populations can easily encode a reversal of sign, as in $R_2 - R_1 < 0$.

Retinotopic coordinates are, however, dimensionally inconsistent with motor coordinates. By contrast, target position coordinates are dimensionally consistent with motor coordinates. That is why recoding of retinotopic coordinates into target position coordinates was necessary before the target position coordinates could be recoded into motor coordinates at the HMI.

D. *Opponent Recoding and Linearity*

Another possibility is suggested by the HMI example. Perhaps the opponency of agonist-antagonist populations can be used without their motor interpretation. Perhaps each RM is recoded into a vector field that is encoded with opponent populations, albeit opponent populations that are not derived from motor outflow or inflow signals (Figure 9.6c). Such a recoding into opponent populations could be achieved by spatial gradients from the RM to the vector field. The URM could, in turn, learn these opponent patterns using the learning mechanism which is found within the HMI (Figure 9.6c).

This scheme also faces a formidable obstacle. Unless the spatial gradients from the RM to the vector field vary *linearly* with RM position, then retinotopic positions R_1, R_2, and R_3 which generate the same *formal* difference vector $R_3 - R_2 = R_2 - R_1$ could generate different patterns of opponent activation at the vector field. Moreover, the same pattern of opponent activation at the vector field could be generated by different vector differences of RM and URM positions. Such a vector field could not generate consistent movement commands.

One can now better appreciate how the HMI solves this problem. Corollary discharges derived from motor outflow signals are used to compute present position signals at the HMI. These present position signals are linearly related to present eye position signals due to the action of the muscle linearization network, or MLN (Chapter 5). Target position signals learn these corollary discharges at the HMI, and the HMI computes a vector whose suprathreshold activities vary linearly with the difference of target position and present position. Then these vectors can be consistently mapped back into retinotopic coordinates to generate movement commands which are corrected by second light error signals (Chapter 3).

We have not discovered any neurally plausible mechanism whereby direct recoding of retinotopic maps RM and URM into difference vectors can achieve these linearity properties. Due to the combined impact of these failures, we have reached the tentative conclusion that retinotopically coded positions are not directly recoded as difference vectors. If this conclusion is correct, then retinotopically coded cells in a predictive region, such as the frontal eye fields, may elsewhere be recoded into target positions before being recoded once again into difference vectors in motor coordinates at an HMI.

Such a recoding into target position coordinates may be implicit rather than explicit. As we will show in Chapter 10, combinations of retinotopic and eye position signals can be distributed across a network in such a way that certain cells act *as if* they are encoded in target position coordinates, even though they may also be excited by many different combinations of retinotopic and eye position signals.

It cannot yet be ruled out that other neural designs than the ones we have considered are capable of directly transforming retinotopic positions into difference vectors. If such a design does exist, then we might anticipate that it solves the functional problems which we have identified, such as coordinated reset of all RMs with a URM, and vector sign reversal using opponent processing. In addition, such a network would most likely inhibit all the stored positions in its predictive RM each time a new pattern of lights was instated there. Otherwise, sequential scanning of a fixed set of light sources could encode each light with a new retinotopic position every time the eye moved. After n eye movements, each nonfoveated light would have n retinotopic encodings within the RM, thereby creating massive confusions in the choice of which light should be foveated next. It therefore seems unlikely that any RM which is not totally reset by a new light input is directly recoded into difference vectors. This STM reset property can be used to indirectly test the nature of the retinotopic recoding into difference vectors in brain regions where all the transformations leading to difference vectors are not under direct experimental control.

If an RM is recoded into an invariant target position map (TPM) before the TPM is used to compute difference vectors, then total reset of the RM by each new light is not necessary, but also is not forbidden. We now turn to an analysis of how an RM may be implicitly recoded into an invariant TPM.

CHAPTER 10
FORMATION OF AN INVARIANT
TARGET POSITION MAP

10.1. Invariant Self-Regulating Multimodal Maps

In Section 1.4, we described properties that it would be desirable for a target position map (TPM) to possess. The most important property is that of map *invariance*; namely, the many-to-one activation of a single spatial locus that corresponds to a prescribed target position, no matter which of the many possible combinations of retinal position and eye position give rise to that target position. In an invariant TPM, after movements of the eye occur with respect to a fixed light source, no change occurs in the spatial locus which the light activates. More generally, if an invariant TPM stores a pattern of n lights, no change occurs in the spatial positions of map activation as the eyes inspect the successive lights. Although the spatial positions of map activation do not change, other more subtle indices may change. For example, habituation may reduce the activation of a target position if it is stored in the map for a long time (Grossberg, 1980, 1982b). Such an habituated target position could gradually lose its ability to attract an observer's attention.

In a noninvariant TPM, by contrast, a different map position is activated by a fixed light each time the observer moves his eyes. A single light can hereby activate a series of target positions. These target loci cannot habituate as a function of the total time that the light has been stored. Using multiple noninvariant encodings of a single target position in a predictive command network (PCN) could cause serious problems, since the very act of saccading to a target position could activate a new spatial locus corresponding to that target position, as well as new loci corresponding to all the remaining target positions, simply because the eyes moved. These multiple activations and reactivations could cause a breakdown in the temporal order code that was moving the eyes (Chapter 9). We therefore restrict our attention to the design of invariant TPMs in this chapter.

As in our discussion of spatial maps in Chapter 6, we will describe more than one possible design of an invariant TPM. Both designs satisfy the theory's functional requirements and both are built up from plausible neural mechanisms. One TPM design depends more heavily on prewired mechanisms. The other design is built up through learning. This latter design has remarkable formal properties. Indeed, it possesses all of the properties which were listed in Section 1.4 as desirable ones for a TPM to have, including invariance, self-regulation, error tolerance, and multimodal self-consistency. Of special interest is the way in which macroscopic functional properties emerge from the interaction of microscopic cellular processes. Notable among the microscopic processes from which an invariant TPM can be synthesized are chemical transmitter systems that possess autoreceptors. Certain catecholaminergic transmitter systems are well known to possess autoreceptors (Cubeddu, Hoffmann, and James, 1983; Dubocovich and Weiner, 1982; Groves and Tepper, 1983; Groves, Fenster, Tepper, Nakamura, and Young, 1981; Niedzwiecki, Mailman, and Cubeddu, 1984; Siever and Sulser, 1984; Tepper, Young, and Groves, 1984). However, this is the first time that they have been used to explain such a high-order functional capability as invariant multimodal map formation. We will show how to combine a known transmitter learning equation and transmitter autoreceptor equation (Grossberg, 1981, 1984) into a new self-regulating transmitter learning equation. When this new transmitter learning equation is obeyed at all the learning synapses of a properly designed neural circuit, it enables the circuit as a whole to learn an invariant TPM. In particular, the autoreceptive part of the new learning equation enables the circuit as a whole to compensate for variable numbers of sampling sources without causing any contradictions in the rules which emerge through learning. This theory of how invariant multimodal maps can self-organize is potentially relevant to a large class of problems concerning the emergence of maps and rules in neurobiology and artificial intelligence.

10.2. Prewired Positional Gradients: The Mean Value Property

Several schemes for generating prewired TPMs are known. They are all based on variants of the following simple idea. Consider for the moment one-dimensional maps; for example, maps of target position in a horizontal direction. Imagine that a one-dimensional retinotopic map (RM) and a one-dimensional eye position map (EPM) map topographically onto a one-dimensional TPM, as in Figure 10.1. Denote the activated position of the RM by R and the activated position of the EPM by E. Our task is to design an TPM which is maximally excited at a single spatial locus, in response to any physical choice of R and E such that $R + E = $ constant. Denote the one-dimensional spatial variable of the TPM by p. We will describe several schemes which imply that the maximally excited spatial locus of the TPM is

$$p = \frac{1}{2}(R + E);\tag{10.1}$$

that is, the mean value of R and E.

The formal constraints governing schemes of this type are easily described. Their neural instantiation is another matter. For example, suppose that activation of position R in the RM causes a spatially distributed input to the TPM of size

$$I_R(p) = Ae^{-\mu(R-p)^2}\tag{10.2}$$

and that activation of position E in the EPM causes a spatially distributed input to the TPM of size

$$I_E(p) = Be^{-\mu(E-p)^2}.\tag{10.3}$$

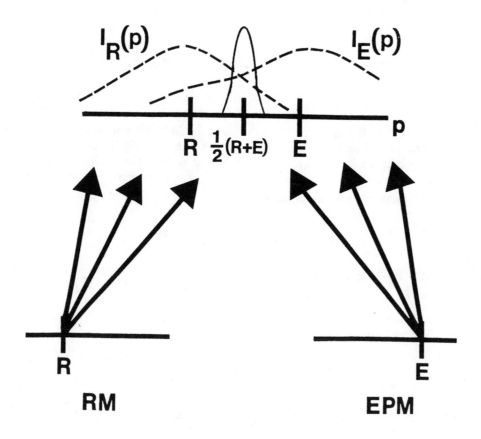

Figure 10.1. Generating a 1-dimensional target position map (TPM) from a 1-dimensional retinotopic map (RM) and eye position map (EPM): Each position R in the RM and E in the EPM activates a broadly distributed gradient of pathways to the TPM. The TPM contrast enhances the total inputs, thereby focusing its activity near position $\frac{1}{2}(R + E)$.

In other words, the RM and the EPM cause Gaussianly distributed inputs to the TPM whose maxima occur at positions $p = R$ and $p = E$, respectively. Such gradients could develop, for example, due to growth of connections from the RM and EPM to the TPM guided by TPM morphogens which undergo significant lateral diffusion within the TPM.

Suppose that the activity pattern caused within the TPM by active R and E loci is given by

$$x_1(p) = I_R(p)I_E(p). \tag{10.4}$$

Alternatively, suppose that the TPM activity pattern is defined by

$$x_2(p) = I_R(p) + I_E(p). \tag{10.5}$$

In other words, the input patterns generate TPM activation either through a multiplicative (shunting, gating) process, as in (10.4), or through an additive process, as in (10.5). The shunting process is more robust, but both processes work within an achievable parameter range.

In the shunting case, equations (10.2)–(10.4) imply that

$$x_1(p) = ABe^{-\mu[(R-p)^2+(E-p)^2]}. \tag{10.6}$$

The position $p = P_1$ at which $x_1(p)$ is maximum is found by minimizing quantity

$$(R - p)^2 + (E - p)^2. \tag{10.7}$$

This minimum occurs at

$$P_1 = \frac{1}{2}(R + E). \tag{10.8}$$

A similar conclusion holds for the additive gradient $x_2(p)$. An important addition constraint holds in the additive case, however, since a maximum occurs at

$$P_2 = \frac{1}{2}(R + E) \tag{10.9}$$

only if the positions R and E are not too far apart relative to the decay rate μ of the Gaussian positional gradients. In particular $y = \mid R - E \mid$ must not be larger than the unique positive root of the equation

$$2e^{\frac{-\mu}{4}y^2} - e^{-\mu y^2} = 1. \tag{10.10}$$

Thus broad positional gradients are needed to admit a wide range of R and E values. No such quantitative constraints on μ exist in the shunting case. However, even in the shunting case, μ must be chosen sufficiently small to guarantee physically realizable gradients which cover the entire TPM.

Gaussian gradients are not the only ones that imply the mean value property in (10.8) and (10.9). Exponential gradients $I_R(p) = Ae^{-\mu|R-p|}$ and $I_E(p) = Be^{-\mu|E-p|}$ could, for example, also be used, as could other gradients that decrease with the distance from the inducing input sources R and E.

Invariant target positions can also be derived from two dimensional RMs and EPMs. Then formulas like (10.2) and (10.3) for $R(p)$ and $E(p)$, respectively, generalize to

$$I_R(p, q) = (A_1 e^{-\mu(R_1-p)^2}, A_2 e^{-\nu(R_2-q)^2}) \qquad (10.11)$$

and

$$I_E(p, q) = (B_1 e^{-\mu(E_1-p)^2}, B_2 e^{-\nu(E_2-q)^2}) \qquad (10.12)$$

and a formula such as (10.4) for $x_1(p)$ generalizes to

$$x_1(p, q) = (A_1 B_1 e^{-\mu[(R_1-p)^2+(E_1-p)^2]}, A_2 B_2 e^{-\nu[(R_2-q)^2+(E_2-q)^2]}). \qquad (10.13)$$

The spatial locus of maximal activity of the activity pattern $x_1(p, q)$ occurs at the position (P_1, Q_1) such that

$$P_1 = \frac{1}{2}(R_1 + E_1) \qquad (10.14)$$

and

$$Q_1 = \frac{1}{2}(R_2 + E_2). \qquad (10.15)$$

In both the one-dimensional and two-dimensional maps, the strongest input constraint is the requirement that eye positions match up, at least approximately, with the corresponding retinal positions. This requirement can be met, for example, by mapping tonic cell output patterns into an EPM using a one-dimensional or three-dimensional position-threshold-slope (PTS) shift map (Chapter 6.3).

If retinal position and eye position are combined one dimension at a time, then an extra processing stage is needed to combine the one-dimensional maps. This final stage only needs to achieve response selectivity, because invariance is already guaranteed by the one-dimensional maps. Several types of coincidence detectors can achieve the desired selectivity, as can an adaptive filter (Chapter 6).

In all versions of a prewired TPM, the final stage must contrast enhance the final activity pattern in order to convert its diffusely distributed activity into a sharply defined target position. In general, many of the mechanisms that go into the design of prewired TPMs are specializations of the general spatial mapping mechanisms that were described in Chapter 6.

It remains to discuss how shunting rules like (10.4) and additive rules like (10.5) could be physically instantiated. The additive rule (10.5) has an obvious neural interpretation. The shunting rule (10.4) deserves serious consideration if only because preliminary data of Anderson, Essick, and Siegel (1984) suggest that the interaction of eye position and retinal position information in the parietal cortex of macaque monkeys may be approximately multiplicative. A presynaptic gating action of EPM synaptic knobs on RM synaptic knobs is a possible shunting mechanism.

10.3.   Self-Organizing Target Position Maps: Multimodal Sampling of a Unimodal Eye Position Map

We now turn to a problem that we find much more engaging: the problem of invariant TPM self-organization. In our treatment of this problem, we will assume that an RM and an EPM exist and act as sources of conditionable pathways which converge upon another EPM. Denote the sampling EPM by EPM_1 and the sampled EPM by EPM_2. We will show how cooperative self-organization of the signalling from the RM and the EPM_1 convert EPM_2 into an invariant TPM. The internal structures of the sampling maps RM and EPM_1 do not need to be topographically organized, but EPM_2 does have an internal topography. Moreover, the design works given any number of sampling maps, not just two. Any number of modalities can join to learn a globally self-consistent rule at the sampled map using the mechanisms that we will describe. We focus on the case of two sampling maps RM and EPM_1 because that is our main application.

Suppose that the RM and the EPM_1 store a retinal position and an initial eye position in short term memory (STM) before a saccade begins. Assume that STM storage persists until after the saccade is over. Also assume that the accuracy of the saccades progressively improves through time due to learning via second light error signals (Chapter 3). In other words, the saccades in question are the visually reactive saccades of the retinotopic command network (RCN). The invariant TPM that we will describe is built up on the shoulders of RCN learning.

We will consider a time frame when these RCN-generated saccades are already quite accurate. After such an accurate saccade terminates, a Now Print gate opens, just like in the HMI (Chapter 9), and allows the RM and the EPM_1 to sample the activity locus within the EPM_2. This EPM_2 activity locus encodes target position *because* the saccade was accurate. It codes target position *invariantly* because it is a unimodal code that is directly derived from final eye position, rather than from a multimodal combination of retinal position and initial eye position.

This kind of many-to-one learning will go on until activating positions within the RM and the EPM_1 can begin to reliably activate EPM_2 positions before a saccade occurs. Once the RM and the EPM_1 can reliably activate the EPM_2, then the EPM_2 will automatically become an invariant TPM.

Then the invariant TPM positions can begin to learn TPM muscle coordinates at the HMI, the HMI vectors can begin to be encoded by an RM, and so on, as in Chapters 4 and 9. Processing stages that learn temporally stable maps can successively support the formation of further temporally stable maps. Thus, intentional movement controls emerge in a developmental progression.

10.4. Double Duty by Sampling Maps and their Neural Interpretation

The retinotopic map RM that samples EPM_2 has the same properties as the RM which is the basis of retinotopic sampling of the adaptive gain (AG) stage in the RCN (Chapter 3). The simplest hypothesis is that these two maps are really the same map, and thus that this RM also controls the direct unconditioned pathway and the indirect conditioned pathway that generate visually reactive saccades. The eye position map EPM_1 that samples the EPM_2 has the same properties as the EPM that updates eye position signals to the SG within the eye position update network, or EPUN (Chapter 7). The simplest hypothesis is that these two maps are also a single map. We therefore interpret EPM_1 as the movement EPM, or EPM_M, that was discussed in Chapter 9.

The sampled map EPM_2 becomes an invariant TPM by virtue of the learning rules whereby RM and EPM_1 interact with it. The map EPM_2 need not have any internally invariant properties. Any reasonably continuous change of activation locus in EPM_2 with final eye position will do. Any of the spatial mapping mechanisms of Chapter 6 satisfy this modest formal requirement. The theory thus suggests that the invariant TPM emerges from a noninvariant EPM.

The posterior parietal cortex is the most likely anatomical site for such an invariant TPM (Hyvärinen, 1982; Lynch, 1980; Motter and Mountcastle, 1981). Hence the model suggests that, at an early developmental stage, the posterior parietal cortex may be sensitive to a unimodal source of final eye position before its cells can encode target position as a function of multimodal visual and initial eye position signals. The model also suggests that the RM and the EPM_1 which sample EPM_2 are no "higher" in the cortical hierarchy than the parietal cortex.

Given this constraint, the RM is best interpreted at the present time as being somewhere on the pathways from superior colliculus and visual cortex to posterior parietal lobe. The EPM_1, and thus the movement EPM, or EPM_M of Section 9.9 may be housed in the parietal cortex, since it is probably not found in visual cortex. This argument makes it seem unlikely that the EPM_M lies in the frontal cortex, where the postural EPM, or EPM_{Pos}, seems to reside. Such an anatomical interpretation of the EPM_M suggests that many cells in parietal cortex are exclusively sensitive to eye position, as opposed to light, even in the adult, and that these cells will be activated by initial eye position rather than by final eye position.

10.5. Associative Learning at Autoreceptive Synaptic Knobs

The learning rule which we will apply joins together two properties of chemical transmitter models (Grossberg, 1981, 1984) into a new self-regulating transmitter learning equation. One property concerns an associative learning rule of the form

$$\frac{d}{dt} z_{ij} = \epsilon S_i [-A z_{ij} + B x_j]. \tag{10.16}$$

In (10.16), z_{ij} is interpreted as the production rate of a chemical transmitter in the synaptic knob(s) of pathway(s) e_{ij} from cell (population) v_i to cell (population) v_j. This is essentially the same learning rule that we used in (6.19) to learn a spatial map. In (10.16), S_i is a presynaptic sampling signal that travels along pathway e_{ij}. If $S_i = 0$, then $\frac{d}{dt} z_{ij} = 0$. Hence a presynaptic signal, rather than the postsynaptic signal of (6.19), turns on the plasticity of this transmitter system. The small parameter ϵ just says that the learning rate can be chosen to be slow even if S_i can become large.

As in our discussion of associative learning in Chapter 6, we also assume that transmitter is released at a rate proportional to $S_i z_{ij}$. This property leads us to consider the second property of chemical transmitter models that we will use. The equation

$$\frac{d}{dt} z_{ij} = C(D - z_{ij}) - S_i z_{ij} - E \sum_{k=1}^{n} S_k z_{kj} \tag{10.17}$$

says that, in the absence of any transmitter release (all $S_k = 0$), z_{ij} accumulates to a target level D. This target level is determined by two factors: a constant production rate (term CD) combined with feedback inhibition (term $-C z_{ij}$) of transmitter z_{ij} onto an intermediate stage of transmitter production. When the sampling signal S_i is turned on, transmitter is released at a rate $S_i z_{ij}$; hence the term $-S_i z_{ij}$. The additional term $-E \sum_{k=1}^{n} S_k z_{kj}$ says that a fraction of the total transmitter released at cell v_j is reabsorbed by autoreceptors into the synaptic knobs of pathway e_{ij}. Once in these knobs, the reabsorbed transmitter inhibits transmitter production via feedback inhibition.

A major effect of autoreceptive inhibition is to normalize the total amount of transmitter impinging upon a postsynaptic cell. To see why this is so, suppose for definiteness that all presynaptic signals $S_i = 1$. Let the total amount of transmitter produced in pathways abutting v_j be denoted by $z_j = \sum_{k=1}^{n} z_{kj}$. Then (10.17) implies that

$$\frac{d}{dt} z_j = nCD - C z_j - (1 + nE) z_j. \tag{10.18}$$

At equilibrium, $\frac{d}{dt}z_j = 0$, so that

$$z_j = \frac{nCD}{1 + C + nE}.$$ (10.19)

By (10.19), $z_j \leq \frac{CD}{E}$ no matter how many pathways impinge upon v_j. Thus the total amount of transmitter does not grow with the total number of pathways. This is the normalization, or conservation, property that we seek.

In our present application, this type of normalization helps to achieve self-regulation of the TPM. In Grossberg (1981), this property was used to explain how very large lesions of the nigrostriatal bundle can cause surprisingly minor behavioral deficits (Stricker and Zigmond, 1976). To see how such sparing can occur in system (10.17), suppose that some pathways p_{ij} to v_j are cut. Then feedback inhibition of transmitter production within the remaining pathways is reduced, thereby amplifying their transmitter production levels in a compensatory fashion.

The transmitter learning rule that we will use combines the transmitter laws (10.16) and (10.17) into the single law

$$\frac{d}{dt}z_{ij} = eS_i[-Fz_{ij} + Gx_j - H\sum_{k=1}^{n} S_k z_{kj}].$$ (10.20)

In (10.20), the constant asymptote D of (10.17) is replaced, due to learning, by a variable asymptote proportional to x_j, as in (10.16). This apparently simple change has profound consequences for the course of learning when equation (10.20) holds at all the cells v_j at which learning occurs. Term $-AS_i z_{ij}$ in (10.16) and term $-S_i z_{ij}$ in (10.17) are absorbed into term $-FS_i z_{ij}$ in (10.20). Term S_i in (10.20) also gates the autoreceptive influx $-H\sum_{k=1}^{n} S_k z_{kj}$. Although this property is of conceptual interest, it did not substantially influence our simulations due to the slow forgetting rate $-eF$.

Given the learning rule (10.20), all of the desired TPM properties arise through self-organization just so long as combinations of RM and EPM$_1$ positions are allowed to sample the correct target eye positions within EPM$_2$. Thus individual cells in the EPM$_2$ can receive simultaneous sampling signals from the RM and the EPM$_1$. By equation (10.20), an RM-activated LTM trace and an EPM$_1$-activated LTM trace can influence one another through autoreceptive interactions at the same sampled cell in EPM$_2$. We will now describe how this interaction influences the self-organization process both mathematically and through computer simulation results.

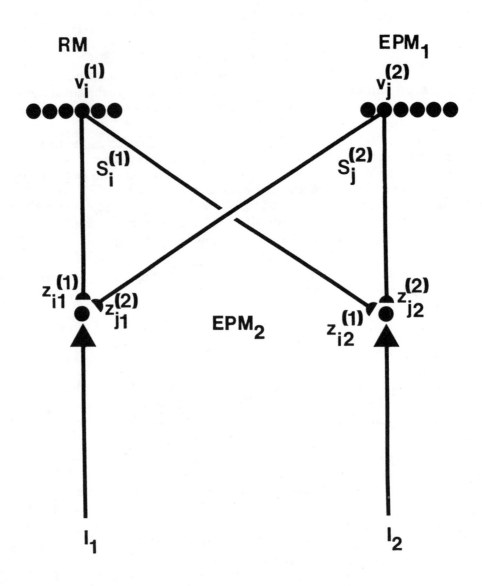

Figure 10.2. Self-organization of an invariant self-regulating target position map due to simultaneous sampling by a retinotopic map (RM) and an eye position map (EPM$_1$) of another eye position map (EPM$_2$): Pairs of sampling cells $v_i^{(1)}$ in RM and $v_j^{(2)}$ in EPM$_1$ conjointly learn the target position patterns (I$_1$, I$_2$) via their LTM traces $z_{ik}^{(1)}$ and $z_{jk}^{(2)}$, respectively, where $k = 1, 2$.

10.6. Multimodal Learning of Invariant Self-Regulating Spatial Maps

Figure 10.2 describes a model in which two fields RM and EPM_1 sample spatial patterns of activity across a field EPM_2. Field RM contains p cells $v_i^{(1)}$, $i = 1, 2, \ldots, p$, and field EPM_1 contains q cells $v_j^{(2)}$, $j = 1, 2, \ldots, q$. To simplify our graphic displays, we have chosen EPM_2 to contain only two cells V_1 and V_2, although the results go through for any number of cells, as Section 10.6 will illustrate. Denote the sampling signal from $v_i^{(1)}$ by $S_i^{(1)}$ and the sampling signal from $v_j^{(2)}$ by $S_j^{(2)}$. The LTM traces from $v_i^{(1)}$ to V_k are denoted by $z_{ik}^{(1)}$, and from $v_j^{(2)}$ to V_k are denoted by $z_{jk}^{(2)}$, $i = 1, 2, \ldots, p$; $j = 1, 2, \ldots, q$; $k = 1, 2$. The activities of V_1 and V_2 are denoted by x_1 and x_2, respectively. The inputs which activate V_1 and V_2 are denoted by I_1 and I_2, respectively. The input pattern (I_1, I_2) represents the target position that is sampled by an appropriate pair $v_i^{(1)}$ and $v_j^{(2)}$ of RM and EPM_1 cells, respectively. We will show how conjoint sampling by pairs of RM and EPM_1 cells leads to learning of this input pattern. Learning is not harmed by increasing the number of cells in RM and EPM_1, despite the fact that such an increase in cells also increases the number of cells in EPM_1 with which each cell in RM is paired, and conversely. Thus no contradictions in rule learning are generated by adding more cells. This example raises the possibility that RM and EPM_1 *in vivo* may directly learn a pattern of corollary discharges at the HMI rather than an invariant TPM.

The equations governing the model are as follows.

EPM_2 Activities

Let

$$\frac{d}{dt}x_1 = -x_1 + I_1 + z_1, \tag{10.21}$$

where z_1 equals the total sampling input from RM and EPM_1 to V_1, namely

$$z_1 = \sum_{i=1}^{p} S_i^{(1)} z_{i1}^{(1)} + \sum_{j=1}^{q} S_j^{(2)} z_{j1}^{(2)}. \tag{10.22}$$

Similarly, let

$$\frac{d}{dt}x_2 = -x_2 + I_2 + z_2, \tag{10.23}$$

where

$$z_2 = \sum_{i=1}^{p} S_i^{(1)} z_{i2}^{(1)} + \sum_{j=1}^{q} S_j^{(2)} z_{j2}^{(2)}. \tag{10.24}$$

Long Term Memory Traces

Let

$$\frac{d}{dt}z_{ik}^{(1)} = \epsilon S_i^{(1)}[-Fz_{ik}^{(1)} + Gx_k - Hz_k] \qquad (10.25)$$

and

$$\frac{d}{dt}z_{jk}^{(2)} = \epsilon S_j^{(2)}[-Fz_{jk}^{(2)} + Gx_k - Hz_k] \qquad (10.26)$$

where $i = 1, 2, \ldots, p$; $j = 1, 2, \ldots, q$; and $k = 1, 2$.

It remains to specify the rule whereby RM and EPM$_1$ signals can sample a consistent target position pattern across EPM$_2$. On every trial, one population $v_i^{(1)}$ in RM and one population $v_j^{(2)}$ in EPM$_1$ is randomly activated. We let $i = i_n$ be the randomly chosen index in $\{1, 2, \ldots, p\}$ of an RM cell and $j = j_n$ be the randomly chosen index in $\{1, 2, \ldots, q\}$ of an EPM$_1$ cell on trial n. In other words,

Sampling Signals

$$S_i^{(1)} = \begin{cases} 1 & \text{if } i = i_n \\ 0 & \text{if } i \neq i_n \end{cases} \qquad (10.27)$$

and

$$S_j^{(2)} = \begin{cases} 1 & \text{if } j = j_n \\ 0 & \text{if } j \neq j_n, \end{cases} \qquad (10.28)$$

where $n = 1, 2, \ldots, N$ and N is the number of learning trials. The inputs to V_1 and V_2 on trial n are denoted by (I_{1n}, I_{2n}). In order to represent target positions, the inputs are chosen to be a function of $i_n + j_n$. For definiteness we consider the following function.

Inputs

$$I_{1n} + I_{2n} = K \qquad (10.29)$$

and

$$I_{2n} = L(i_n + j_n), \qquad (10.30)$$

where K and L are positive constants. In other words, both I_{1n} and I_{2n} are linear functions of the total sampling index $i_n + j_n$, and I_{2n} increases as I_{1n} decreases.

Figure 10.3 describes how the LTM traces from RM and EPM$_1$ to EPM$_2$ build up as a function of how many cells in RM and EPM$_1$ are allowed to sample EPM$_2$. Each figure represents a superposition of RM and EPM$_1$ LTM values. In Figure 10.3b, only 40 cells in RM and EPM$_1$ sample EPM$_2$. In Figure 10.3d, the number of sampling cells in each field is increased to 80, and in Figure 10.3f to 160. Notice that increasing the number of cells, and hence the number of sampling combinations, in going from Figure 10.3b to 10.3d to 10.3f has no significant effect on the LTM values of the previous maps. In other words, the learning process is self-regulatory.

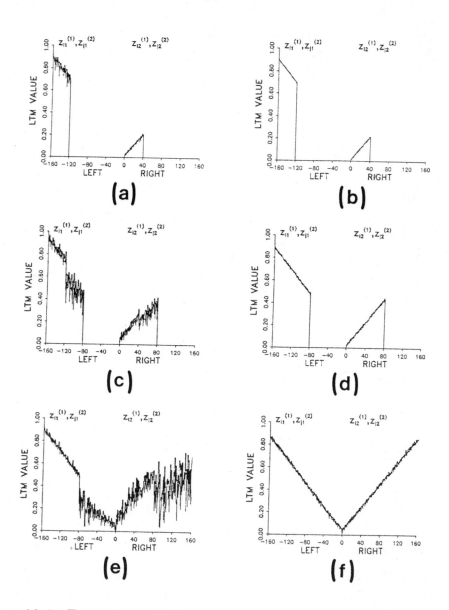

Figure 10.3. Expansion of LTM maps due to increase of the number of cells in the RM and the EPM_1 which sample the EPM_2: (a) Intermediate stage of learning using 40 sampling cells in the RM and the EPM_1; (b) Final stage of learning using 40 cells in each sampling field; (c) Intermediate stage of learning using 80 sampling cells in each field; (d) Final stage of learning using 80 cells; (e) Intermediate stage using 160 cells; (f) Final stage using 160 cells.

Figures 10.3b, d, and f illustrate the final, or asymptotic, LTM values that are obtained after many learning trials. Figures 10.3a, c, and e illustrate intermediate stages of learning. Figure 10.3a describes an intermediate LTM pattern prior to the final LTM pattern in Figure 10.3b. Using the pattern of final LTM values in Figure 10.3b as initial LTM values, an expanded field of sampling inputs then began to learn. Figure 10.3c shows a learning stage intermediate between Figures 10.3b and 10.3d. Then the field of sampling inputs was expanded again. Figure 10.3e shows a learning stage intermediate between Figures 10.3d and 10.3f. One can clearly see how new parts of the LTM maps build up in Figures 10.3a, c, and f.

We now quantify how well the map learning process in Figure 10.3 satisfies the properties of map invariance and self-regulation. Let m equal the number of sampling cells in each of the maps RM and EPM_1. In the following simulations, we chose $m = 40, 80$, and 160. In order to assess map invariance, we first define the mean values of all the LTM traces which abut each sampled cell in EPM_2. We compare these mean values with the sampled input patterns and with each LTM combination that corresponds to the same target position.

Thus we let

$$M_{k1}^{(m)} = \frac{1}{c(k)} \sum_{i+j=k} (z_{i1}^{(1)} + z_{j1}^{(2)}) \tag{10.31}$$

and

$$M_{k2}^{(m)} = \frac{1}{c(k)} \sum_{i+j=k} (z_{i2}^{(1)} + z_{j2}^{(2)}). \tag{10.32}$$

where $c(k)$ is the number of combinations of i and j such that $i + j = k$. In particular,

$$c(k) = \begin{cases} k - 1 & \text{if } k = 2, 3, \ldots, m \\ 2m - k + 1 & \text{if } k = m + 1, m + 2, \ldots, 2m. \end{cases} \tag{10.33}$$

Each summand in (10.31) equals the total LTM trace $z_{i1}^{(1)} + z_{j1}^{(2)}$ from $v_i^{(1)}$ in RM and $v_j^{(2)}$ in EPM_1 such that $i + j = k$. If RM and EPM_1 can cooperate to learn the EPM_2 patterns, then after sufficiently many learning trials, each summand $z_{i1}^{(1)} + z_{j1}^{(2)}$ in (10.31) should approximate $I_1 = K - L(i+j)$, by (10.29) and (10.30), and each summand $z_{i2}^{(1)} + z_{j2}^{(2)}$ in (10.32) should approximate $I_2 = L(i + j)$, by (10.30), for all i and j such that $i + j = k$. Consequently the following standard deviations should be small.

Invariant Map

Let

$$U_k^{(m)} = \left[\sum_{i+j=k} \left[(z_{i1}^{(1)} + z_{j1}^{(2)} - M_{k1}^{(m)})^2 + (z_{i2}^{(1)} + z_{j2}^{(2)} - M_{k2}^{(m)})^2 \right] \right]^{\frac{1}{2}} \tag{10.34}$$

and

$$V_k^{(m)} = \left[\left(\frac{M_{k1}^{(m)}}{M_k^{(m)}} - \frac{K - Lk}{K}\right)^2 + \left(\frac{M_{k2}^{(m)}}{M_k^{(m)}} - \frac{Lk}{K}\right)^2\right]^{\frac{1}{2}} \qquad (10.35)$$

where

$$M_k^{(m)} = M_{k1}^{(m)} + M_{k2}^{(m)}. \qquad (10.36)$$

Figures 10.4 and 10.5 show that both standard deviations are small for each choice of $m = 40, 80, 160$ and all k within the chosen range. The standard deviations $U_k^{(m)}$ in (10.34) show that each combination of retinal position and eye position comes close to the mean value corresponding to the target position. This measure shows that the map exhibits invariance, but it does not show that this invariant map actually learns the input pattern. The standard deviations $V_k^{(m)}$ in (10.35) show that the mean values corresponding to different target positions do learn the input patterns which they sample, up to a scaling factor.

To establish map self-regulation, we must show that the LTM maps are insensitive to the size m of the sampling sets in RM and EPM$_1$. Our computer simulations using the following standard deviations establish this property.

Self-Regulating Map

The numbers

$$W_k^{(M,m)} = \left[(M_{k1}^{(M)} - M_{k1}^{(m)})^2 + (M_{k2}^{(M)} - M_{k2}^{(m)})^2\right]^{\frac{1}{2}} \qquad (10.37)$$

should be small for every pair of sampling set sizes m and M such that $M > m$ and $k = 2, 3, \ldots, 2m$. In Figure 10.6 we plot $W_k^{(M,m)}$ where $m = 40$ and $M = 80$ or 160. The small values of $W_k^{(M,m)}$ demonstrate map self-regulation.

Figure 10.7 illustrates that the map learning process is just as effective if the initial LTM values are randomly chosen numbers between 0 and 1, rather than the zero initial LTM values of Figure 10.3a. Again similar LTM maps emerge. These figures thus show the stability with which the LTM traces form invariant self-regulating asymptotic LTM patterns.

The numerical parameters used to generate Figures 10.3–10.7 are listed below for completeness. The learning rate parameter ϵ in (10.25) and (10.26) was chosen so small that the potentials x_1 and x_2 in (10.21) and (10.23) were always in an approximate equilibrium with respect to the inputs and LTM traces. Hence we set $\frac{d}{dt}x_1 = \frac{d}{dt}x_2 = 0$ and substituted the equations

$$x_1 = I_1 + z_1 \qquad (10.38)$$

and

$$x_2 = I_2 + z_2 \qquad (10.39)$$

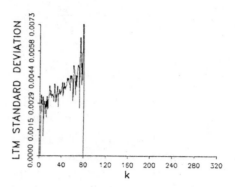

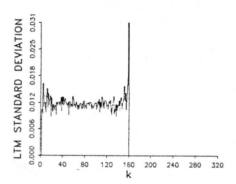

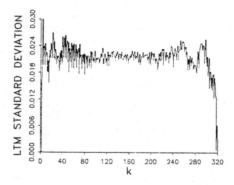

Figure 10.4. Standard deviation $U_k^{(m)}$ in equation (10.34) which measures map invariance: Each picture plots $U_k^{(m)}$ as a function of k with a different value of $m = 40$, 80, or 160.

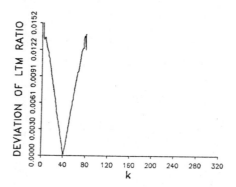

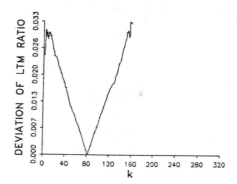

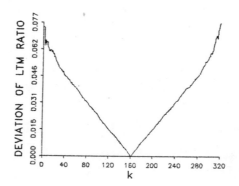

Figure 10.5. Standard deviation $V_k^{(m)}$ in equation (10.35) which measures map invariance: Each picture plots $V_k^{(m)}$ as a function of k with a different value of $m = 40$, 80, or 160.

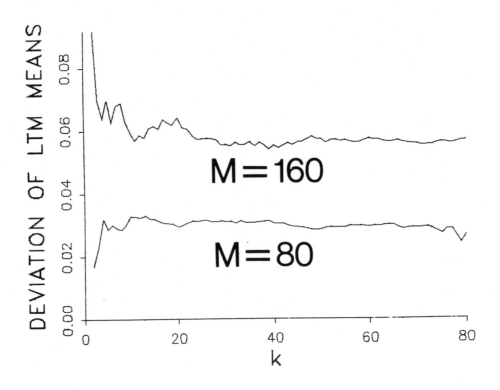

Figure 10.6. Standard deviation $W_k^{(M,40)}$ in equation (10.36) which measures map self-regulation: Each picture plots $W_k^{(M,40)}$ as a function of k with $M = 80$ or 160.

into the LTM equations (10.25) and (10.26). In these LTM equations, we chose

$$F = .2, \tag{10.40}$$

$$G = 1, \tag{10.41}$$

$$H = 2. \tag{10.42}$$

We also chose

$$p = q = 160 \tag{10.43}$$

as the total number of sampling cells in RM and in EPM_1. In the input functions (10.29) and (10.30), we let

$$L = \frac{2}{p+q} = \frac{1}{160} \tag{10.44}$$

and

$$M = 2(1 + L) = \frac{161}{80}. \tag{10.45}$$

Consequently input I_1 in (10.29) varied from $\frac{1}{160}$ to 2 and input I_2 in (10.30) varied from 2 to $\frac{1}{160}$ across learning trials. The total number of learning trials used in Figure 10.3 was $5(10)^5$, divided among the $(160)^2$ possible combinations of randomly chosen sampling pairs. For initial conditions, we chose $x_1(0) = x_2(0) = 0$. We also chose all initial LTM traces equal to zero (Figure 10.3) or equal to randomly chosen numbers between 0 and 1 (Figure 10.7).

10.7. Multimodal Learning of an Invariant Self-Regulating Target Position Map

In order to study formation of a topographic TPM, we replaced the two population EPM_2 of the preceding example with a multicellular EPM_2 network. In order to achieve manageable computation times, we let RM, EPM_1, and EPM_2 each have 40 cells, or cell populations. The activity of the kth cell in EPM_2 was defined by

$$\frac{d}{dt} x_k = -x_k + I_k + z_k, \tag{10.46}$$

$k = 1, 2, \ldots, r$, where

$$z_k = \sum_{i=1}^{p} S_i^{(1)} z_{ik}^{(1)} + \sum_{j=1}^{q} S_j^{(2)} z_{jk}^{(2)}. \tag{10.47}$$

The LTM equations for $z_{ik}^{(1)}$ and $z_{jk}^{(2)}$ are the same as in (10.25) and (10.26) with the addition that $i = 1, 2, \ldots, p, j = 1, 2, \ldots, q$, and $k = 1, 2, \ldots, r$.

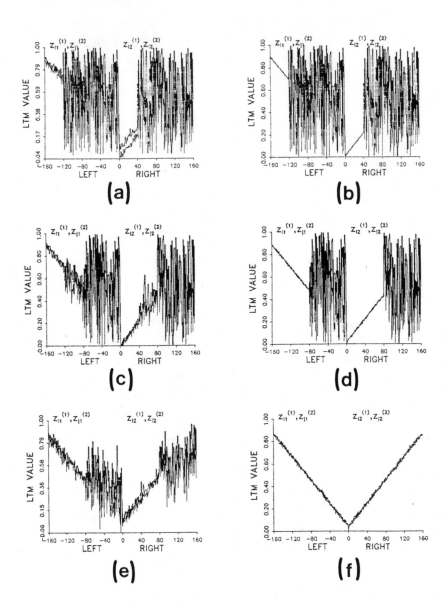

Figure 10.7. Expansion of LTM maps due to increase of the number of cells in the RM and the EPM_1 which sample the EPM_2: Initial LTM values are chosen randomly between 0 and 1 instead of equal to zero, as in Figure 10.3. The final learned LTM values in Figure 10.3 and this figure agree, thereby illustrating the stability of this invariant self-regulating map learning process.

In our simulations, $p = q = r = 40$. The main difference between this example and the previous one is that here the EPM_2 represented target eye positions by spatially focussed peaks. To represent this spatial map, we defined i_n and j_n as before, let

$$k_n = \left[\left| \frac{(i_n + j_n)r}{p+q} \right|\right] \tag{10.48}$$

and chose the input to cell v_k in EPM_2 on trial n to equal

$$I_{kn} = e^{\frac{-(k-k_n)^2}{\lambda}}, \tag{10.49}$$

where $\| w \|$ denotes the largest integer less than or equal to w. Equation (10.49) says that the maximal activation of EPM_2 on trial n occurs at position $k = k_n$. Other activations of EPM_2 on trial n are Gaussianly distributed around position $k = k_n$. Position k_n represents the target position attained by the nth saccade. In (10.48), we scaled k_n using the factor $r(p+q)^{-1}$ to keep it between 1 and the number of cells r within the EPM_2.

Figure 10.8 plots the LTM surfaces generated by this learning model. As before, invariant map learning was excellent. We quantified how well an invariant map was learned as follows. After the $5(10)^5$ learning trials were over, we fixed the LTM values. We then randomly chose 10,000 combinations of cells in the RM, the EPM_1, and the EPM_2. As before, we let $i = i_n$ be the index of the RM population and $j = j_n$ be the index of the EPM_1 population on the nth choice. In addition, we let $k = m_n$ be the index of the EPM_2 population on the nth choice. In terms of these choices, we compared the relative sizes of LTM traces and inputs on the nth random choice using the function

$$Y_n = \left| \frac{z^{(1)}_{i_n m_n} + z^{(2)}_{i_n m_n}}{Z^{(n)}} - \frac{I_{m_n n}}{I^{(n)}} \right|, \tag{10.50}$$

where

$$Z^{(n)} = \sum_{k=1}^{40} (z^{(1)}_{i_n k} + z^{(2)}_{j_n k}), \tag{10.51}$$

$$I^{(n)} = \sum_{k=1}^{40} I_{m_n k}, \tag{10.52}$$

$$I_{m_n k} = e^{\frac{-(m_n - k_n)^2}{\lambda}}, \tag{10.53}$$

and k_n is defined in terms of i_n and j_n by (10.48). Then we computed the average size of the values Y_n in terms of the function

$$Y = \frac{1}{10,000} \sum_{n=1}^{10,000} Y_n. \tag{10.54}$$

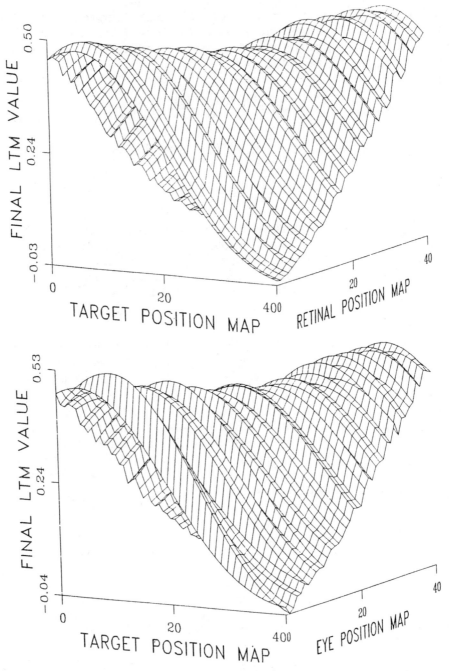

Figure 10.8. Final LTM values when randomly chosen RM and EPM$_1$ positions sample activity gradients distributed as Gaussians across a spatial topography defined in equation (10.49): The graphs depict the spatial distributions of LTM values across EPM$_2$ corresponding to each RM and EPM$_1$ position.

In our simulations, $Y = .0515$. Since the LTM traces and inputs varied between 0 and 1, this error represents excellent learning of the invariant map.

10.8. Associative Pattern Learning

Some mathematical insight can be gleaned into how multimodal map learning occurs by noticing that system (10.21)–(10.26) has the properties of a completely nonrecurrent associative learning network (Grossberg, 1969c, 1972b, 1982a). The stable pattern learning properties of these networks also hold in the present case. These properties enable one to understand how the correct *relative* LTM pattern values are learned by each sampling cell. The correct self-regulating *absolute* LTM values are learned due to the action of the autoreceptors.

In order to clarify these associative learning properties, we define two types of variables.

Total Activity Variables

Let

$$I = I_1 + I_2, \tag{10.55}$$

$$x = x_1 + x_2, \tag{10.56}$$

$$z_{ij1} = z_{i1}^{(1)} + z_{j1}^{(2)}, \tag{10.57}$$

$$z_{ij2} = z_{i2}^{(1)} + z_{j2}^{(2)}, \tag{10.58}$$

and

$$z_{ij} = z_{ij1} + z_{ij2}. \tag{10.59}$$

Relative Activity Variables

Let

$$\theta_1 = \frac{I_1}{I}, \tag{10.60}$$

$$\theta_2 = \frac{I_2}{I}, \tag{10.61}$$

$$X_1 = \frac{x_1}{x}, \tag{10.62}$$

$$X_2 = \frac{x_2}{x}, \tag{10.63}$$

$$Z_{ij1} = \frac{z_{ij1}}{z_{ij}}, \tag{10.64}$$

and

$$Z_{ij2} = \frac{z_{ij2}}{z_{ij}}. \tag{10.65}$$

Our goal is to indicate how relative pattern learning occurs. On a trial when $v_i^{(1)}$ is active in RM and $v_j^{(2)}$ is active in EPM$_1$, the relative LTM traces Z_{ij1} and Z_{ij2} in (10.64) and (10.65) measure how well RM and EPM$_1$ have cooperated to learn the relative inputs θ_1 and θ_2 in (10.60) and (10.61). We will show that the relative LTM pattern (Z_{ij1}, Z_{ij2}) is attracted to the relative input pattern (θ_1, θ_2) via the relative STM pattern (X_1, X_2) of (10.62) and (10.63).

On a learning trial when $v_i^{(1)}$ and $v_j^{(2)}$ are active, z_1 in (10.22) and z_2 in (10.24) reduce to

$$z_1 = z_{ij1} \tag{10.66}$$

and

$$z_2 = z_{ij2}, \tag{10.67}$$

where z_{ij1} and z_{ij2} are defined in (10.57) and (10.58), respectively. Consequently, (10.21) and (10.23) reduce to

$$\frac{d}{dt}x_1 = -x_1 + I_1 + z_{ij1} \tag{10.68}$$

and

$$\frac{d}{dt}x_2 = -x_2 + I_2 + z_{ij2}. \tag{10.69}$$

Adding (10.68) and (10.69) implies that

$$\frac{d}{dt}x = -x + I + z_{ij}. \tag{10.70}$$

For similar reasons on such a learning trial, addition of (10.25) and (10.26) implies that

$$\frac{d}{dt}z_{ij1} = e[-(F + 2H)z_{ij1} + 2Gx_1] \tag{10.71}$$

and

$$\frac{d}{dt}z_{ij2} = e[-(F + 2H)z_{ij2} + 2Gx_2], \tag{10.72}$$

from which it follows by a further addition of (10.71) and (10.72) that

$$\frac{d}{dt}z_{ij} = e[-(F + 2H)z_{ij} + 2Gx]. \tag{10.73}$$

We use these equations to derive equations for the relative STM and LTM traces. The basic tool is the elementary formula for the derivative of a ratio:

$$\frac{d}{dt}\left(\frac{f}{g}\right) = \frac{1}{g}\left[\dot{f} - \frac{f}{g}\frac{d}{dt}g)\right], \tag{10.74}$$

which we apply to the ratios $X_1 = \frac{x_1}{x}$, $X_2 = \frac{x_2}{x}$, $Z_{ij1} = \frac{z_{ij1}}{z_{ij}}$, and $Z_{ij2} = \frac{z_{ij2}}{z_{ij}}$. We find the familiar pattern learning equations

$$\frac{d}{dt}X_k = P_{ijk}(Z_{ijk} - X_k) + Q_k(\theta_k - X_k) \tag{10.75}$$

and

$$\frac{d}{dt}Z_{ijk} = R_{ijk}(X_k - Z_{ijk}), \tag{10.76}$$

$k = 1, 2$, where the coefficients are the nonnegative functions

$$P_{ijk} = \frac{z_{ij}}{x_k}, \tag{10.77}$$

$$Q_k = \frac{I}{x_k}, \tag{10.78}$$

and

$$R_{ijk} = \frac{2\epsilon Gx}{z_{ijk}}. \tag{10.79}$$

Term $Q_k(\theta_k - X_k)$ in (10.75) describes read-in of the input pattern θ_k into STM X_k. This term causes X_k to approach θ_k. Term $P_{ijk}(Z_{ijk} - X_k)$ describes read-out of LTM into STM. It causes X_k to approach Z_{ijk}. Thus the relative STM trace X_k is torn between the tendency to represent new, as yet unlearned, patterns θ_k and to read-out old remembered patterns Z_{ijk}. Term $R_{ijk}(X_k - Z_{ijk})$ in (10.76), on the other hand, describes read-in of STM into LTM. This term causes Z_{ijk} to approach X_k. In all, the STM and LTM patterns mutually attract each other, while the STM pattern is attracted to the input pattern:

$$Z_{ijk} \leftrightarrow X_k \rightarrow \theta_k. \tag{10.80}$$

The net effect of these attractive tendencies is that the LTM pattern is attracted towards the input pattern:

$$Z_{ijk} \rightarrow \theta_k. \tag{10.81}$$

This is true given any fixed but random choice of i and j through time. The simulations demonstrate that, in response to a randomly chosen sequence of (i, j) pairs through time, these learning tendencies fit together to synthesize a globally consistent, invariant, self-regulating TPM.

The role of autoreceptors in enabling the network to self-regulate is indicated by an examination of the LTM traces of equation (10.25) at equilibrium. At equilibrium, $\frac{d}{dt}x_1 = 0$. Then (10.21) becomes

$$x_1 = I_1 + z_1. \tag{10.82}$$

Consider $z_{i1}^{(1)}$ in (10.25) by letting $k = 1$. If we substitute for x_1 in this equation, we get

$$\frac{d}{dt}z_{i1}^{(1)} = \epsilon S_i^{(1)}\left[-Fz_{i1}^{(1)} + G(I_1 + z_1) - Hz_1\right]. \qquad (10.83)$$

At equilibrium, $\frac{d}{dt}z_{i1}^{(1)} = 0$, which by (10.83) implies that

$$Fz_{i1}^{(1)} + (H - G)z_1 = GI_1. \qquad (10.84)$$

We assume that the LTM decay rate F is very small. Then (10.84) implies that

$$z_1 \cong \frac{G}{H - G}I_1. \qquad (10.85)$$

Thus the relative size of H to G determines the scaling factor that converts inputs into LTM values. This scaling factor does not influence the goodness-of-fit measured by $V_k^{(m)}$ in (10.35).

On the nth learning trial, $z_1 = z_{i_n 1}^{(1)} + z_{j_n 2}^{(2)}$ due to equations (10.27) and (10.28). Thus for all large choices of n, when the network is close to equilibrium, (10.85) implies

$$z_{i_n 1}^{(1)} + z_{j_n 2}^{(2)} \cong \frac{G}{H - G}I_1. \qquad (10.86)$$

Given that the network can approach an approximate equilibrium as n becomes sufficiently large, equation (10.86) has the following implications. First, it implies that $H > G$. Computer simulations show that system variables can diverge if $H - G$ becomes too small. Second, equation (10.86) shows that the equilibrium value of each LTM trace $z_{i1}^{(1)}$ depends upon the equilibrium values of all LTM traces $z_{j2}^{(2)}$ with which it is paired. In particular, each $z_{i1}^{(1)}$ adjusts its equilibrium value to compensate for the addition or deletion of LTM values $z_{j2}^{(2)}$, as in Figure 10.3. Thus equation (10.86) describes a sharing of adaptive load quite different from that described in Chapter 3. The present type of load sharing is the property of self-regulation that we seek. The problem remains open of mathematically proving that this nonlinear system of stochastic differential equations always approaches an approximate equilibrium as $n \to \infty$ if $H - G$ is sufficiently large, ϵ is sufficiently small, and the input indices i_n and j_n are randomly chosen.

CHAPTER 11
VISUALLY REACTIVE, MULTIMODAL, INTENTIONAL, AND PREDICTIVE MOVEMENTS: A SYNTHESIS

11.1. Avoiding Infinite Regress: Planned Movements Share Reactive Movement Parameters

In this Chapter, we tie together the design principles and mechanisms which we have introduced in the preceding chapters. This synthesis quantifies a developmental sequence in which obligatory saccadic reactions to flashing or moving lights on the retina are supplemented by attentionally mediated movements towards motivationally interesting or intermodal sensory cues. These movements are supplemented once again by predictive saccades which form part of planned sequences of complex movement synergies that can totally ignore the sensory substrate on which they are built.

The analysis of such a complex system would be hopeless in the absence of sufficient design constraints. The previous chapters illustrate our contention that an analysis of development and learning is essential to discover sufficiently many constraints. This chapter continues such an analysis until it discloses a small number of closely related global network designs that are capable of simultaneously satisfying all of the constraints.

The primacy of learning constraints is perhaps most urgently felt when one squarely faces the problem of infinite regress. On what firm computational foundation can adaptive calibrations be based? If parameters in several subsystems can all be changing due to different types of learning signals, then what prevents them from confounding each other's learning by causing a global inconsistency within the system? An analysis of how the problem of infinite regress may be solved shows how to hierarchically organize motor learning circuits so that each circuit can benefit from and build upon the learning of a more primitive learning circuit. This hierarchical organization of learning problems can be profitably compared to the hierarchical organization whereby simple motor synergies in the spinal cord can be temporally organized by descending cortical commands (Grillner, 1975; Grossberg, 1969d, 1974).

The need to solve the problem of infinite regress is evident in our method of calibrating a target position command in muscle coordinates at the head-muscle interface, or HMI (Chapter 4). We have suggested that an active target position map (TPM) population will sample whatever eye position corollary discharges are read-into the HMI after the eye comes to rest. These eye position signals may or may not correspond to the target position that is active within the TPM. The TPM will eventually sample the correct eye position only if an independent learning mechanism enables the eye to accurately foveate retinal lights.

We have suggested that this independent learning mechanism forms part of the RCN, or retinotopic command network (Chapter 3), whereas the HMI forms part of the VCN, or vector command network (Chapter 4).

One goal of this chapter is to complete our analysis of the interactions that occur between these two types of networks.

The RCN learning mechanism utilizes a multisynaptic pathway that probably includes the superior colliculus (SC) and the visual cortex (Huerta and Harting, 1984). This pathway is hypothesized to be activated by flashing and moving lights on the retina (Frost and Nakayama, 1983), and to be functional at an early stage of development. The VCN learning mechanisms, notably the TPM and HMI, are hypothesized to process attentionally modulated neocortical commands. These attentionally modulated VCN commands may be able to inhibit the relatively simple motion-sensitive signals of the RCN at a later developmental stage, but before they can do so, they first need to be calibrated using the motion-sensitive SC pathway as a reliable computational substrate. The first two problems that shall be considered in this chapter are how this calibration problem is solved and how attention can modulate cortical movement commands.

11.2. Learning and Competition from a Vector-Based Map to a Light-Based Map

The motion-sensitive system uses second light error signals to improve its foveating capability (Chapter 3). The HMI uses the learned accuracy of the motion-sensitive saccades in order to compute accurate difference vectors in muscle coordinates, which can then be transformed into a retinotopic map, or RM (Chapter 6). It remains to show how such an RM can generate accurate saccadic movements. Two main possibilities exist, and we suggest that both may be used *in vivo*. In one possibility, the RM learns to read-out commands to the saccade generator (SG) using the output pathways of the motion-sensitive RCN system. We suggest that this pathway is used by attentionally modulated commands from the parietal cortex, at least in monkeys and humans. In the other possibility, the RM controls its own output pathways through which it learns its own correct movement parameters. We suggest that this pathway is used by predictive commands from the frontal eye fields (FEF) in monkeys and humans. Each possibility implies a distinct constellation of functional and structural properties which can be empirically tested.

First we study how an RM in the VCN can learn to activate the RCN output pathways, and to thereby generate accurate saccades using the adaptive gains which had previously been learned within the RCN. This analysis resolves the following paradox: How does the VCN both learn from and inhibit the RCN? In order for the RM to become associated with the correct RCN output pathways, these pathways must be *excited* during the learning phase. In order for VCN commands to supplant RCN commands, the RM must be able to *inhibit* RCN output pathways during later performance trials. How can excitation during learning give rise to inhibition during performance?

The sampled RCN output pathways also form an RM. Thus our problem is to study learning of an $RM \rightarrow RM$ associative transform. In order to avoid notational confusion, we denote the RM within the VCN by RM_V and the RM within the RCN by RM_R.

Before learning occurs, each RM_V population gives rise to conditionable pathways which are distributed nonspecifically across the RM_R, because it is not known *a priori* which RM_R population will be associated with which RM_V population. The LTM traces in these pathways are initially small. While the RCN is still learning how to make accurate saccades, the LTM traces within the $RM_V \rightarrow RM_R$ conditionable pathways remain broadly distributed and small, because each RM_V population can become associated with many different RM_R populations. Several reasons for this exist. Until accurate saccades persistently occur, the TPM cannot form with precision (Chapter 10) because each fixed combination of retinal position and initial eye position can sample a different final position whenever a foveation error occurs. Each TPM population can, in turn, sample many corollary discharge patterns at the HMI due to foveation errors. Thus, across learning trials, each *fixed* combination of TPM and corollary discharge inputs to the HMI can activate many different vectors there and, by extension, many different RM_V populations. Thus each RM_V population can sample many different RM_R populations until learning within the RCN stabilizes. Consequently the $RM_V \rightarrow RM_R$ associative transform will remain broadly distributed and weak until the RCN becomes capable of reliably generating correct foveations.

Competitive interactions are assumed to occur among the RM_R populations in order to choose a winning population for storage in short term memory (STM). Such a population's activity must be stored in STM until after the saccade terminates, so that it can sample any second light error signals that may then be registered (Chapter 2). During the learning trials when foveation errors still regularly occur within the RCN, the $RM_V \rightarrow RM_R$ signals, being weak, lose the competition for STM storage to the first light-activated movement signals. The RM_V consequently does not interfere with the initial stages of learning within the RCN.

By contrast, after the RCN becomes capable of generating correct foveations, the LTM traces of each RM_V population begin to sample the same RM_R population on all future learning trials. The LTM traces of these pathways become strong due to the cumulative effect of these consistent learning trials, while the LTM traces of other, less favored, pathways become weak. The $RM_V \rightarrow RM_R$ associative map thereby becomes more topographic as some of its LTM traces become large due to the cumulative effects of consistent learning on successive saccadic trials. After the LTM traces become sufficiently large, a conditioned signal from RM_V to RM_R can successfully compete with a first light-activated movement signal within the RCN. When this happens, attentionally amplified VCN commands can take precedence over motion-sensitive RCN commands.

In order for this scheme to work, the RM_R must occur at a stage that is prior to the RCN's error signal pathway to the adaptive gain (AG) stage, or cerebellum (Chapter 3). Then the $RM_V \rightarrow RM_R \rightarrow AG \rightarrow SG$ pathway can use the cerebellar gain that was previously learned in response to second light error signals of RCN vintage (Figure 11.1).

This example shows in several ways how a suitably designed network hierarchy can avoid infinite regress by exploiting previously learned movement parameters. The RCN helps the VCN to learn its TPM, to calibrate its HMI, and to sample accurately calibrated movement commands using its AG stage adaptive gains.

11.3. Associative Pattern Learning and Competitive Choice: Non-Hebbian Learning Rule

This section mathematically demonstrates the properties which were intuitively explained within the previous section. Suppose that a network $F^{(1)}$ sends broadly distributed conditionable pathways to a disjoint network $F^{(2)}$. We have in mind, of course, the special case in which $F^{(1)} = RM_V$ and $F^{(2)} = RM_R$, but our discussion is more general. Denote the cells of $F^{(1)}$ by $v_j^{(1)}$ and the cells of $F^{(2)}$ by $v_i^{(2)}$. The cells $F^{(1)} = \{v_j^{(1)}\}$ are generically called *sampling cells* and the cells $F^{(2)} = \{v_i^{(2)}\}$ are generically called *sampled cells*.

For simplicity, let each cell population $v_j^{(1)}$ emit the sampling signal S_j within the axons e_{ji} from $v_j^{(1)}$ to all cells $v_i^{(2)}$ in $F^{(2)}$. Let a long term memory (LTM) trace z_{ji} be computed at the synaptic knobs of each pathway e_{ji}. Suppose that z_{ji} computes a time-average of the signal S_j times the postsynaptic potential $x_i^{(2)}$ of $v_i^{(2)}$. It has been proved, under general mathematical conditions, that the pattern of LTM traces $(z_{j1}, z_{j2}, ..., z_{jn})$ learns a weighted average of the STM patterns $(x_1^{(2)}, x_2^{(2)}, ..., x_n^{(n)})$ that occur across $F^{(2)}$ while S_i is active (Grossberg, 1968b, 1969c, 1972b, 1982a). This is the same theorem about associative pattern learning that we used to clarify the learning of an invariant TPM in Chapter 10. In the present example, a different version of the same learning laws shows how a topographic associative map can be learned.

To see how this can happen, suppose for definiteness that $F^{(2)}$ chooses at most one activity $x_i^{(2)}$ for storage in STM at any given time, as in Section 2.6. Suppose that the population $v_{i_j}^{(2)}$ with $i = i_j$ in $F^{(2)}$ is stored in STM at times when population $v_j^{(1)}$ is active in $F^{(1)}$. Since S_j is active during time intervals when the particular STM trace $x_{i_j}^{(2)}$ is chosen for STM storage, the relative LTM trace $z_{ji_j}(\sum_{k=1}^n z_{jk})^{-1}$ monotonically approaches 1 as learning proceeds. In other words, only the LTM trace z_{ji_j} becomes large, as all the other traces $z_{j1}, z_{j2}, ..., z_{jn}$ become small. This is a non-Hebbian form of learning, because both conditioned increases *and* conditioned decreases in LTM traces z_{ji} can occur due to pairing of

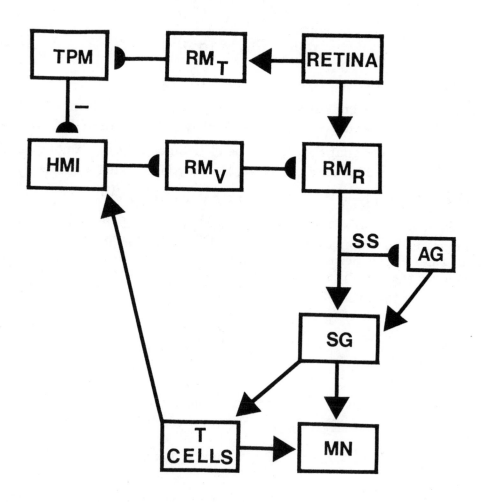

Figure 11.1. Interactions between the retinotopic command network (RCN) and the vector command network (VCN): The coupling between these subsystems enable the motorically encoded vectors in the head-muscle interface (HMI) of the VCN to be retinotopically recoded within the retinotopic map (RM_R) of the RCN. HMI vectors can then use the unconditioned movement pathway $RM_R \rightarrow SG$ and the conditioned movement pathway $RM_R \rightarrow AG \rightarrow SG$ of the RCN to generate accurate eye movements. Abbreviations: SS = sampling signals, AG = adaptive gain stage, SG = saccade generator, T cells = tonic cells, MN = motoneurons, TPM = target position map, RM_T, RM_V, and RM_R = retinotopic maps.

S_j and $x_i^{(2)}$. A simple learning equation with this property is

$$\frac{d}{dt}z_{ji} = \epsilon S_j(-z_{ji} + x_i^{(2)}). \qquad (11.1)$$

Performance of the learned pattern of LTM traces occurs as follows. Suppose that the signal that reaches each population $v_i^{(2)}$ from $v_j^{(1)}$ equals $S_j z_{ji}$. In other words, S_j is multiplicatively gated by the LTM trace z_{ji} before the gated signal $S_j z_{ji}$ perturbs $v_i^{(2)}$. Since only z_{ji_j} among all the LTM traces $z_{j1}, z_{j2}, \ldots, z_{jn}$ is large, the only large gated signal is $S_j z_{ji_j}$. Consequently, only $v_{i_j}{}^{(2)}$ is significantly activated by $v_j^{(1)}$.

To illustrate how all the inputs to $F^{(2)}$ influence its dynamics through time, let us approximate the choice-making behavior of $F^{(2)}$ by an algebraic rule. This is permissible in the present case because the LTM traces, which are the variables of primary interest, fluctuate through time much more slowly than the STM traces $x_i^{(2)}$ or their inputs I_i. Thus, let

$$J_i = I_i + \sum_{j=1}^{m} S_j z_{ji} \qquad (11.2)$$

equal the total input to $v_i^{(2)}$ at any time, where I_i is a light-induced motion-sensitive input and $\sum_{j=1}^{m} S_j z_{ji}$ is the total conditioned input from $F^{(1)}$. Also let

$$x_i^{(2)} = \begin{cases} 1 & \text{if } J_i > \max\{\delta, J_k : k \neq i\} \\ 0 & \text{otherwise} \end{cases} \qquad (11.3)$$

be the rule whereby $F^{(2)}$ activities are chosen and stored in STM. In (11.3), parameter $\delta > 0$ estimates the quenching threshold (QT) of $F^{(2)}$ (Section 2.6). By (11.3), $v_i^{(2)}$ is chosen and stored with the normalized activity 1 if its input exceeds the QT and is the largest total input received by $F^{(2)}$. Equation (11.3) approximates a network with broad lateral inhibitory interactions and signal functions selected to make a global choice (Section 2.6).

Before learning occurs, all the LTM traces are small and uniformly distributed across $F^{(2)}$. Consequently the maximal J_i is determined by the maximal I_i. The choice behavior of $F^{(2)}$ is then controlled by the motion-sensitive inputs I_i, as in Chapter 3. Suppose that at most one signal S_j is large at any time (because only one RM_V population is activated by the HMI at any time). Also suppose, as above, that activity in $v_{i_j}{}^{(2)}$ is paired with activity in $v_j^{(1)}$, so that only z_{ji_j} becomes large due to associative learning. In particular, equation (11.1) implies that z_{ji_j} approaches 1 as a result of learning and all z_{ji} approach zero, $i \neq i_j$. These conclusions follow from the conjoint action of several properties. For one, $S_j = 0$ implies that $\frac{d}{dt} z_{ji} = 0$; no learning occurs unless the sampling signal S_j is active. If $S_j > 0$ when $x_{i_j} = 1$, then (11.1) implies that z_{ji_j} approaches 1. If $S_j > 0$ when $x_i = 0$, $i \neq i_j$, then (11.1) implies that all z_{ji} approach zero, $i \neq i_j$.

Suppose, moreover, that each S_j becomes larger than the maximal possible input size I_i whenever S_j is positive. The size of S_j may, in particular, be amplified by attentional gain control or by incentive motivational signals (Section 2.6). After learning occurs, consider a performance trial during which the sampling signal S_j is on while a motion-sensitive input I_i is on in a different $F^{(2)}$ channel ($i \neq i_j$). Because $z_{ji_j} \cong 1$ and all $z_{ji} \cong 0$, $i \neq i_j$, it follows by (11.2) that

$$J_{ij} \cong S_j z_{ji_j} \cong S_j \qquad (11.4)$$

and that

$$J_i \cong I_i, i \neq i_j. \qquad (11.5)$$

Consequently,

$$J_{ij} > J_i, i \neq i_j. \qquad (11.6)$$

By (11.3), it follows that

$$x_{ij} = 1 \qquad (11.7)$$

whereas all

$$x_i = 0, i \neq i_j. \qquad (11.8)$$

In other words, after learning occurs, the VCN-activated population $v_{i_j}{}^{(2)}$ wins the STM competition over the RCN-activated population $v_i^{(2)}$ despite the fact that $v_i^{(2)}$ wins the STM competition over $v_{i_j}^{(2)}$ before learning occurs.

By winning the STM competition, population $v_{i_j}{}^{(2)}$ also stabilizes the memory within its LTM trace z_{ji_j}. This property also follows from the learning equation (11.1). When $S_j = 0$, it follows that $\frac{d}{dt} z_{ji_j} = 0$, so that no learning *or forgetting* occurs unless the sampling signal S_j is active. Suppose that when $S_j = 0$, z_{ji_j} starts out equal to 1 due to prior learning. If z_{ji_j} can cause $x_{i_j}{}^{(2)}$ to quickly win the STM competition, then also $x_{i_j}{}^{(2)} = 1$ at these times. By (11.1), even if $S_j > 0$,

$$\frac{d}{dt} z_{ji_j} = S_j(-1 + 1) = 0. \qquad (11.9)$$

Consequently, once LTM trace z_{ji_j} learns the value 1, it reinforces its memory of this value during subsequent performance. Note, however, that the LTM trace has not lost its plasticity. It is in a dynamical equilibrium with the STM activation that it causes.

In summary, after learning of the associative transform $F^{(1)} \to F^{(2)}$ occurs, $F^{(1)}$ can control STM decisions within $F^{(2)}$, even though $F^{(1)}$ had no influence over these STM decisions before learning occurred. Moreover, $F^{(1)}$ can maintain its control in a stable fashion due to the feedback exchange between STM and LTM that occurs in equations (11.1) and (11.3).

This model describes a critical period that ends when its LTM traces achieve a dynamical equilibrium with its STM traces. In the absence of further learning-contingent structural changes within the network, such a model predicts that new learning can occur in the adult if the correlations between sampling populations $v_j^{(1)}$ and sampled populations $v_i^{(2)}$ are systematically changed using artificially large inputs I_i, despite the absence of any apparent plasticity before such a change takes place. Artificially large direct inputs to $F^{(2)}$ are needed to overcome the competitive advantage of $F^{(1)}$ signals after learning takes place. Additional memory buffering interactions, modulated by the catecholaminergic transmitter norepinephrine, have been predicted to occur in more complex associative mapping models (Grossberg, 1976b, 1980, 1984) and have received some experimental support (Kasamatsu and Pettigrew, 1976; Pettigrew and Kasamatsu, 1978). In such models, a learned feedback map $F^{(2)} \to F^{(1)}$ is also predicted to exist. No data are yet available on which to base the judgment of whether such a dynamic LTM buffer also exists between the RM_V and the RM_R networks.

11.4. Light Intensity, Motion, Attentional, and Multimodal Interactions within the Parietal Cortex

The previous two sections have shown how the VCN can feed into the RCN. We begin this section by noting that the RCN can also feed into the VCN, as in Figure 11.1. Indeed, when the target position map (TPM) of the VCN is trying to gain control over the RM_R, it does so by correlating the *same* retinotopic position within the RM_V and the RM_R. In other words, from an early stage of development, the TPM, no less than the RM_R, is also sensitive to light-induced intensity and motion changes on the retina. The RM that feeds into the TPM, which is denoted by RM_T in Figure 11.1, registers these light-sensitive activations and passes them on to the TPM. The high correlation between activations of the *same* retinotopic positions within the RM_T and the RM_R leads to the growth of large LTM traces within the $RM_V \to RM_R$ associative transform.

The TPM never loses its sensitivity to light-induced changes on the retina. As development progresses, however, other modulatory influences can also begin to play upon the RM_T and the TPM. These include multimodal interactions, notably auditory inputs (Section 1.15), and attentionally modulated signals. In Section 11.2, for example, we discussed how a TPM-activated population v_{ij} can win the STM competition within the RM_R over a population v_i, $i \neq i_j$, that is directly activated by a light-sensitive input I_i. This can only occur if multimodal or attentional inputs can bias the TPM to activate a target position that does not correspond to the retinotopic position v_i. Such mismatches must not be allowed to frequently occur until after the $RM_V \rightarrow RM_R$ map is learned, because they would undermine the transform learning process. Fortunately, such mismatches *cannot* occur until after the $RM_V \rightarrow RM_R$ transform is learned, because this transform must be learned before intentional movements can generate a mismatch at the RM_R via the $RM_V \rightarrow RM_R$ transform. Infinite regress is thus once again averted.

In this section, we describe some of the multimodal and attentional mechanisms that can influence which TPM population will be chosen to activate the $TPM \rightarrow HMI \rightarrow RM_V \rightarrow RM_R$ pathway. Concerning the important problem of multimodal interactions, we will make only some brief observations.

A light-activated invariant TPM is computed in head coordinates. So too is a TPM based on auditory signals. Once both types of TPMs have been formed, strong correlations between sounds and lights can be the basis for learning an associative transform from sound-activated target positions to light-activated target positions, and possibly an inverse transform from vision to audition. This transform can be learned using the same associative laws that enabled the $RM_V \rightarrow RM_R$ transform to be learned.

After this transform is learned, the target position of a sound can compete for STM activation with the discordant target position of a light at all TPMs where both types of signals are registered (Figure 11.2). The target position of a sound can also amplify the activation of the target position of a light into which it is associatively mapped. Meredith and Stein (1983) have reported both competitive and cooperative interactions due to light and sound stimuli within the deeper laminae of the superior colliculi of cats and hamsters. Within our theory, such an interaction manifests itself via the circuit

$$(\text{auditory } TPM) \rightarrow (\text{visual } TPM) \rightarrow HMI \rightarrow RM_V \rightarrow RM_R \quad (11.10)$$

in Figures 11.1 and 11.2.

As in the associative transform described in Section 11.3, an intermodal associative transform tends to stabilize its prior learning via a dynamically maintained critical period (Knudsen, 1983, 1984). Although this discussion does not address the complex issue of how binaural signals are used to localize an object in space, any more than it describes how binocular disparity cues are used for visual localization, the following conclusion is robust: Whatever be the fine structure of these TPMs, if they are both computed in head coordinates, then multimodal associative

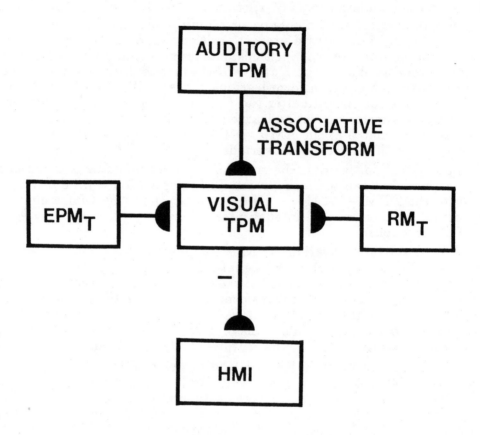

Figure 11.2. An auditory target position map (TPM) can be associatively mapped upon a visual TPM because the two maps are dimensionally consistent.

transformations can form with a precision that covaries with the degree to which their sampling and sampled map positions are correlated.

11.5. Nonspecific and Specific Attentional Mechanisms

Two types of attentional mechanisms are suggested to occur in the neocortical regions that control saccadic movements. Both types of mechanisms were derived from postulates concerning classical conditioning and instrumental conditioning (Grossberg, 1973, 1975; Grossberg and Levine, 1975) before relevant cortical data began to be reported (Motter and Mountcastle, 1981; Mountcastle, Anderson, and Motter, 1981; Wurtz, Goldberg, and Robinson, 1982). This is thus another area where theory and data seem to be rapidly converging.

The most elementary attentional mechanism is a nonspecific alteration of the gain, or sensitivity, across a neural network. This operation leads to either amplification or attenuation of all responses within the network. Such a nonspecific modulation of sensitivity is controlled by a parameter called the *quenching threshold* (QT) of the network (Section 2.6). Any of several network parameters can, in principle, cause state-dependent changes of the QT. A large QT imposes a high criterion for cell activation. A very large QT can totally desensitize the network to all inputs. A low QT enables even small inputs to activate their cells. A typical mechanism for controlling the QT is a nonspecific signal that shunts the interneuronal pathways within the network.

A nonspecific type of attentional reaction has been reported in the posterior parietal cortex (Mountcastle, Anderson, and Motter, 1981). If, for example, the QT of the auditory TPM became large and/or the QT of the visual RM_T became small during attention to visual cues, then auditory inputs would have great difficulty competing to activate the HMI. By contrast, if the QT of the visually-activated RM_T became large and the QT of the auditory TPM became small during attention to auditory cues, then auditory inputs could more easily activate the HMI.

A more specific type of attentional modulation is also needed to effectively control classical conditioning and instrumental conditioning. These specific attentional signals are learned incentive motivational signals from midbrain reward and punishment centers (Section 2.6). The conditioning model developed in Grossberg (1975, 1982b, 1982c, 1984) shows how the sensory representations of motivationally charged cues can be differentially enhanced by incentive motivational signals before the locations of the enhanced representations are encoded in a TPM. Analogous cue-specific enhancements have been reported in the posterior parietal cortices of monkeys who were trained to perform eye movement tasks to receive juice as a reward (Wurtz, Goldberg, and Robinson, 1982).

If a target position receives a large incentive motivational signal, then it can more effectively compete with factors like retinal light intensity or retinal movement for STM storage within a cortical TPM. If a target position receives a multimodal combination of auditory and visual signals, then it can more effectively compete with a source of only visual signals.

In addition, nonspecific gain change may alter the salience of different modalities through time. At any given moment, a complex interplay of retinal light intensity signals, retinal motion signals, specific intermodal signals, specific motivational signals, and nonspecific modality-selective attentional signals will help to determine which activated target positions within the TPM will win the competition to activate the HMI. In addition to these input factors, the learned factors which group familiar sensory patterns into object representations will also influence the intensity with which these representations activate their corresponding target positions (Carpenter and Grossberg, 1985b; Grossberg, 1980, 1984). As in life, the more interesting and complex are the objects being viewed, the more complex will be the activity patterns across the TPM that enable us to visually explore them.

11.6. Multiple Retinotopic Maps

We can now begin to gather together constraints derived in earlier chapters to refine the macrocircuit diagram of Figure 11.1. We will do this in stages using figures that omit processes which are not immediately being discussed. Where important circuit variations are consistent with functional requirements, we will note them in order to stimulate experiments capable of deciding between them.

Figure 11.3 depicts a refinement of Figure 11.1. Figure 11.3 contains two macrostages that were not included in Figure 11.1: a pair of retinotopic maps, RM_{R1} and RM_{R2}, instead of a single retinotopic map RM; and a pair of target position maps, TPM_1 and TPM_2, instead of a single target position map TPM. The retinotopic map RM_{R2} plays the role of RM_R and the target position map TPM_1 plays the role of TPM. First, we describe the role of the new retinotopic map RM_{R1}.

Figure 2.4 summarizes the functional role of the RM_{R1}. In Figure 2.4, two successive network stages are used to process light-activated signals from the retina. The first stage, the RM_{R1}, chooses the retinotopic position that receives the most favorable combination of retinal intensity and motion factors at any time. As in Figure 2.4, the RM_{R1} gives rise to second light error signals (ES) which act at the adaptive gain (AG) stage, or cerebellum. In both Figures 2.4 and 11.3, the RM_{R1} activates the next retinotopic map, the RM_{R2}, at which the light that is chosen by the RM_{R1} is stored in STM. The RM_{R2} gives rise to the conditioned pathways along which sampling signals (SS) learn adaptive gains within the AG stage in response to second light error signals. The chosen light must thus be stored in STM until after the saccade is over, so that its conditioned pathways can sample the second light error signals.

As in Figure 11.1, the RM_V in Figure 11.3 samples the RM_{R2}, so that it can learn to transmit an attentionally modulated choice of retinotopic position to the RM_{R2}. Due to $RM_V \rightarrow RM_{R2}$ signals, the choice which is stored within the RM_{R2} might differ from the choice which was made by the RM_{R1}. The RM_{R2} chooses the largest signal which it receives before storing it in STM, as in equation (11.3). Attentional and intentional

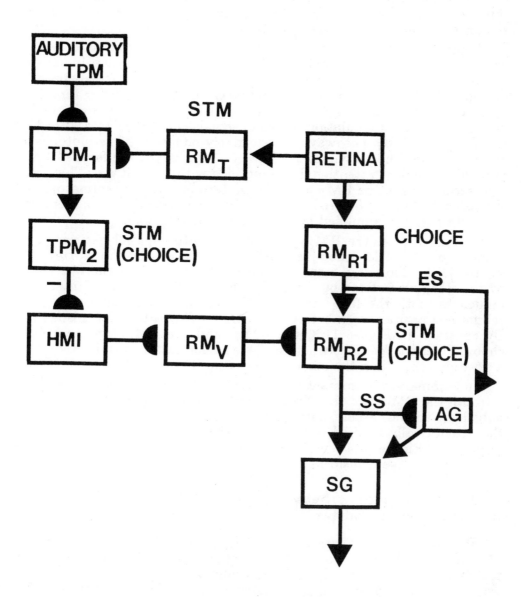

Figure 11.3. Refinement of the circuit in Figure 11.1: A pair of retino-topic maps RM_{R1} and RM_{R2} replace RM_R and a pair of target position maps TPM_1 and TPM_2 replace TPM. See text for details. Abbreviations: ES = error signal.

factors may hereby override visually reactive factors within the RM_{R2}, as in Section 11.3. However, sufficiently vigorous reaction to a moving stimulus may override an insufficiently amplified attentional focus. Despite this fact, visual factors remain the exclusive source of second light error signals from the RM_{R1} to the AG stage.

Figure 11.4 describes a variation on Figure 11.3 that is consistent with functional requirements. In Figure 11.4, a multisynaptic pathway $RM_{R1} \rightarrow RM_T \rightarrow RM_{R2}$ replaces the direct $RM_{R1} \rightarrow RM_{R2}$ pathway of Figure 11.3. This multisynaptic pathway plays the following functional role. In both Figures 11.3 and 11.4, the RM_T is a retinotopic map at which attentional modulation of visual signals can occur. In Figure 11.4, the $RM_{R1} \rightarrow RM_T$ pathway can selectively enhance the retinotopic position that was chosen within the RM_{R1}. As a result, the favored RM_{R1} population is also "attentionally" amplified within the RM_T. The TPM_1 thus receives from the RM_T a spatial pattern of activated retinotopic positions such that the favored RM_{R1} position can effectively compete with positions that are amplified by other attentional factors.

In Figure 11.4, the RM_{R2} receives the entire spatial pattern of positions from the RM_T, not just the position chosen by the RM_{R1}, as in Figure 11.3. Thus if a retinotopic position other than the one chosen by the RM_{R1} is favored by the RM_T, then, in the absence of intermodal influences, both the RM_V and the RM_{R2} will tend to choose the same retinotopic position even before the $RM_V \rightarrow RM_{R2}$ transform is learned. By contrast, in Figure 11.3, the RM_{R2} and the RM_V can more easily choose different positions whenever attentional factors within RM_T favor a position other than the one chosen by the RM_{R1}.

In summary, the interactions in Figure 11.4 strengthen the tendency for both the RM_V and the RM_{R2} to choose the same positions whenever only light-activated cues enter the movement decision, whether or not the attentionally favored positions are the retinally favored ones. This property of Figure 11.4 tends to further stabilize learning of the $RM_V \rightarrow RM_{R2}$ associative transform.

11.7. Interactions between Superior Colliculus, Visual Cortex, and Parietal Cortex

We interpret the stages RM_{R1}, RM_{R2}, and RM_T in Figures 11.3 and 11.4 in terms of interactions between superior colliculus (SC), visual cortex, and parietal cortex. These retinotopic maps interact with other network stages that possess unambiguous anatomical interpretations. Such linkages constrain the anatomical interpretation of the retinotopic maps themselves. For example, the TPM_1 is assumed to occur in the parietal cortex. Both the RM_{R1} and the RM_{R2} project to the AG stage, which is assumed to occur in the cerebellum. The RM_{R1} gives rise to visually activated error signals, which are assumed to reach the cerebellum via climbing fibers. The RM_{R2} gives rise to visually activated sampling signals, which are assumed to reach the cerebellum via mossy fibers. The

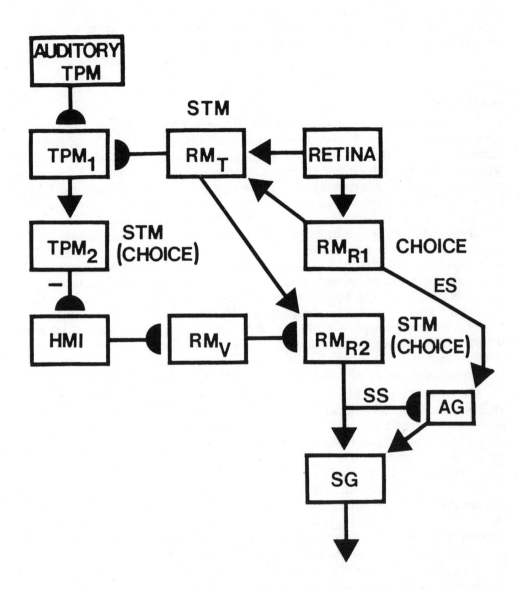

Figure 11.4. A variation on the circuit in Figure 11.3: The direct $RM_{R1} \rightarrow RM_{R2}$ projection of Figure 11.3 is replaced by an indirect projection in which the RM_{R1} projects to the RM_T which, in turn, projects to the RM_{R2}. The text describes the functional benefits of using such an indirect pathway.

RM_{R1} activates the RM_{R2}, whether monosynaptically or multisynaptically, but not conversely. The RM_{R2}, but not the RM_{R1}, stores a choice in STM from a time before a saccade begins until a time after a saccade ends. The RM_{R2}, but not the RM_{R1} or RM_T, projects to the saccade generator (SG). The RM_{R2} also receives inputs that are sensitive to corollary discharges. The RM_T, but not the RM_{R1}, processes retinotopic position signals that are attentionally modulated. Last but not least, each of the regions RM_{R1}, RM_{R2}, and RM_T is a *retinotopic* map; hence, it possesses enough internal topography to differentially process many distinct map positions.

These properties suggest that the RM_T is either part of the parietal cortex, or is in a part of the prestriate cortex that directly projects to parietal cortex. Because all of the maps are retinotopic maps, the deep layers of the SC, which are coded in motor coordinates, seem to be ruled out as a possible interpretation. Thus any SC role in computing RM_{R1}, RM_T, or RM_{R2} would seem to be restricted to the superficial layers of the SC (Huerta and Harting, 1984; Wurtz and Albano, 1980). The deeper SC layers, including the quasi-visual cells (Section 4.2), are interpreted to occur somewhere between the RM_{R2} and the SG in Figures 11.3 and 11.4. A likely location of the RM_{R1} is within the superficial SC layers. The following facts are consistent with this interpretation. The superficial SC layers receive a topographically organized retinal input. The superficial SC layers also project to several areas of visual cortex, as well as to the parietal cortex (compare $RM_{R1} \rightarrow RM_T$ in Figure 11.4). If this interpretation of the RM_{R1} is correct, then a positional choice based upon retinal light intensity and motion factors is made somewhere along the pathways between the superficial SC, the visual cortex, and the parietal cortex.

Given that the RM_T is interpreted to be in parietal cortex or in an adjacent prestriate cortical region, the reader may wonder why the retina is shown projecting directly to the RM_T in Figure 11.4. The projection from the retina to the RM_T is recognized to be multisynaptic *in vivo*, but we are not herein analysing the many processing stages used for visual form, depth, and color perception (Cohen and Grossberg, 1984a, 1984b; Grossberg and Mingolla, 1985a, 1985b) or for visual object recognition (Carpenter and Grossberg, 1985b; Grossberg and Stone, 1985a). The circuit in Figure 11.4 is a lumped representation of the visual factors that now play a role in our eye movement theory. The minimal network can and will be expanded as recent models of visual cortex are used to generate locations of movement commands in the theory.

It remains to anatomically interpret the RM_{R2} stage. Although this stage is the most functionally distinctive one—receiving as it does retinotopically recoded signals due to corollary discharges, projecting via mossy fibers to the cerebellum, and storing chosen lights in STM throughout a saccade—the available neural data do not seem to force an unambiguous anatomical interpretation. We consider the anatomical localization of the RM_{R2} to be a problem of major importance for neurobiologists interested in the saccadic system. Just as several anatomical stages intervene between the retina and the RM_T *in vivo*, the single macrostage RM_{R2} may consist of several closely interacting nuclei of cells *in vivo*.

11.8. Multiple Target Position Maps within Parietal Cortex and Frontal Eye Fields

The single TPM in Figure 11.1 is expanded into two successive TPMs, namely TPM_1 and TPM_2, in Figure 11.4. These successive TPMs play a role that is similar in important respects to the successive TPMs that were used to regulate sequences of predictive saccades in Figure 10.3. Map TPM_1 in both Figures 10.3 and 11.4 is an invariant TPM which can simultaneously encode several active target positions. In Figure 11.4, the activity level at each target position is the resultant of a combination of light-activated, multimodal, incentive motivational, and attentional gain control signals. In Figure 10.3, such factors interact with predictive mechanisms to read-out sequences of learned movement synergies. In both Figure 10.3 and Figure 11.4, the map TPM_2 chooses the target position from TPM_1 which achieves the largest activity based upon all of these influences. The chosen target position is stored in STM until after the saccade is over, so that it can then sample the corollary discharge at its HMI. In Figure 11.4, we interpret the TPM_1 on-center cells to be formal analogs of the light-sensitive attentionally modulated cells of the posterior parietal cortex (Yin and Mountcastle, 1977), and the on-center cells in TPM_2 to be formal analogs of the saccade cells in the posterior parietal cortex (Lynch, 1980; Motter and Mountcastle, 1981).

The TPMs of the parietal cortex (Figure 11.4) are assumed, however, to differ from the TPMs that control predictive saccades (Figure 10.3) in a crucial way: The parietal TPMs are incapable of storing temporal order information in STM. As we saw in Chapter 10, the ability to effectively store temporal order information in STM requires specialized auxiliary mechanisms that enable a match-mediated nonspecific rehearsal wave to sequentially read-out and reset the STM activity pattern within the TPM_1. We assume that this type of reset mechanism is found in the frontal eye fields (FEF) and is a version of a frontal cortex architecture that is specialized to organize "the temporal ordering of recent events" (Milner and Petrides, 1984, p.403). In addition to the machinery that is needed to regulate storage and sequential read-out of STM in a predictive system, we suggest that the predictive STM patterns may be encoded in long term memory (LTM) as motor plans, or chunks. These motor plans may be read-into STM from LTM in the absence of sensory cues. Both the regulatory STM machinery and the LTM chunking and read-out machinery are assumed to be part of the predictive design. Applications of this type of temporal ordering machinery to the processing of language and other types of motor control sequences are described in Grossberg (1978a, 1978b, 1985c) and Grossberg and Stone (1985a, 1985b).

11.9. Learning Multiply-Activated Target Position Maps

The previous sections have suggested that one TPM system is needed at which intermodal, motivational, and light-related factors can compe-

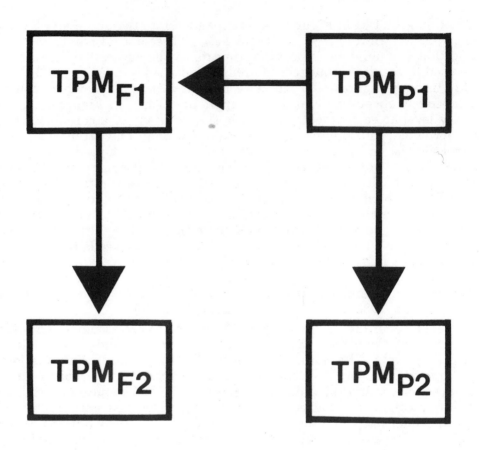

Figure 11.5. A possible circuit for connecting an attentionally modulated target position map (TPM_{P1}) with a predictive target position map (TPM_{F1}): Using this arrangement, the TPM_{F1} can automatically inherit both the target position coordinates and the attentional modulations of the TPM_{P1}. Both TPMs could, in principle, be implicitly built up from their own separate sources of retinotopic and eye position signals.

titively struggle to define an attentional focus capable of directing an eye movement. A second TPM system is needed at which predictive sequences of eye movements can be performed and can be learned, perhaps as part of more general motor plans. Neural data suggest, moreover, that the former TPM system is centered in the parietal cortex, whereas the latter TPM system is centered in the frontal eye fields (FEF). Consideration of how these two types of TPM systems interact leads to further constraints on system design. In order to unambiguously discuss these two TPM systems, we denote the parietal TPM stages by TPM_{P1} and TPM_{P2} and the frontal TPM stages by TPM_{F1} and TPM_{F2}.

A major issue concerns how these TPMs form. In Chapter 10, we considered several ways in which an invariant TPM can arise. In the subsequent discussion, we will fix ideas by assuming that the TPM_{P1} forms through a process of self-organization, as in Section 10.6. *Whatever* mechanism gives rise to the TPM_{P1}, once the TPM_{P1} develops, it can *automatically* generate the TPM_{F1}. If a topographic map exists from the TPM_{P1} to the TPM_{F1}, then the cells in the TPM_{F1} inherit the invariant target positions that are encoded by the corresponding cells in TPM_{P1} (Figure 11.5). Moreover, all of the attentional factors that weight the importance of target positions in TPM_{P1} can also weight the target positions in TPM_{F1}. Thus the specialized intermodal and motivational mechanisms that feed directly into TPM_{P1} can automatically influence the TPM_{F1} without necessitating the replication of these mechanisms at the TPM_{F1}. Although we consider this an attractive possibility, the TPM_{F1} could also implicitly form from combinations of RM_T and EPM signals, as in Chapter 10. Such a TPM would not, however, benefit from parietal forms of attentional modulation.

It is also conceivable that retinotopic inputs to the FEF are directly recoded into difference vectors. Such a direct recoding would, however, have to surmount the functional problems described in Section 9.10. In the present exposition, we explicitly consider the case in which the FEF possesses its own TPM_{F1}. With this exposition in hand, the above variations can also be understood.

From the TPM_{P1}, the target position with the largest weight, or activity, can generate a movement command via the TPM_{P2}. From the TPM_{F1}, the whole pattern of active target positions can be sequentially read-out in order of decreasing activity, and can be gradually encoded on successive performance trials into long term memory as part of a unitized motor plan for future predictive performances. Once it is recognized that these two types of TPM systems exist, several design issues come into focus concerning how it is decided which of these TPM systems will learn or perform eye movements at any given time.

Further consideration needs to be given to how the TPM_{P1} is formed. In Chapter 10, we considered a self-organization model in which a single retinal position (RM) and a single initial eye position (EPM_1) can sample a single target eye position (EPM$_2$) on every learning trial. Eventually, pairs of signals from the RM and the EPM_1 to the EPM_2 learn to generate individual target position activations at the EPM_2, thereby converting it into a TPM. In the adult TPM_{P1}, by contrast, we assume several target positions can simultaneously be active at any time. In order to ensure the applicability of the model in Chapter 10, one could alternatively suppose that just one target position can win the attentional competition at any time. This assumption is equivalent to lumping TPM_{P1} and TPM_{P2} into a single stage. This may, in fact, be true in sufficiently simple organisms.

This assumption is inadequate for our purposes, however. Then the TPM_{P1} could not map to the TPM_{F1}, because the TPM_{F1}, as a predictive mechanism, must be able to simultaneously store several target positions in STM. We would therefore have to ask how the TPM_{F1} could self-organize in response to multiple retinotopic sampling inputs. We would thus have to solve the same functional problem for the TPM_{F1} if we try to escape this problem at the TPM_{P1}. Moreover, if the TPM_{P1} can store only one target position at a time, then we would have lost the desirable property that attentional modulation within the TPM_{P1} alters the temporal ordering of predictive movements from the TPM_{F1}. Consequently, we now face the issue of how the TPM_{P1} can self-organize in the presence of multiple retinotopic sampling signals. The manner in which this issue is forced upon us illustrates how available design constraints can severely limit the number of hypotheses that one can reasonably entertain.

Two types of solutions are known. They are, moreover, experimentally testable. In the first solution, we suggest that the problem causes no new difficulties for the following reason. On any given saccadic trial, a single initial eye position (EPM_1) can combine with several retinotopic positions (RM) to sample a single target eye position (EPM_2). Only one combination of retinotopic position with initial eye position is the correct one, and this combination will consistently sample its correct target eye position on all learning trials, thereby generating a cumulative effect on the corresponding LTM traces. On the average, the other retinotopic positions will be randomly chosen with respect to the correct retinotopic position across sampling trials. Their LTM traces will tend to encode as many erroneous LTM increments as decrements, thereby tending to cancel their net LTM change due to erroneous correlations across learning trials. If only this property of random error distribution prevents map relearning errors from accumulating, then an electrode input that persistently activates the same false target eye position at EPM_2 after each saccade should cause a massive learned distortion in the adult TPM_{P1}.

In the second solution, TPM_{P1} map learning occurs only during a developmentally plastic critical period. This critical period terminates before such diverse attentional influences as multimodal and motivational factors can begin to override retinal light intensity and motion factors. During such a critical period, the RM_{R1} in Figure 11.4 can strongly bias the RM_T to differentially amplify its preferred light position. The input from the RM_T to the TPM_{P1} then approximates the choice of a single retinotopic position. After the TPM_{P1} is formed in this way, the critical period ends, and future multiple activations of the RM_T cannot cause map errors to be learned. If this model is valid, then approximate choices should occur within the RM_T at an early developmental stage, and electrode activations of an adult TPM_{P1} should not recode its target positions.

11.10. Multiple Parietal and Frontal Eye Field Vector Systems

Given that two TPM systems exist, it is necessary to consider whether they compute neural vectors using their own head-muscle interfaces (HMI) or whether they share a single HMI. The results in Chapter 4 showed how a TPM can convert its target positions into vectors at an HMI via a learning process. These results imply that only a single target position at a time can sample an HMI. If two or more target positions simultaneously sampled an HMI, then each target position would learn only a fractional part of the target eye position, by equations (4.1) and (4.2). Thus either each TPM system has its own HMI (Figure 11.6a), or each TPM system activates the same HMI at different times (Figure 11.6b), or only the TPM_{F2} projects to an HMI, which is reached by the TPM_{P1} via the TPM_{F1} (Figure 11.6c). In the last case, the TPM_{P1} would have to equal the TPM_{P2} in order for the TPM_{P2} to be able to activate a single (nonpredictive) vector. Then we would be reduced once again to considering a network in which the TPM_{F1} would have to self-organize in response to multiple sampling inputs from a retinotopic map (RM) and a source of initial eye movements (EPM_1). The parietal TPM_{P1} system could not then attentionally weight the order of predictive FEF saccades. We therefore reject this option and consider the two cases in which each TPM system can directly access an HMI.

Experimental data which support this conclusion were reported by Schiller and Sandell (1983), who showed that vector compensation using a Mays and Sparks (1980) light-electrode arrangement (Section 4.2) can occur after extirpation of the FEF, or of the SC, while stimulating the other. In our theory, the SC-controlled vector compensation is interpreted to include a TPM system, namely TPM_{P1} in the parietal cortex.

It remains to decide whether the TPM_P and TPM_F systems share a single HMI or whether each possesses its own HMI. We favor the latter alternative on general grounds because it provides the predictive movement system with a greater independence from interference by irrelevant sensory cues. We also favor this latter alternative for specific reasons. For example, if only one HMI existed, then the TPM_P and TPM_F systems would need to be able to competitively inhibit each other's output signals before these signals reached the shared HMI, since only one TPM can be allowed to sample the HMI at any time. Given that the TPM_{P2} and the TPM_{F2} are most likely to include large neocortical or subcortical regions, this would necessitate the ability of two large and topographically organized neural regions to nonspecifically shut each other off. Whereas this is not formally impossible, it is much easier for the two systems to compete nonspecifically at a smaller neural region, such as the SC or the SG. It is not inconceivable that, as a predictive movement capability evolved through phylogeny, a single HMI-based system evolved into a multiple HMI-based system. By considering the more difficult multiple HMI case

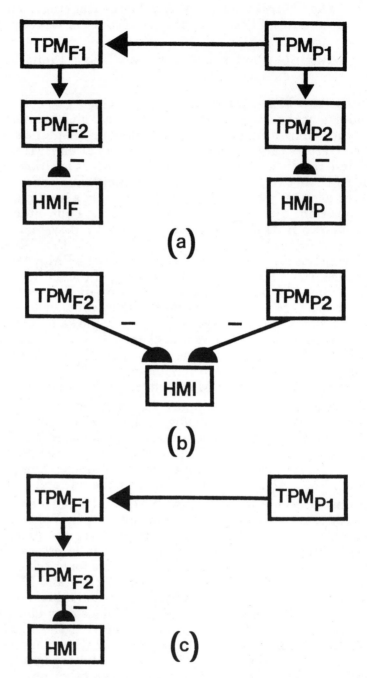

Figure 11.6. Some possible circuits for attaching a head-muscle interface (HMI) to a target position map (TPM): The text discusses some advantages in using separate HMIs in the attentional (HMI$_P$) and predictive (HMI$_F$) systems.

herein, many of the properties which arise using a simpler single HMI case are also implicitly analysed.

A multiple HMI-based system is also supported by the data of Mays and Sparks (1980) and of Schiller and Sandell (1983). The data of Mays and Sparks (1980) show that HMI vectors get read out through the quasi-visual (QV) cells of the SC. Suppose that the RM_R stage in Figure 11.4 feeds into the QV cells, or includes the QV cells. Then extirpation of the SC would prevent the HMI in Figure 11.4 from reading-out its movement commands. If the TPM_F system fed its signals into this same HMI, then SC lesions would prevent the read-out of FEF saccades. The data of Schiller and Sandell (1983) suggest that this is false, at least in monkeys. Bruce and Goldberg (1984) have provided additional evidence that the FEF can generate vector commands. They showed that electrical stimulation of certain FEF cells could generate saccades of a fixed size and direction, independent of the initial eye position.

11.11. Learning Neural Vectors and Adaptive Gains in a Predictive Movement System

Henceforth we assume that two HMI systems exist, corresponding to the two TPM systems TPM_P and TPM_F. We denote these HMIs by HMI_P and HMI_F, respectively, as in Figure 11.6a. We now consider what new learning issues are raised by the existence of a separate HMI_F system. The main issues concern how target positions are converted into muscle coordinates by the learned $TPM_{F2} \rightarrow HMI_F$ transform, and how vector commands from the HMI_F gain control of adaptive gains at the AG stage that can generate accurate foveations.

The problem in its most severe form arises if the TPM_F system, unlike the TPM_P system of Figure 11.4, does not sample the RM_{R2}. Then the TPM_F system cannot use the adaptive gains which the RM_{R2} controls via the AG stage. It is theoretically possible for the TPM_F system to sample the RM_{R2}, but it would have to do so in a way that does not also inhibit sampling by the TPM_P system. In particular, the TPM_F system would have to sample the RM_{R2} at a stage subsequent to the stage at which the TPM_P system samples the RM_{R2}, so that TPM_F signals would not competitively preempt sampling of the RM_{R2} by the TPM_P system. Such a convergence of visually reactive, TPM_P, and TPM_F commands at the RM_{R2} could, however, cause a high probability of erroneous command choice during sequences of predictive saccades. Erroneous command choices during predictive saccades can be minimized if the predictive movement system can nonspecifically inhibit all visually reactive and TPM_P signals. This cannot happen if the TPM_F system can sample the RM_{R2}, because the sampled pathways must be activated by visually reactive signals. In order for the predictive movement system to nonspecifically inhibit other sources of movement commands, it must feed into the SG at a stage subsequent to the RM_{R2}, so that it can nonspecifically inhibit $RM_{R2} \rightarrow SG$ movement signals without inhibiting its own movement signals.

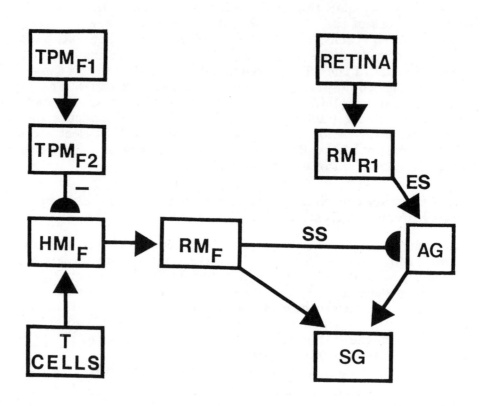

Figure 11.7. A circuit in which the predictive system controls its own unconditioned and conditioned movement pathways. Abbreviations: ES = error signal, SS = sampling signal.

We therefore consider a model in which the TPM_F system controls its own unconditioned $HMI_F \to RM_F \to SG$ and conditioned $HMI_F \to RM_F \to AG \to SG$ movement pathways to the SG, as in Figure 11.7. This model faces and meets the full force of the infinite regress problem. If the adaptive gains controlled by the RM_{R2} are not used to achieve accurate predictive saccades, then how does the predictive command network (PCN) learn its adaptive gains? No learning difficulties arise if the vectors used by the PCN via the HMI_F are accurately calibrated. Any adequate solution of how sequences of predictive saccades are controlled must include a solution of this problem. If HMI_F vectors are accurately calibrated, then predictive commands from the PCN can cause unconditioned movements via the pathway $HMI_F \to RM_F \to SG$ in Figure 11.7. Second light error signals, registered via the Retina $\to RM_{R1} \to AG$ pathway, can then alter the adaptive gains within the $RM_F \to AG \to SG$ pathway, using the mechanisms of Chapter 3. Thus the retinotopic command network (RCN) helps to calibrate the PCN using its second light error signal subsystem. We now indicate how the RCN also helps to calibrate the vectors computed within the HMI_F of the PCN. Thus the RCN acts in two ways to overcome the infinite regress problem that might otherwise be faced by the PCN.

The main requirements are (1) the $TPM_{F2} \to HMI_F$ transform is correctly learned before the HMI_F can begin to generate predictive commands, and (2) the $TPM_F \to HMI_F$ transform is not unlearned due to performance errors caused by HMI_F-generated saccades before the $HMI_F \to RM_F \to AG \to SG$ pathway can learn the correct adaptive gains. Both requirements are achieved by making an assumption concerning the type of saccade-driven gate (Section 9.7) that turns on learning within the HMI_F.

The best performance is achieved if the SG is broken up into two subsystems: One subsystem SG_R receives unconditioned and conditioned movement signals from the RM_{R2}, and thus also from the HMI_P (Figure 11.8). The other subsystem SG_F receives unconditioned and conditioned movement signals from the HMI_F via the RM_F. Both subsystems are assumed to possess their own complement of burster cells and pauser cells that send convergent signals to tonic cells and motoneurons (Section 7.8). We assume that the learning gate within the HMI_F is turned on either by onset of pauser activity or by offset of burster activity within the SG_R. We also assume that the same class of SG_R cells turns on the learning gate within the HMI_P (Figure 11.8). Thus the learned transformation of target position into motor coordinates is assumed to be regulated by RM_{R2}-controlled gating signals in *both* HMIs. Since the RM_{R2} can learn to generate correct saccades using second light error signals (Chapter 3), it can generate correct target eye positions for learning at the HMIs.

In order for the TPM_{F2} to sample the RM_R-generated target positions at the HMI_F, the TPM_{F1} must be capable of activating the TPM_{F2} before RM_R-generated saccades occur. Thus the TPMs of the FEF must be sensitive to lights at a developmental stage prior to the emergence of predictive saccades. This property implies that factors other than volition

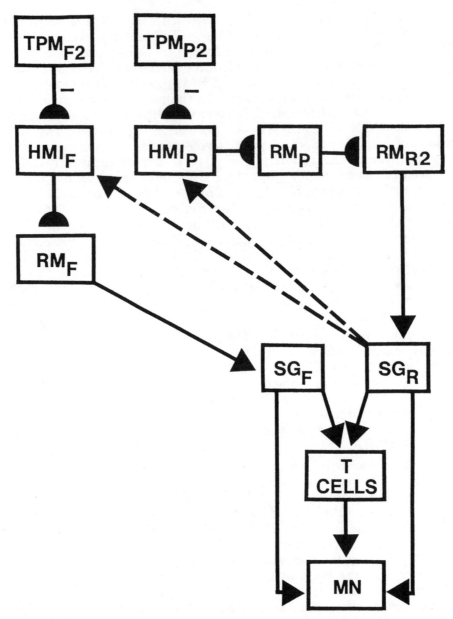

Figure 11.8. Regulation of target position learning within both the parietal head-muscle interface (HMI$_P$) and the frontal head-muscle interface (HMI$_F$) by the same source of gating signals. This source is the saccade generator (SG$_R$) that is activated by the retinotopic command network (RCN). This scheme enables vectors in the HMI$_F$ to be correctly calibrated before the predictive command network (PCN) begins to compete with the RCN. Abbreviations: SG$_F$ = frontally activated saccade generator. The gating pathways are marked with dashed lines.

can enable the TPM_{F1} to activate the TPM_{F2} (Section 9.4). In particular, we assume that specific output signals from the TPM_{P1} to the TPM_{F1} give rise to inhibitory interneurons capable of shutting off the tonic gating cells which inhibit TPM_{F1} output signals (Figure 11.9). A volitional signal can also shut off these cells, as in Section 9.4. We assume furthermore that such a volitional signal opens an output gate which enables the HMI_F to activate the SG_F (Figure 11.9).

11.12. Frontal Eye Field Control of Voluntary Saccadic Eye Movements and Posture: Cell Types

These assumptions imply that the FEF system can learn correct vectors in response to light-sensitive inputs, but can only generate saccades in response to an act of volition. These properties are consistent with the conclusion of Bruce and Goldberg (1984, p.439) that "frontal eye field cells discharge before purposive saccadic eye movements." Bruce and Goldberg (1984) described *visuomovement cells* which begin to discharge in response to a visual stimulus and continued to respond until after a saccade began, and *movement cells* which responded just before and during a saccade. These cells were studied during an experiment in which the monkey was trained not to respond to a peripheral target until the fixation light was turned off over a second later. The visuomovement cells continued to discharge throughout the presaccadic interval even if the target presentation was brief (100 msec.). Thus these visuomovement cells were capable of storing the target position in STM until after the saccade began.

These experimental properties are consistent with the assumptions that visuomovement cells occur in the TPM_{F1}, movement cells occur in the TPM_{F2}, and a volitional signal enables the stored command in the TPM_{F1} to be read into the TPM_{F2}, thereby generating a voluntary saccade.

The FEF also contains cells that discharge after saccadic eye movements (Bizzi, 1968; Bizzi and Schiller, 1970; Goldberg and Bushnell, 1981). These post-saccadic cells respond only after saccades of fixed dimensions. Bruce and Goldberg (1984, p.440) noted that "Because they respond after both spontaneous and visually elicited saccades, it seems likely that they are driven by an efference copy from the brainstem saccade generator." Our theory suggests that three types of post-saccadic cell may be found in the FEF, or in closely associated neural regions. One type may be part of the eye position map (EPM) within the tension equalization network (TEN) of Chapter 8. These EPM cells are activated by tonic cells of the SG after a saccade terminates. They are driven by an efference copy from the brainstem saccade generator, and respond only after saccades of fixed dimensions are over. Their functional role is to read out the learned postural gains that prevent postsaccadic drift.

A second type of post-saccadic cell may exist in the FEF if the HMI_F is housed within the FEF. Such cells would relay gating signals from the SG_R to the HMI_F (Figure 11.8). These cells would be active after both spontaneous and visually elicited saccades. They could, however, respond after saccades of variable size, since their function is to enable the TPM_{F2}

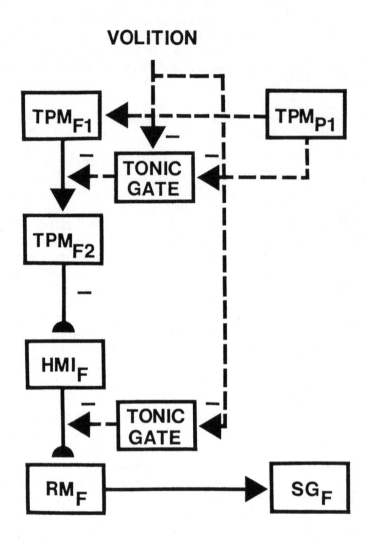

Figure 11.9. Gating signals which regulate the predictive, or frontal, command system: Volitional signals can enable read-out of the TPM_{F1} and of the HMI_F signals to occur. Attentionally modulated sensory signals, say from the TPM_{P1}, can also enable read-out of the TPM_{F1} to occur. In this way HMI_F vectors can be calibrated even if movement commands from the HMI_F are not released. The gating pathways are marked with dashed lines.

to learn whatever target eye position was attained by the previous saccade. It may be that the SG_R directly gates the HMI_F without the intervention of HMI_F interneurons. Then the activity of axons, rather than cell bodies, would be predicted to possess these functional properties.

The TPM_{F2} cells which we have identified with FEF movement cells (Bruce and Goldberg, 1984) may also occasionally respond like a type of post-saccadic cell. Suppose that the TPM_{F1} has been storing several target positions in STM while spontaneous or visually elicited saccades are taking place. The TPM_{F2} and the HMI_F can process such target positions because the TPM_{F2} must be able to learn its target eye positions at the HMI_F in response to visually activated movement commands (Section 11.11). Thus after a saccade takes place, a rehearsal wave may occur enabling the TPM_{F1} to read a new target position into the TPM_{F2}. Such a TPM_{F2} cell would occur after the saccade was over. Hence the cell would appear to be a "post-saccadic cell." This cell might not cause the next saccade unless the volitional gate is opened (Figure 11.9). Hence its role in controlling a future voluntary saccade could be mistaken for a reaction to a past visually reactive saccade. Such a cell would not encode an efference copy from the SG. Rather, it would encode the target position of a possible voluntary saccade. To distinguish this type of "post-saccadic cell" from an EPM cell which controls the read-out of postural gain, one could use the Bruce and Goldberg (1984) paradigm to discover whether the cell can also function as a movement cell in an experiment that requires voluntary saccades.

11.13. Coupled Vector and Adaptive Gain Learning

A possible variation of the circuit design described in Figures 11.8 and 11.9 is also worthy of experimental study. If the gating rules summarized in Figure 11.9 are imposed, then the PCN can achieve a significant competence even if the SG is not broken into two subsystems. The gating rules in Figure 11.8 enable the TPM_{F2} to calibrate accurate vectors at the HMI_F before the HMI_F can begin to generate predictive saccades. Thus, when HMI_F-generated saccades emerge, the vectors computed within the HMI_F are already accurately calibrated, whereas the adaptive gains of the conditioned pathway $HMI_F \rightarrow RM_F \rightarrow AG \rightarrow SG$ are not yet accurately calibrated. Consequently saccadic errors will occur. In Figure 11.8, we prevented these errors from causing the relearning of inaccurate vectors by using the SG_R to shut off vector learning in the HMI_F when predictive saccades are being made.

We now observe that new vector learning may be permitted to occur in the predictive mode. The learning of incorrect target positions within the HMI_F which is caused by foveation errors will tend to be compensated by learning within the AG stage *if* the HMI_F starts out with accurately calibrated vectors. For example, suppose that an undershoot error occurs. Then the vector which caused the saccade will learn a larger adaptive gain (Chapter 3), but the TPM_{F2} will learn to generate a smaller vector in response to the same retinal position on a later saccadic trial (Chapter

4). On successive undershoot trials, progressively smaller vectors and progressively larger gains will be learned hand-in-hand. Finally, a time is reached at which either the saccades cannot get shorter, or the larger adaptive gains by themselves will start to cause longer, and therefore more correct, saccades. At such a time, the adaptive gains are larger than they were at the outset, and are hence better able to prevent undershoot errors, but the vectors read-out by the TPM are too small. As large vectors begin to be learned, the adaptive gains will grow even larger to prevent further undershoot errors. Thereafter, relearning of correct vectors and of large enough adaptive gains to prevent undershoot errors go hand-in-hand until accurate saccades are generated.

This coupled vector-gain learning process is not yet fully understood. It may help to stabilize learning within the PCN even in organisms wherein HMI_F learning is gated by the SG, but not by a specialized SG_R subsystem.

11.14. Gating of Learning, Movement, and Posture

The network to which our analysis of sensory-motor learning has led us is now a large and complex one. It includes circuits whose physiological and anatomical properties help to explain and predict data from the retina, superior colliculus, peripontine reticular formation, oculomotor nuclei, cerebellum, visual cortex, parietal cortex, and frontal eye fields. Underlying this complexity are a few general circuit designs—such as head-muscle interfaces, eye position maps, target position maps, and adaptive gain stages—which are utilized in multiple network locations. The placement of these circuits into different network positions endows them with different functional capabilities. The reader need only recall the many uses of eye position maps, including their possible role in generating an invariant TPM (Chapter 10), to appreciate this fact. Thus a significant part of the intelligence embodied within these large circuits lies in the genetic and developmental rules which control the correct placement of a few standardized circuit designs.

Another part of the intelligence of such a system lies in the gating rules which synchronize the switching on and off of the correct subsystems through time. Such gating rules have arisen repeatedly during the preceding chapters. They must be simple enough to generate correct switching decisions based upon locally computable signals. They give rise to global intelligence due to the manner in which they are connected to network subsystems. In particular, they are organized to achieve synchronous switching between movement and postural subsystems, and to modulate learning within each of these subsystems (Chapter 9). The present section summarizes and further develops the gating rules that are needed to prevent contradictory movement or postural signals from being generated during the saccade cycle.

Figures 11.10–11.13 describe the main types of gates that are needed in our theory. In all of the figures, gating pathways are denoted by dashed lines. The gates that regulate sequential read-out of target positions

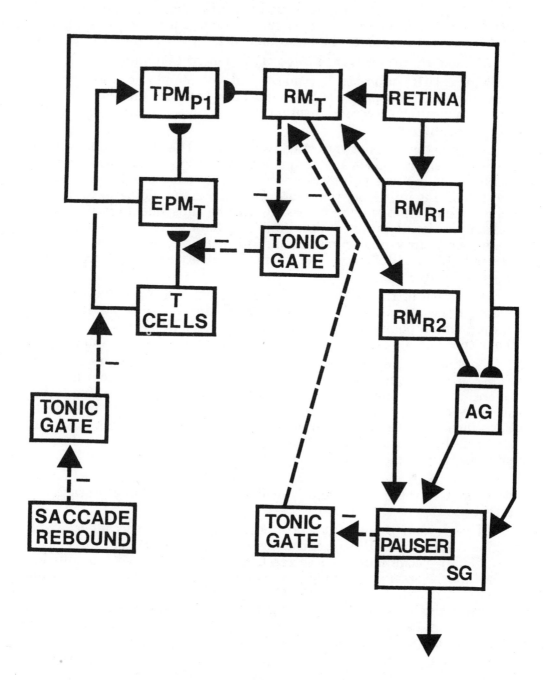

Figure 11.10. Gating of map reset events by signals from the saccade generator (SG). See text for details. Gating pathways are marked by dashed lines.

within the PCN will not be discussed, because they were already dealt with in Chapter 9. Figures 11.10–11.12 show that just a few types of gating actions suffice to regulate the entire network.

A. *Read-in, Reset, and Storage of Movement Commands*

Figure 11.10 indicates how movement commands activate the network, how they reset previous commands, and how they are stored in STM long enough after a saccade terminates to sample adaptive gains at the SG stage (Chapter 2).

Suppose that the network starts out at rest. The pauser population in the SG is then on. This is an omnipauser population that is on between all saccades and is turned off by all saccades. Because these pausers are on, they inhibit the inhibitory tonic gate. The RM_T is therefore free to respond to lights that impinge upon the retina. (In the subsequent discussion, we will suppose for definiteness that inhibitory tonic gates modulate network stages. Excitatory phasic gates could, in principle, do the same job, as Figure 11.13 will illustrate. Such thematic variations will be determined experimentally.)

Activation of the RM_T has three major effects. First, the RM_T can instate a new retinotopic position into the RM_{R2}. By so doing, it inhibits any retinotopic position that was previously stored by the RM_{R2}, as well as the output signals from the RM_{R2} to the SG and to the AG stage.

Second, the RM_T enables a new initial eye position to be read into the EPM_T, by inhibiting the tonic gate that kept the T cells from doing so before. This eye position is stored in STM within the EPM_T. Due to this sequence of events, the RM_{R2} is inhibited before the EPM_T can be reset. Consequently, the new eye position at the EPM_T cannot initiate a saccade staircase by inputting a new eye position signal to the SG before the previous retinotopic signal is shut off (Section 7.6).

Third, both the new RM_T position and the new EPM_T position can now input to the TPM_{P1}, which leads to choice and STM storage of a target position at the TPM_{P2}.

These events prepare the network to initiate a new saccade by instating new retinotopic (RM_{R2}), initial eye position (EPM_T), and target position (TPM_{P2}) commands. These reset events also occur with a sufficient delay after a previous saccade has ended to allow the RM_{R2}, EPM_T, and other systems which sample the AG stage to benefit from any second light error signals that the RM_{R1} might generate there. All of these events are regulated by two tonic gates, both of which are controlled, directly or indirectly, by populations in the SG.

Figure 11.10 also notes that a different type of gate is needed in order to learn an invariant TPM_{P1}. Such a gate is opened only after a saccade occurs, in response to the activation of saccade rebound cells. This gate enables the RM_T retinotopic position and the EPM_T initial eye position to sample the target eye position that is attained by the saccade (Section 10.5). Saccade rebound cells can arise as the off-cells of a gated dipole opponent process (Grossberg, 1972c, 1980, 1984), whose on-cell input source

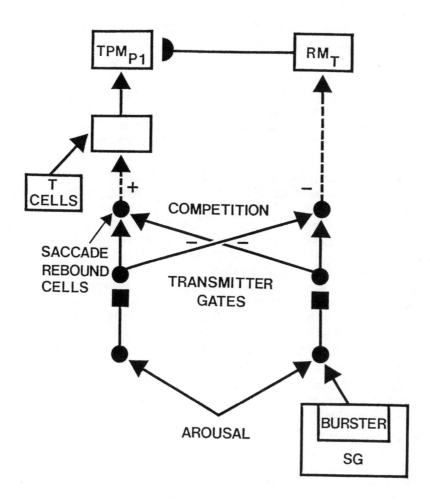

Figure 11.11. A possible mechanism giving rise to the saccade rebound cells of Figure 11.10. A tonically-aroused opponent process, called a gated dipole, can inhibit the retinotopic map RM_T via its on-channel and excite the gate in the T cell$\rightarrow TPM_{P1}$ pathway via its off-channel. A burster population in the saccade generator (SG) can excite the on-channel. Offset of the burster generates a transient output burst from the off-channel. Habituation of the slowly accumulating transmitter gates within the gated dipole regulates its on and off responses.

is an SG burster cell population (Figure 11.11). In fact, the on-cells of such a gated dipole can replace the disinhibitory pauser gate in Figure 11.10 by an inhibitory burster gate (Figure 11.11).

B. Read-Out and Competition of Movement Commands

Figure 11.12 describes gating actions that regulate the flow of movement commands to the saccade generator (SG). The critical gate in this figure is an inhibitory tonic gate which acts at a stage somewhere between (or within) the RM_{R2} and the SG. We hypothesize that this gate exists within the substantia nigra (Hikosaka and Wurtz, 1983) and therefore interpret its site of action as the deep layers of the superior colliculus (SC). We also assume that several different movement sources can act upon this gate.

The RM_{R2} can inhibit the gate, and thereby enable its stored retinotopic position to activate the SG, other things being equal. Two properties govern our choice of the RM_{R2} as a possible source of gate inhibition. First, the RM_{R2} stores a choice in STM, and hence is active throughout a saccade. Thus the gate stays off throughout an RM_{R2}-activated saccade and thereby enables the SG to fully react to the RM_{R2} movement command. Second, the RM_{R2} is part of the retinotopic command network (RCN). The RM_{R2} can therefore be activated by attended lights before the developmental stage occurs during which the invariant TPM_{P1} forms. The RCN can thus generate and correct the visually reactive saccades on which invariant TPM formation, vector calibration within the HMI, and other later learning processes are based.

The TPM_{P2} is also assumed to inhibit the tonic gate. This enables attentionally modulated multimodal inputs, in addition to visually reactive visual inputs, to generate saccades via the $TPM_{P2} \rightarrow HMI_P \rightarrow RM_P \rightarrow RM_{R2} \rightarrow SG$ pathway.

Finally, we assume that the RM_F can powerfully excite the tonic gate. This excitation can counteract inhibition from the RM_{R2} and the TPM_{P2}. Thus, when the volitional gate in the FEF opens (Chapter 9) and a vector from HMI_F activates the RM_F, this voluntary command can inhibit other movement commands as it activates its own pathway to the SG_F. This hypothesis is consistent with the fact that the FEF projects to the SC via the substantia nigra (Hikosaka and Wurtz, 1983).

Figure 11.12 also describes another possible way in which the FEF movement system can compete with the SC movement system. Suppose that RM_F commands excite the bursters of SG_F and the pausers of SG_R, and possibly that RM_{R2} commands excite the bursters of SG_R and the pausers of SG_F. If the pausers of SG_R could be kept on by RM_F excitation even in the presence of inhibition from SG_R long lead bursters, then the FEF could dominate SC commands even within the peripontine reticular formation (Section 7.8). We do not know any data relevant to this possibility. The circuit can work without this mechanism.

One general conclusion from Figures 11.10–11.12 is that SG cells such as tonic cells, bursters, and pausers may interact with far-flung neocortical cells, no less than with nearby cells of the SG circuit.

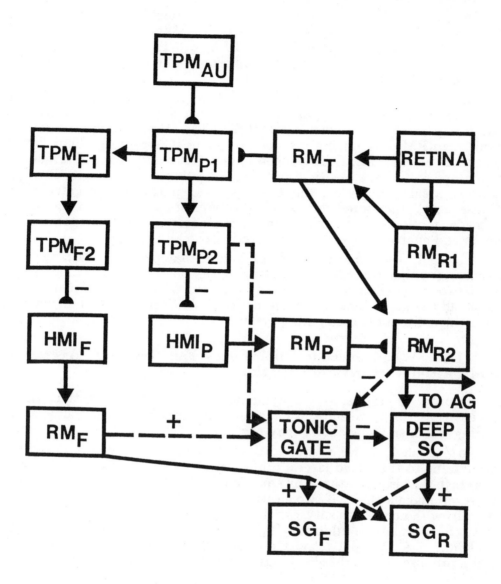

Figure 11.12. Gating processes that regulate the flow of movement commands to the saccade generator (SG). See text for details. Gating pathways are indicated by dashed lines.

C. *Gating of Posture and Learning*

In Figure 11.13, the postural eye position map (EPM_{Pos}) is allowed to store eye positions only between saccades. While a saccade is being performed, the tonic gate inhibits the EPM_{Pos}. Thus the EPM_{Pos} reads out the adaptive gains which prevent postsaccadic drift only during the postural state (Chapter 8).

In Figure 11.13, we have assumed for simplicity that the same tonic gate acts upon the EPM_{Pos} and upon vector outputs from the HMI_P and the HMI_F. Outputs leave each HMI for STM storage within its retinotopic map RM only during the postural state (Chapter 4). Thus before a saccade begins, each HMI can compute a vector difference of target position and initial eye position and store it retinotopically in its RM. As soon as a saccade begins, the $HMI \rightarrow RM$ pathways are gated shut. Consequently the stored retinotopic positions are not changed due to the saccadic motion. After the saccade terminates, the output gates open again and enable new vectors to be retinotopically stored.

Figure 11.13 also includes a tonic gate that prevents learning from occurring within the HMI except during the postural state (Chapter 4). In networks wherein a saccade generator subsystem like SG_R does not exist, all the gating actions in the figure could, in principle, be governed by a single SG-controlled gating system.

11.15. When Saccade Choice May Fail: Saccadic Averaging and Partial Vector Compensation

In order to emphasize the dynamic nature of the interactions which we have described, we end this chapter by considering some circumstances during which saccadic choice may partially fail.

In Section 11.3, we suggested that choice of one retinotopic position occurs due to the broad lateral inhibitory signals and signal functions at the stage that is caricatured by equation (11.3). Such a network may not, however, make a choice if two electrodes simultaneously activate a pair of its cells with equal intensity, or with intensities that are greater than the strength of its lateral inhibitory signals. Under these circumstances, both cells may retain partial activity and may thus generate a saccade that is a compromise, or weighted average, of the individual saccadic commands (Schiller and Sandell, 1983).

In Chapter 9 and Figures 11.3, 11.4, 11.8, and 11.9, we suggested that only one target position at a time can normally be stored within a TPM_2; then only one vector at a time can be computed at the corresponding HMI. By contrast, the process of STM reset and STM storage at a TPM_2 takes some time. It may be possible for one light to be partially stored within the TPM_2 when another, more salient, light occurs. Such a second light may be able to instate itself in the TPM_2 before the previous light can be fully stored. In this case, a partial vector compensation may occur that is rapidly followed by a second, more complete, vector compensation (Young, 1981).

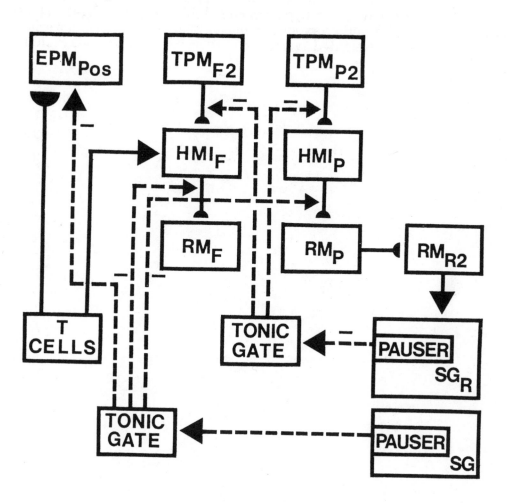

Figure 11.13. Gating processes that regulate reset events during posture. See text for details. Gating pathways are indicated by dashed lines.

Finally, only one saccade is usually generated by the retinotopic command network (RCN), or the predictive command network (PCN), but not both. On the other hand, simultaneously active electrodes placed in both subsystems may either bypass their inhibitory gates (Figure 11.12) or may override the inhibitory signals due to these gates. Then a saccade may occur that is a weighted average of both saccadic commands (Schiller and Sandell, 1983).

CHAPTER 12

ARE THERE UNIVERSAL PRINCIPLES OF SENSORY-MOTOR CONTROL?

In the preceding chapters, we have identified a set of functional problems, notably problems of self-calibration, which need to be solved by sensory-motor systems. We have also suggested neural circuits which are competent to solve these problems. In cases where several qualitatively different circuit solutions are capable of solving a functional problem, and where available data do not unambiguously favor one solution, we have developed enough properties of the solutions to differentiate them in future experiments. Although it was not feasible to describe all possible anatomical and physiological variations of these solutions, we have selected examples which clearly articulate the basic functional issues. These examples should make it easier to interpret functionally related data in variations which we did not explicitly develop.

Many of the functional problems that we have addressed are not restricted to the saccadic eye movement system. This fact raises the question of whether similar neural designs may be used to control other sensory-motor systems than the saccadic system. In a general sense, the answer to this question clearly seems to be "yes." Many of the circuits which we have suggested are naturally decomposed into functionally specialized macrostages, such as the adaptive gain stage (Chapter 3), which are utilized in multiple circuits due to their specialized processing capabilities. Moreover, different sensory-motor systems must communicate via commands that are dimensionally consistent. In particular, our discussion of how intermodality circular reactions are learned (Section 1.3) suggested that several sensory-motor systems compare target position with present position in order to generate their movement commands. In addition, functional problems such as learning the correct gains for movements vs. postures, and compensating for changes in muscle plant characteristics, beset many sensory-motor systems other than the saccadic system. The need to learn motor synergies, rather than individual muscle commands, and to change coordinates between different sensory, motor, and vector stages are also shared by many sensory-motor systems.

Differences between the saccadic control system and other goal-oriented sensory-motor systems may be sought in finer, but nonetheless important, distinctions, such as (I) the distinction between the control of continuous vs. ballistic movements, and (II) the distinction between the control of motor organs that are regularly perturbed by unexpected loads vs. motor organs that are not regularly perturbed by unexpected loads. The first distinction might lead to differences in how target positions and present positions are generated and compared through time, and how each system computes and compensates for self-motion vs. world-motion. The second distinction might lead to differences in automatic load compensation mechanisms and to modified uses of inflow and outflow signals. It remains for future experimental and theoretical work to determine how many of the neural designs which we have suggested for the saccadic system are modified for use in other sensory-motor systems, and how many need to be supplemented by qualitatively new neural designs.

Psychological Review, 1988, **95**, 49–90
©1988 American Psychological Association

CHAPTER 13

NEURAL DYNAMICS OF PLANNED ARM MOVEMENTS: EMERGENT INVARIANTS AND SPEED-ACCURACY PROPERTIES DURING TRAJECTORY FORMATION

Daniel Bullock† and Stephen Grossberg‡

Abstract

A real-time neural network model, called the Vector Integration to Endpoint, or VITE, Model, is developed and used to quantitatively simulate behavioral and neural data about planned and passive arm movements. Invariants of arm movements emerge through network interactions rather than through an explicitly precomputed trajectory. Motor planning occurs in the form of a Target Position Command, or TPC, which specifies where the arm intends to move, and an independently controlled GO command, which specifies the movement's overall speed. Automatic processes convert this information into an arm trajectory with invariant properties. These automatic processes include computation of a Present Position Command, or PPC, and a Difference Vector, or DV. The DV is the difference of the PPC and the TPC at any time. The PPC is gradually updated by integrating the DV through time. The GO signal multiplies the DV before it is integrated by the PPC. The PPC generates an outflow movement command to its target muscle groups. Opponent interactions regulate the PPC's to agonist and antagonist muscle groups. This system generates synchronous movements across synergetic muscles by automatically compensating for the different total contractions that each muscle group must undergo. Quantitative simulations are provided of Woodworth's Law, of the speed-accuracy trade-off known as Fitts' Law, of isotonic arm movement properties before and after deafferentation, of synchronous and compensatory "central error correction" properties of isometric contractions, of velocity amplification during target switching, of velocity profile invariance and asymmetry, of the changes in velocity

† Supported in part by the National Science Foundation (NSF IST-84-17756).

‡ Supported in part by the Air Force Office of Scientific Research (AFOSR F49620-86-C-0037 and AFOSR F49620-87-C-0018) and the National Science Foundation (NSF IST-84-17756).

profile asymmetry at higher movement speeds, of the automatic compensation for staggered onset times of synergetic muscles, of vector cell properties in precentral motor cortex, of the inverse relationship between movement duration and peak velocity, and of peak acceleration as a function of movement amplitude and duration. It is shown that TPC, PPC, and DV computations are needed to actively modulate, or gate, the learning of associative maps between TPC's of different modalities, such as between the eye-head system and the hand-arm system. By using such an associative map, looking at an object can activate a TPC of the hand-arm system, as Piaget noted. Then a VITE circuit can translate this TPC into an invariant movement trajectory. An auxiliary circuit, called the Passive Update of Position, or PUP, Model, is described for using inflow signals to update the PPC during passive arm movements due to external forces. Other uses of outflow and inflow signals are also noted, such as for adaptive linearization of a nonlinear muscle plant, and sequential read-out of TPC's during a serial plan, as in reaching and grasping. Comparisons are made with other models of motor control, such as the mass-spring and minimum-jerk models.

13.1. Introduction: Are Movement Invariants Explicitly Planned?

The subjective ease with which we carry out simple action plans—rotating a wrist-watch into view, lifting a coffee cup, or making a downstroke while writing—masks the enormously complex integrative apparatus needed to achieve and maintain coordination among the thousands of sensors, neurons, and skeleto-motor units that contribute to any act's planning and execution. Moreover, recent studies of the kinematics of planned arm movements (Abend, *et al.*, 1982; Atkeson and Hollerbach, 1985; Howarth and Beggs, 1981) have shown that the integrative action of all these separate contributors produces velocity profiles whose global shape is remarkably invariant over a wide range of movement sizes and speeds. This raises a fundamental question for the theory of sensory-motor control, and for the neurosciences in general: How can the integrated activity of thousands of separate elements produce globally invariant properties?

Two broad species of answers to this question can be contemplated. The first includes theories that posit the existence of a high level stage involving explicit computation and internal representation of the invariant, in this case the velocity profile, as a whole. This representation is then used as a basis for performing the desired action. Such theories have been favored recently by many workers in the field of robotics, and at least one theory of this type has already been partially formulated to accommodate kinematic data on human movements: the "minimized Cartesian jerk theory" (Hogan, 1984; Flash and Hogan, 1985), which is a special case of global optimization analysis. The second species of answers includes theories in which no need arises for explicit computation and representation of the invariant trajectory as a whole (Sections 13.7 and 13.16). In models associated with such theories, a trajectory with globally invariant properties emerges in real-time as the result of events distributed across many interacting sensory, neural, and muscular loci.

This article describes a theory of arm trajectory invariants that conforms to the latter ideal (Bullock and Grossberg, 1986). Our analysis suggests that trajectory invariants are best understood not by focusing on velocity profiles as such, but by pursuing more fundamental questions: What principles of adaptive behavioral organization constrain the system design that governs planned arm movements? What mechanisms are needed to realize these principles as a real-time neural network? Our development of this topic proceeds via analyses of learned eye-hand coordination, synchronization among synergists, intermediate position control during movement, and variable velocity control. These analyses disclose a neural network design whose qualitative and quantitative operating characteristics match those observed in a wide range of experiments on human movement. Because velocity profile invariance, as well as speed-dependent changes in velocity profile asymmetry ignored by prior models (Section 13.12), are among the neural network's emergent operating characteristics, our work shows that neither an explicit trajectory nor a kinematic invariant need be explicitly represented within a motor control system at any time. Thus our work supports a critical insight of workers in the mass-spring modeling tradition, that movement kinematics need not be explicitly pre-programmed. By the same token, our results reject a mass-spring model in its customary form and argue against models based upon optimization theory. Instead we show how a movement control system may be adaptive without necessarily optimizing an explicit cost function.

To further support these conclusions, we use the neural model to quantitatively simulate Woodworth's Law and Fitts' Law, the empirically derived speed-accuracy tradeoff function relating error magnitudes, movement distances and movement durations; isotonic arm movement properties before and after deafferentation (Bizzi, Accornero, Chapple, and Hogan, 1982, 1984; Evarts and Fromm, 1978; Polit and Bizzi, 1978); synchronous and compensatory "central error correction" properties of isometric contractions (Freund and Büdingen, 1978; Ghez and Vicario, 1978; Gordon and Ghez, 1984, 1987a, 1987b,); velocity amplification during target switching (Georgopoulos, Kalaska, and Massey, 1981); velocity profile invariance and asymmetry (Abend, Bizzi, and Morasso, 1982; Atkeson and Hollerbach, 1985; Georgopoulos, Kalaska, and Massey, 1981; Beggs and Howarth, 1972; Morasso, 1981; Soechting and Lacquaniti, 1981); the changes in velocity profile asymmetry at higher movement speeds (Beggs and Howarth, 1972; Zelaznik, Schmidt, and Gielen, in press); vector cell properties in precentral motor cortex (Evarts and Tanji, 1974; Georgopoulos, Kalaska, Caminiti, and Massey, 1982; Georgopoulos, Kalaska, Crutcher, Caminiti, and Massey, 1984; Kalaska, Caminiti, and Georgopoulos, 1983; Tanji and Evarts, 1976); the inverse relationship between movement duration and peak velocity (Lestienne, 1979); and peak acceleration as a function of movement amplitude and time (Bizzi, Accornero, Chapple, and Hogan, 1984). In addition, the work reported here extends a broader program of research on adaptive sensory-motor control (Grossberg, 1978a, 1986a, 1986b; Grossberg and Kuperstein, 1986), which enables functional and mechanistic comparisons to be made between the neural systems governing arm and eye movements, suggests how eye-hand coordination is accomplished, and provides a foundation for work on mechanisms of trajectory realization which compensate for the mechanical effects generated by variable loads and movement velocities (Bullock and Grossberg, 1988b).

13.2. Flexible Organization of Muscle Groups into Synergies

In order to move a part of the body, whether an eye, head, arm, or leg, many muscles must work together. For example, muscles controlling several different joints—shoulder, elbow, wrist, and fingers—may contract or relax cooperatively in order to perform a reaching movement. When groups of muscles cooperate in this way, they are said to form a synergy (Bernstein, 1967; Kelso, 1982).

Muscle groups may be incorporated into synergies in a flexible and dynamic fashion. Whereas muscles controlling shoulder, elbow, wrist, and fingers may all contract or relax synergetically to produce a reaching movement, muscles of the fingers and wrist may form a synergy to perform a grasping movement. Thus, one synergy may activate shoulder, elbow, wrist, and finger muscles to reach towards an object, and another synergy may then activate only finger and wrist muscles to grasp the object while maintaining postural control over the shoulder and elbow muscles. Groups of fingers may move together synergetically to play a chord on the piano, or separate fingers may be successively activated in order to play arpeggios.

One of the basic problems of motor control is to understand how neural control structures quickly and flexibly reorganize the set of muscle groups that are needed to synergetically cooperate in the next movement sequence. Once one squarely faces the problem that many behaviorally important synergies are not hard-wired, but are rather dynamically coupled and decoupled through time in ways that depend upon the actor's experience and training, the prospect that the trajectories of all synergists are explicitly preplanned seems remote at best. In support of a dynamic conception of synergy formation, Buchanan, Almdale, Lewis, and Rymer (1986) conclude from their experiments on isometric contractions of human elbow muscles that "The complexity of these patterns raises the possibility that synergies are determined by the tasks and may have no independent existence."

13.3. Synchronous Movement of Synergies

When neural commands organize a group of muscles into a synergy, the action of these muscles often occurs synchronously through time. It is partly for this reason that the complexity of the neural commands controlling many movements often goes unnoticed. These movements seem to occur in a single gesture, rather than as the sum of many asynchronous components.

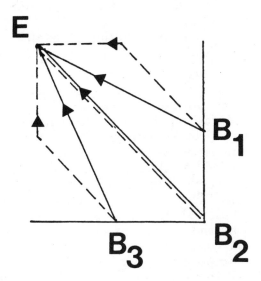

Figure 13.1. Consequences of two motor-control schemes. Dashed lines: Movement paths generated when a synergist producing vertical motion and a synergist producing horizontal motion contract in parallel and at equal rates to effect movements from various beginning points (Bs) to the common endpoint E. Solid lines: Movement paths generated when the synergists' contraction rates are adjusted to compensate for differences in the lengths of the vertical and horizontal components of the movement.

In order to understand the type of control problem that must be solved to generate synchronous movement, consider a typical arm movement of reaching forward and across the body midline with the right hand in a plane parallel to the ground. Suppose for simplicity that the synergist acting at the shoulder is responsible for across-midline motion, that the synergist acting at the elbow is responsible for forward motion, and that the hand is to be moved from points B1, B2, or B3 to point E. Figure 13.1 illustrates the effects of two distinct control schemes that might be used to produce these three movements. In the first scheme, the two synergists begin their contractions synchronously, contract at the same rate, and cease contracting when their respective motion component is complete. This typically results in asynchronous contraction terminations, and in bent-line movements, because the synergist responsible for the longer motion component takes longer to complete its contribution. With this scheme, approximately straight-line motions and synchronous contraction terminations occur only in cases like the B2–E movement, for which the component motions happen to be of equal length. In the second scheme, the two synergists contract, not at equal rates, but at rates that have been adjusted to compensate for any differences in length of the component motions. This results in synchronous contraction terminations. Normal arm movement paths are similar to those implied by the second control scheme (e.g., Morasso, 1981) and experimental studies (Freund and Büdingen, 1978) have shown that contraction rates are made unequal in a way that compensates for inequalities of distance.

What types of adaptive problems are solved by synchronization of synergists? Figure 13.1 provides some insight into this issue. Without synchronization, the direction of the first part of the movement path may change abruptly several times before the direction of the last part of the movement path is generated (Figure 13.1). This creates a problem because transporting an object from one place to another with the arm may destabilize the body unless one can predict, and anticipatorily compensate for, the arm movement's destabilizing effects, which are always directional. In the same way, many actions require that forces be applied to surfaces in particular directions. The first control scheme makes the direction in which force is applied difficult to predict and control. Both of these problems are eliminated by the approximately straight-line movement paths which become possible when synergists contract synchronously. Finally, if the various motions composing a movement failed to end synchronously, it would become difficult to ensure smooth transitions between sequentially ordered movements.

In summary, the untoward effects of asynchrony place strong constraints on the mechanisms of movement control: Across the set of muscles whose synergistic action produces a multi-joint movement, contraction durations must be roughly equal, and, because contraction distances are typically unequal, contraction rates must be made unequal in a way that compensates for inequalities of distance.

13.4. Factoring Target Position and Velocity Control

Inequalities of distance are translated into neural commands as differences in the total amounts of contraction by the muscles forming the synergy, and thereby into mechanical terms as the total amounts of change in the angles between joints (Hollerbach, Moore, and Atkeson, 1986). In order to compensate for differences in contraction, information must be available that is sufficient to compute the total amounts of contraction that are required. Thus a representation of the initial contraction level of each muscle must be compared with a representation of the target, expected, or final contraction level of the muscle. A primary goal of this article is to specify how this comparison is made. Although information about target position and initial position are both needed to control the total contraction of a muscle group, these two types of information are computed and updated in different ways, a fact that we believe has caused much confusion about whether only target position needs to be coded (Section 13.7). In particular, we reject the common assumption (Adams, 1971) that the representation of initial contraction used in the comparison is based on afferent feedback from the limbs. We propose instead that it is based primarily on feedback from an outflow command integrator that is located along the pathway between the precentral motor cortex and the spinal motorneurons.

Another source of confusion has arisen because target position information is needed to form a trajectory. This is the type of information which invites concepts of motor planning and expectation. However tempting it may be to so infer, concepts of motor planning and expectation do *not* imply that the *whole trajectory* is *explicitly* planned.

A second aspect of planning enters into trajectory formation which also does not imply the existence of explicit trajectory planning. This aspect is noticed by considering that the hand-arm system can be moved between fixed intital and target positions at many different velocities. When, as a result of a changed velocity, the overall movement duration changes, the component motions occurring around the various joints must nonetheless remain synchronous. Since fixed differences in initial and target positions can be converted into synchronous motions at a wide range of velocities, there must exist an independently controlled velocity, or GO signal (Section 13.11). The independent control of target position commands, or TPCs, and velocity commands, or GO signals, is a special case of a general neural design which has been called the *factorization of pattern and energy* (Grossberg, 1978a, 1982a).

13.5. Synchrony versus Fitts' Law: The Need for a Neural Analysis of Synergy Formation

Our discussion of synchronous performance of synergies has thus far emphasized that different muscles of the hand-arm system may need to contract by different amounts in equal time in order to move a hand through a fixed distance. When movement of a hand over different distances is considered, a striking contrast between behavioral and neural properties of movement becomes evident. This difference emphasizes that synergies are assembled and disassembled through time in a flexible and dynamic way.

Fitts' Law (Fitts, 1954; Fitts and Peterson, 1964) states that movement time (MT) of the arm is related to distance moved (D) and to width of target (W) by the equation

$$MT = a + b\log_2(\frac{2D}{W}), \tag{13.1}$$

where a and b are empirically derived constants. Keele (1981) has reviewed a variety of experiments showing that Fitts' Law is remarkably well obeyed despite its simplicity. For example, the law describes movement time for linear arm movements (Fitts, 1954), rotary movements of the wrist (Knight and Dagnall, (1967), back-and-forth movements like dart throwing (Kerr and Langolf, 1977), head movements (Jagacinski and Monk, 1985), movements of young and old people (Welford, Norris, and Schock, 1969), and movements of monkeys as well as humans (Brooks, 1979).

Equation (13.1) asserts that movement time (MT) increases as the logarithm of distance (D) moved, other things being equal. The width parameter W in (13.1) is interpreted as a measure of movement accuracy (Section 13.27). Although movement distance and time may covary on the behavioral level that describes the aggregate effect of many muscle contractions, such a relationship does not necessarily hold on the neural level, where individual muscles may contract by variable amounts, or "distances", in order to achieve synchronous contraction within a constant movement time.

A fundamental issue is raised by this comparison of behavioral and neural constraints. This issue can be better understood through consideration of the following gedanken example. When each of two fingers is moved separately through different distances, each finger may separately obey Fitts' Law. Then the finger which moves a larger distance should take more time to move, other things being equal. In contrast, when the two fingers move the above distances as part of a single synergy, then each finger should complete its movement in the same time in order to guarantee synergetic synchrony. Thus either one of the fingers must violate Fitts' Law, or it must reach its target with a different level of accuracy. Kelso, Southard, and Goodman (1979) and Marteniuk and MacKenzie (1980) have experimentally studied this type of synchronous behavior in experiments on one or two handed movements, and have documented within-synergy violations of Fitts' Law.

Such examples suggest that Fitts' Law holds for the aggregate behavior of the largest collection of motor units which form a synergy during a given time interval. Fitts' Law need not hold for all subsets of the motor units which comprise a synergy. These subsets may, in principle, violate Fitts' Law by travelling variable distances in equal time in order to achieve synchrony of the aggregate movement. To understand how Fitts' Law can be reconciled with movement synchrony thus requires an analysis of the neural control mechanisms which flexibly bind muscle groups, such as those controlling different fingers, into a single motor synergy. If such a binding action does not involve explicit planning of a complete trajectory, yet does require activation of a target position command and a GO command, then neural machinery must exist which is capable of *automatically* coverting such commands into complete trajectories with synchronous and invariant properties. One of the primary tasks of this article is to describe the circuit design of this neural machinery and to explain how it works.

13.6. Some General Issues in Sensory-Motor Planning: Multiple Uses of Outflow versus Inflow Signals

Before beginning a mechanistic analysis of these circuits, we summarize several general issues about motor planning to place the model developed in this article within a broader conceptual framework. In Sections 13.8–13.13 and 13.27–13.29, a number of key experiments are reviewed to more sharply constrain the theoretical analysis. In Sections 13.21–13.28 computer simulations of these data properties are reported.

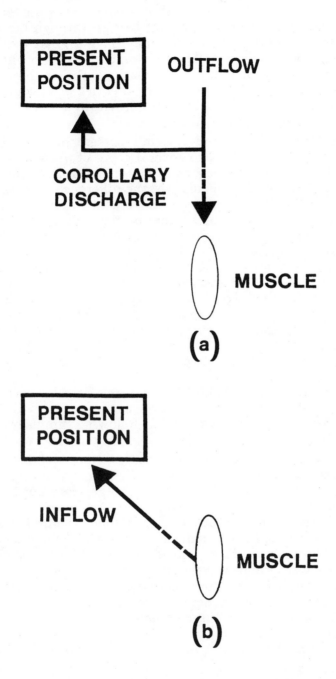

Figure 13.2. Both outflow and inflow signals contribute to the brain's estimate of the limb's present position, but in different ways.

Neural circuitry automates the production of skilled movements in several mechanistically distinct ways. Perhaps the most general observation is that animals and humans perform marvelously dexterous acts in a world governed by Newton's Laws, yet can go through life without ever learning Newton's Laws, and indeed may have a great deal of difficulty learning them when they try. The phenomenal world of movements is a world governed by motor plans and intentions, rather than by kinematic and inertial laws. A major challenge to theories of biological movement control is to explain how we move so well within a world whose laws we may so poorly understand.

The computation of a hand or arm's present position illustrates the complexity of this problem. Two general types of present position signals have been identified in discussions of motor control: *outflow* signals and *inflow* signals. Figure 13.2 schematizes the difference between these signal sources. An outflow signal carries a movement command from the brain to a muscle (Figure 13.2a). Signals that branch off from the efferent brain-to-muscle pathway in order to register present position signals are called *corollary discharges* (Helmholtz, 1866; von Holst and Mittelstaedt, 1950). An *inflow* signal carries present position information from a muscle to the brain (Figure 13.2b). A primary difference between outflow and inflow is that a change in outflow signals is triggered only when an observer's brain generates a new movement command. A new inflow signal can, in contrast, be generated by passive movements of the limb. Evidence for influences of both outflow (Helmholtz, 1866) and inflow (Ruffini, 1898; Sherrington, 1894) has accumulated over the past century. Disentangling the different roles played by outflow and inflow signals has remained one of the major problems in motor control. This is a confusing issue because both outflow and inflow signals are used in multiple ways to provide different types of information about present position. The following summary itemizes some of the ways in which these signals are used in our theory.

Although one role of an outflow signal is to move a limb by contracting its target muscles, the operating characteristics of the muscle plant are not known *a priori* to the outflow source. It is therefore not known *a priori* how much the muscle will actually contract in response to an outflow signal of prescribed size. It is also not known how much the limb will move in response to a prescribed muscle contraction. In addition, even if the outflow system somehow possessed this information at one time, it might turn out to be the wrong information at a later time, because muscle plant characteristics can change through time due to development, aging, exercise, changes in blood supply, or minor tears. Thus the relationship between the size of an outflow movement command and the amount of muscle contraction is, in principle, undeterminable without additional information which characterizes the muscle plant's actual response to outflow signals.

To establish a satisfactory correspondence between outflow movement signals and actual muscle contractions, the motor system needs to compute reliable present position signals which represent where the outflow command tells the muscle to move, as well as reliable present position signals which represent the state of contraction of the muscle. Corollary discharges and inflow signals can provide these different types of information. Grossberg and Kuperstein (1986) have shown how a comparison, or match, between corollary discharges and inflow signals can be used to modify, through an automatic learning process, the total outflow signal to the muscle in a way that effectively compensates for changes in the muscle plant. Such automatic gain control produces a linear correspondence between an outflow movement command and the amount of muscle contraction even if the muscle plant is nonlinear. The process which matches outflow and inflow signals to linearize the muscle plant response through learning is called *adaptive linearization* of the muscle plant. The cerebellum is implicated by both the theoretically derived circuit and experimental evidence as the site of learning (Albus, 1971; Brindley, 1964; Fujita, 1982a, 1982b; Grossberg, 1969a, 1972a; Ito, 1974, 1982, 1984; Marr, 1969; McCormick and Thompson, 1984; Optican and Robinson, 1980; Ron and Robinson, 1973; Vilis and Hore, 1986; Vilis, Snow, and Hore, 1983).

Given that corollary discharges are matched with inflow signals to linearize the relationship between muscle plant contraction and outflow signal size, outflow signals can also be used in yet other ways to provide information about present position. In Sections 13.17–13.23, it is shown how outflow signals are matched with target position signals to generate a trajectory with synchronous and invariant properties. Thus outflow signals are used in at least three ways, and all of these ways are automatically registered: They send movement signals to target muscles; they generate corollary discharges which are matched with inflow signals to guarantee linear muscle contractions even if the muscle plant is nonlinear; and they generate corollary discharges which are matched with target position signals to generate synchronous trajectories with invariant properties.

Inflow signals are also used in several ways. One way has already been itemized. A second use of inflow signals is suggested by the following gedanken example. When you are sitting in an armchair, let your hands drop passively towards your sides. Depending upon a multitude of accidental factors, your hands and arms can end up in any of infinitely many final positions. If you are then called upon to make a precise movement with your arm-hand system, this can be done with the usual exquisite accuracy. Thus the fact that your hands and arms start out this movement from an initial position which was not reached under active control by an outflow signal does not impair the accuracy of the movement.

A wealth of evidence suggests, however, that comparison between target position and present position information is used to move the arms. Moreover, as will be shown below, this present position information is computed from outflow signals. In contrast, during the passive fall of an arm under the influence of gravity, changes in outflow signal commands are not responsible for the changes in position of the limb. This observation identifies the key issue: How is the outflow signal updated due to passive movement of a limb so that the next active movement can accurately be made? Since the final position of a passively falling limb cannot be predicted in advance, it is clear that inflow signals must be used to update present position when an arm is moved passively by an external force.

This conclusion calls attention to a closely related issue that must be dealt with to understand the neural bases of skilled movement: How does the motor system know that the arm is being moved passively due to an external force, and not actively due to a changing outflow command? Such a distinction is needed to prevent inflow information from contaminating outflow commands when the arm is being actively moved. The motor system must use internally generated signals to make the distinction between active movement and passive movement, or postural, conditions. Computational gates must be open and shut based upon whether these internally generated signals are on or off (Grossberg and Kuperstein, 1986).

A third role for inflow signals is needed due to the fact that arms can move at variable velocities while carrying variable loads. Because an arm is a mechanical system embedded in a Newtonian world, an arm can generate unexpected amounts of inertia and acceleration when it tries to move novel loads at novel velocities. During such a novel motion, the commanded outflow position of the arm and its actual position may significantly diverge. Inflow signals are needed to compute mismatches leading to partial compensation for this uncontrolled component of the movement.

Such novel movements are quite different from our movements when we pick up a familiar fountain pen or briefcase. When the object is familiar, we can predictively adjust the gain of the movement to compensate for the expected mass of the object. This type of automatic gain control can, moreover, be flexibly switched on and off using signal pathways that can be activated by visual recognition of a familiar object. Inflow signals are used in the learning process which enables such automatic gain control signals to be activated in an anticipatory fashion in response to familiar objects (Bullock and Grossberg, 1988b).

This listing of multiple uses for outflow and inflow signals invites comparison between how the arm movement system and other movement systems use outflow and inflow signals. Grossberg and Kuperstein (1986) have identified and suggested neural circuit solutions to analogous problems of sensory-motor control within the specialized domain of the saccadic eye movement system. Several of the problems to which we will suggest circuit solutions in our articles on arm movements have analogs with the saccadic circuits developed by Grossberg and Kuperstein (1986). Together these investigations suggest that several movement systems contain neural circuits that solve similar general problems. Differences between these circuits can be traced to functional specializations in the way these movement systems solve their shared problems of movement.

For example, whereas saccades are ballistic movements, arm movements can be made under both continuous and ballistic control. Whereas the eyes normally come to rest in a head-centered position, the arms can come to rest in any of infinitely many positions. Whereas the eyes are typically not subjected to unexpected or variable external loads, the arms are routinely subjected to such loads. Whereas the eyes typically generate a stereotyped velocity profile between a fixed pair of initial and target positions, the arms can move with a continuum of velocity profiles between a fixed pair of initial and target positions. Our analyses show how the arm system is specialized to cope with all of these differences between its behaviors and those of the saccadic eye movement system.

13.7. Neural Control of Arm Position Changes: Beyond the STE Model

A number of further specialized constraints on the mechanisms controlling planned arm movements are clarified by summarizing shortcomings of the simplest example of a "mass-sping" model of movement generation, which we will call the Spring-To-Endpoint (STE) model, to distinguish it from other members of the potentially large family of models that exploit "mass-spring" properties of biological limbs (e.g., Bizzi, 1980; Cooke, 1980; Feldman, 1974, 1986; Humphrey and Reed, 1983; Kelso and Holt, 1980; Sakitt, 1980). As Nichols (1985) and Feldman (1986) have recently noted, past discussions of mass-spring properties have mistakenly lumped together quite different proposals regarding how such properties might be exploited during trajectory formation. Our treatment in this section is meant to serve a pedagogical function, and our criticisms pertain only to the STE Model which is explicitly specified in this section. In particular, no part of our critique denies that the peripheral motor system has mass-spring properties that may be critical to overall motor function. Indeed, in Bullock and Grossberg (1988b), we analyse neural command circuits which exploit mass-spring muscle properties to generate well-controlled movements.

The components of the STE (Spring-To-Endpoint) Model for movement control can be summarized as follows. Imagine that the eye fixates some object that lies within reach. To touch the object, it is necessary to move the tip of the index finger from its current position to the target position on the object's nearest surface. The STE Model suggests that this is accomplished by simply replacing the arm position command that specifies the arm's present posture with a new arm position command that specifies the posture the arm would have to assume in order for the index finger to touch the chosen object surface.

Instatement of the new arm position command is suggested to generate the desired movement as follows. The arm is held in any position by balancing the muscular and other forces (e.g., gravity) that are currently acting on the limb. Instatement of a new command changes the pattern of outflow signals that contract the arm muscles. A step change in the pattern of contraction creates a force imbalance that causes the limb to spring in the direction of the larger force at a rate proportional to the force difference. The limb comes to rest when all the forces acting on it are once again balanced. Despite its elegance, the STE Model exhibits several deficiencies which highlight properties that an adequate control system needs to have. We briefly summarize two fundamental problems: (1) confounding of speed and distance control, and (2) inability to quickly terminate movement at an intermediate position.

The first problem, the speed-distance confound, follows from the dependence of movement rate on the force difference, which in turn depends on the distance between the starting and final positions. This might at first seem to be a desirable property, because it appears to compensate for different distances in the manner needed to ensure synchronization of synergists (Section 13.3). However, consider also the need to vary the speed of a fixed movement. An actor seeking to perform the same movement at a faster speed would have to follow a two-part movement plan: Early in the movement, instate a virtual target position that is well beyond the desired end point and along a line drawn from the initial through the true target position. This command will create a very large initial force imbalance and launch the limb at a high speed. Then, at some point during the movement, instate the true target position command, and let the arm coast to the final position. This example illustrates that the STE Model requires a complex and neurally implausible scheme for achieving variable speed control for movements of fixed length.

Cooke (1980) suggests that variable speed control by an STE Model can be achieved by abruptly changing the stiffness of agonist and antagonist muscles to achieve differences in distance and speed. This model has not yet been shown to produce velocity profiles with the parametric properties of the data (Section 13.12). In addition, Houk and Rymer (1981) and Feldman (1986) have shown that the stiffness of individual muscles is typically maintained at a nearly constant level.

A second problem with the STE Model concerns the critical need to quickly abort an evolving movement and stabilize current arm position. Such a need arises, for example, when an animal wishes to freeze upon detection of a predator who uses motion cues to locate prey. It also arises when an action, such as transporting a large mass, begins to destabilize an animal's overall state of balance. At such times, it is often adaptive to quickly freeze and maintain the current arm position. This is an easy task if the movement command is never much different from the arm's present position. Freezing could then be quickly achieved by preventing further changes in the currently commanded position. In an STE Model, this simple freeze strategy is unavailable, because a large discrepancy exists between present arm position and the target position command throughout much of the trajectory. To implement a freezing response using the STE Model, the system would somehow have to quickly determine and instate a new target position command capable of maintaining the arm's present position. But this is precisely the type of information whose relevance is denied by the STE Model.

13.8. Gradual Updating of PPC's during Trajectory Formation

Several lines of experimental evidence point to deficiencies of the STE Model. One line of evidence, due to Bizzi and his colleagues, demonstrates that a type of gradual updating of the movement command occurs which is inconsistent with the STE model. Earlier studies from the Bizzi lab partially supported the STE model.

The experiments of Polit and Bizzi (1978) studied monkeys who were trained to move their forearms, without visual feedback of hand position, from a canonical starting position to the position of one of several lights. The monkeys' arm movements were studied both before and after a dorsal rhizotomy was performed to remove all sensory feedback from the arm. Before deafferentation, the monkey could move its hand to the target's position without visual feedback, even if its accustomed position with respect to the arm apparatus was changed. After deafferentation, so long as the spatial conditions of training were maintained—in particular the canonical starting orientation and position with respect to the known target array—the animal remained able to move its hand to the target position. However, if the initial position of the upper arm and elbow of the deafferented arm was passively shifted from the position used throughout training, then the animal's forearm movements terminated at a position shifted by an equal amount away from the target position. Thus the movement of the forearm did not compensate for the change in initial position of the upper arm. Instead the same final synergy of forearm-controlling muscles was generated in both cases.

The fact that deafferented monkeys moved to shifted positions emphasized the critical role of the target position command in setting up the movement trajectory. The fact that normal monkeys could compensate for rotation in a way that deafferented monkeys could not indicated an additional role for inflow signals when the arm is moved passively by an external force (Section 13.29).

The later experiments of Bizzi, Accornero, Chapple, and Hogan (1982, 1984) carried out an additional manipulation. The results of these experiments are inconsistent with the STE assumption that the arm's motion is governed exclusively by the spring-like contraction of its muscles towards the position specified by a new target position command. In these experiments, the monkey was again deprived of visual and inflow feedback, and placed in its canonical starting position. In addition, its deafferented arm was surreptitiously held at the target position, then released at variable intervals after activation of the target light. Under these circumstances, the arm travelled back towards the canonical starting position, before reversing direction and proceeding to the target. The arm travelled further backward toward the starting position the sooner it was released after target activation. Moreover, when the arm was moved to the target position and then released in the absence of any target presentation, it sprang back to its canonical starting position. Bizzi *et al.* (1984, p.2742) concluded that "the CNS had programmed a slow, gradual shift of the equilibrium point, a fact which is not consistent with the 'final position control' [read STE] hypothesis."

The Bizzi *et al.* (1984) description of their results as a "gradual shift of the equilibrium point" carries the language of the STE Model into a context where it may cause confusion. From a mathematical perspective, the intermediate positions of a movement trajectory are not, by definition, equilibrium points. In order to explicate the Bizzi *et al.* (1984) data, we show how three quantities are computed and updated through time: a target position command (TPC) which is switched on once and for all before the movement; an outflow movement command, called the present position command (PPC), which is continously updated until it matches the TPC; and the arm position which closely corresponds to the PPC. We use these concepts below to explain data from the Bizzi lab in both normal and deafferented conditions.

We call a movement for which a single TPC (target position command) is switched on before the movement begins an *elementary* movement. Once it is seen how a single TPC can cause gradual updating of the PPC (present position command), movements can also be analysed during which a sequence of TPC's is switched on, either under the control of visual feedback or from a movement planning network which can store and release sequences of TPC's from memory with the proper order and timing (Grossberg and Kuperstein, 1986).

Our analysis of how the PPC is gradually updated during an elementary movement partially supports the Bizzi *et al.* (1984) description of a "gradual shift in equilibrium point" by showing that the arm remains in approximate equilibrium with respect to the PPC, even though none of these intermediate arm positions is an equilibrium point of the system. The only equilibrium point of the system is reached when both the neural control circuit and the arm itself both reach equilibrium. That happens when the PPC matches the TPC, thereby preventing further changes in the present position command and allowing the arm to come to rest.

These conclusions refine, rather than totally contradict, the main insight of the STE Model. Instead of concluding that the arm springs to the position coded by the TPC, we suggest that the spring-like arm tracks the series of positions specified by the PPC as it approaches the TPC. This conception of trajectory formation contrasts sharply with that suggested by Brooks (1986, p.138) in response to the Bizzi data. Brooks inferred that "animals learn not only the end points and their stiffness, but also a series of intermediate equilibrium positions. In other words, they learn an internal 'reference' trajectory that determines the path to be followed and generates torques appropriately to reduce mismatch between the intended and actual events." In a similar fashion, Hollerbach (1982, p.192) suggested that we practice movements to "learn the basic torque profiles." In contrast, we suggest that the read-out of the TPC is learned, but that the gradual updating of the PPC is automatic. A number of auxiliary learning processes are also needed to update the PPC after passive movements due to an external force (Section 13.30), to adaptively linearize the response of a nonlinear muscle plant (Grossberg and Kuperstein, 1986), and to adaptively compensate for the inertial effects of variable loads and velocities (Bullock and Grossberg, 1988b). These additional learning processes enable the automatic updating of the PPC to generate controllable movements without requiring that the entire trajectory be learned.

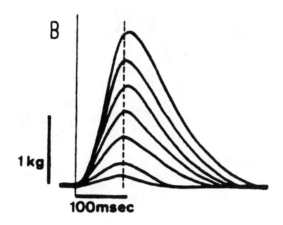

Figure 13.3. Curves for subjects' approach to various targeted force levels. Targeted (peak) levels are reached at nearly the same time, indicating duration invariance across different force "distances". Only the initial part of each curve represents active movement. Post-peak portions represent passive relaxation back to base-line. Reprinted with permission from Freund and Büdingen (1978).

13.9. Duration Invariance during Isotonic Movements and Isometric Contractions

Further information concerning the gradual updating process whereby PPC's match a TPC can be inferred from the detailed spatiotemporal properties of arm trajectory formation. Freund and Büdingen (1978) have studied "the relationship between the speed of the fastest possible voluntary contractions and their amplitudes for several hand and forearm muscles under both isotonic and isometric conditions. These experiments showed the larger the amplitude, the faster the contraction. The increase of the rate of rise of isometric tension or of the velocity of isotonic movements with rising amplitude was linear. The slope of this relationship was the same for three different hand and forearm muscles examined ... the skeleto-motor speed control system operates by adjusting the velocity of a contraction to its amplitude in such a way that the contraction time remains approximately constant ... this type of speed control is a necessary requirement for the synchrony of synergistic muscle contractions" (p.1).

Two main issues are raised by this study. First, it must be explained why, "comparing isotonic movements and isometric contractions, the time from onset to peak was similar in the two conditions" (p.7). Figure 13.3 shows the fastest voluntary isometric contractions of the extensor indicis muscle. Second, it must be explained why the force develops gradually in time with the shapes depicted in Figure 13.3. Below it is shown that both

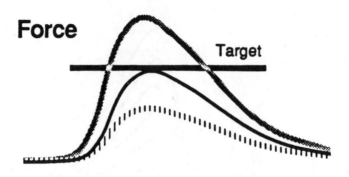

Figure 13.4. Overshooting (gray curve), hitting (black curve), and undershooting (dashed line) a force-level target (horizontal line) in an isometric task. Reprinted with permission from Gordon and Ghez (1987b).

duration invariance and the force development through time are emergent properties of the PPC updating process (see Section 13.22).

13.10. Compensatory Properties of the PPC Updating Process

Ghez and his colleagues (Ghez and Vicario, 1978; Gordon and Ghez, 1984, 1987a, 1987b) have confirmed the duration invariance reported by Freund and Büdingen (1978) in an isometric paradigm which also disclosed finer properties of the PPC updating process. These authors suggest that "compensatory adjustments add to preprogrammed specification of rapid force impulses to achieve more accurately targeted responses" (Gordon and Ghez, 1987b).

In their isometric task, subjects were instructed to maintain superposition of two lines on a CRT screen. The experimenter could cause one of the lines to jump to any of three positions. Subjects could exert force on an immobile lever to move the other line towards the target line. Equal increments of force produced equal displacements of the line. Thus more isometric force was needed to move the line over a larger distance to the target line.

Figure 13.4 defines the major variables of their analysis. The force target is represented by the solid black horizontal line. If the subject performs errorlessly—that is, reaches target without overshoot—the value of the peak force will equal the value of the force target, as in the black curve. Overshoots and undershoots in force are represented by the gray and dashed curves, respectively. Figure 13.5 plots the data of Gordon and Ghez (1987b) in a way that illustrates duration invariance. The horizontal line through the data points shows that force rise time is essentially

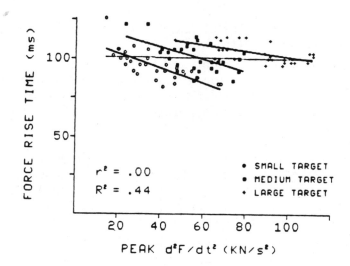

Figure 13.5. Duration invariance across three force target levels. Oblique lines indicate an inverse relation between rise time (duration) and peak acceleration across trials with the same force target level. These trends overlay a direct relation between target level and peak acceleration. Reprinted with permission from Gordon and Ghez (1987b).

independent of peak force acceleration $\left(\frac{d_2 F}{dt_2}\right)$ for all the target distances.

Gordon and Ghez (1987b) separately analysed the data for each of the three target distances, and thereby derived the three oblique lines in Figure 13.5. They interpreted these lines as evidence for an "error correction" process because a negative correlation exists between peak acceleration and the force rise time, or duration. Thus, if the acceleration for a small target distance was too high early in a movement, the trajectory was "corrected" by shortening the rise time. Had this compensation not occurred, the high acceleration could have produced a peak force appropriate for a larger target distance.

Gordon and Ghez (1987b) assumed that trajectories are preplanned and that their peak accelerations are a signature indicating which trajectory has been preplanned. It is from this perspective that they interpreted the compensatory effect shown in Figure 13.5 as an "error correction" process. In contrast, we suggest in Sections 13.13 and 13.21 that this compensatory effect is one of the automatic properties whereby PPC's are gradually updated. We hereby provide an explanation of the compensatory effect that avoids invoking a special mechanism of "error correction" for a movement which does not generate an error in achieving its target. In addition, this explanation provides a unified analysis of the Bizzi *et al.* (1984) data on isotonic movements and the Gordon and Ghez (1987b) data on isometric contractions.

13.11. Target Switching Experiments: Velocity Amplification, GO Signal, and Fitts' Law

Our explanation of the Freund and Büdingen (1978) and Gordon and Ghez (1987a) data considers how a single GO signal, which initiates and drives all movements to completion, ensures duration invariance when applied to all components of the synergy defined by a TPC. Georgopoulos, Kalaska, and Massey (1981) have collected data which provide further evidence pertinent to the hypothesized interaction of a GO signal with the process which instates a TPC and thereby updates the PPC. In their experiments, monkeys were trained to move a lever from a start position to one of eight target positions radially situated on a planar surface. Then the original target position was switched to a new target position at variable delays after presentation of the first target.

Part of the data confirm the fact that "the aimed motor command is emitted in a continuous, ongoing fashion as a real-time process that can be interrupted at any time by the substitution of the original target by the new one. The effects of this change on the ensuing movement appear promptly, without delays beyond the usual reaction time" (p.725). Figure 13.6 depicts movement paths found during the target switching condition. We explain these data in terms of how instatement of a second TPC can rapidly modify the future updating of the PPC.

In addition, Georgopoulous *et al.* (1981) found a remarkable amplification of peak velocity during the switched component of the movement: "the peak velocity attained on the way to the second target was generally much higher (up to threefold) than that of the control ... these high velocities cannot be accounted for exclusively by a mechanism that adjusts peak velocity to the amplitude of movement ... The cause of this phenomenon is unclear" (pp.732-733). In Section 13.25, we explain this phenomenon in terms of the independent control, or factorization, of the GO mechanism and the TPC-switching mechanism that was described in Section 13.4. In particular, the GO signal builds up continuously in time. When the TPC is switched to a new target, the PPC can be updated much more quickly because the GO signal which drives it is already large. The more rapid updating of the PPC translates into higher velocities.

These target switching data call attention to a more subtle property of how a GO signal energizes PPC updating, indeed a property which has tended to mask the very existence of the GO signal: How can a GO signal which was activated with a previous TPC interact with a later TPC without causing errors in the ability of the PPC to track the later TPC? How does the energizing effect of a GO signal transfer to any TPC? A solution of this problem is suggested in Section 13.18.

The fact that peak velocity is amplified without affecting movement accuracy during target switching implies a violation of Fitt's Law, as Massey, Schwartz, and Georgopoulous (1985) have noted. Our mechanistic analy-

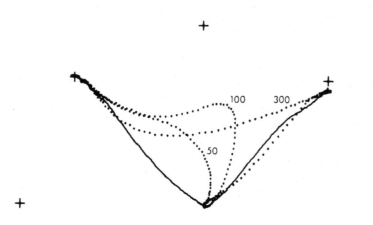

Figure 13.6. Monkeys seamlessly transformed a movement initiated toward the 2 o'clock target into a movement toward the 10 o'clock target when the latter target was substituted 50 or 100 msec. after activation of the 2 o'clock target light. Reprinted with permission from Georgopoulos *et al.* (1981).

sis of synergetic binding via instatement of a TPC and of subsequent PPC updating energized by a previously activated GO signal provides an explanation of this Fitts' Law violation as well as of Fitts' Law itself (Section 13.28).

Our model also suggests an explanation of why the position of maximal curvature and the time of minimal velocity are correlated during two-part arm movements (Abend, Bizzi, and Morasso, 1982; Fetters and Todd, 1987; Viviani and Terzuolo, 1980). This correlation arises in the model if the second TPC is switched on only after the PPC approaches the first TPC. In the Georgopoulous *et al* (1981) experiment, in contrast, the second TPC is switched on due to the second light before the arm reaches the first target. An unanswered question of considerable interest is whether a second GO signal is switched on gradually with the second TPC in the Abend *et al* (1982) paradigm, or whether the reduction in velocity at the turning point is due entirely to nulling of the difference between the PPC and the first TPC while the GO signal maintains an approximately constant value. These alternatives can be tested by measuring the velocities and accelerations subsequent to the position of the turning point.

13.12. Velocity Profile Invariance and Asymmetry

Many investigators have noted that the velocity profiles of simple arm movements are approximately bell-shaped (Abend, Bizzi, and Morasso, 1982; Atkeson and Hollerbach, 1985; Beggs and Howarth, 1972; Georgopoulous, Kalaska, and Massey, 1981; Howarth and Beggs, 1971; Morasso, 1981; Soechting and Lacquaniti, 1981). Moreover the shape of the bell, if rescaled appropriately, is approximately preserved for movements that vary in duration, distance, or peak velocity. Figure 13.7 shows rescaled velocity profiles from the experiment of Atkeson and Hollerbach (1985). These velocity profiles were generated over a fixed distance at several different velocities. Thus both the duration scale and the velocity scale were modified to superimpose the curves shown in Figure 13.7.

On the other hand, Beggs and Howarth (1972) showed that "at high speeds the approach curves of the practised subjects are more symmetrical than at low speeds" (p.451), and Zelaznik, Schmidt, and Gielen (in press) have shown that at very high speeds the direction of asymmetry has actually reversed. Thus the trend documented by Beggs and Howarth continues beyond the range of speeds they sampled. Since velocity profiles associated with slow movements are more asymmetric than those associated with fast movements, they cannot be exactly superimposed. All the velocity profiles shown in Figure 13.7 are taken from slow (1–1.6 sec) movements, and exhibit the sort of more gradual deceleration than acceleration that Beggs and Howarth (1972) reported for such movements.

Asymmetry, its degree, and changes in its direction are of major theoretical importance. For example, the Minimum-Jerk Model of Hogan (1984) predicts symmetric velocity profiles. More generally, superimposability of velocity profiles after time-axis rescaling is a defining characteristic of "generalized motor program" models (Hogan, 1984; Meyer, Smith, and Wright 1982; Schmidt, Zelaznik, and Frank, 1978), which therefore cannot explain how the degree of velocity profile asymmetry varies with overall movement speed. In contrast, our model shows how the gradual updating of the PPC can generate velocity profiles which exhibit the type of speed-dependent asymmetry that is found in the data (Section 13.23).

Both the existence of asymmetry in velocity profiles and the dependence of degree and direction of asymmetry upon movement speed indicate the need for an analysis of the neural dynamics whereby a trajectory unfolds in real-time. In contrast, the Hogan (1984) model's global optimization criterion forces strict superimposability of rescaled velocity profiles because it does not represent a process of temporal unfolding. Beggs and Howarth (1972) suggested that the asymmetry reflects a learned strategy of approaching the target as quickly as possible before making corrective movements near the target. For example, these corrective movements could be made under visual guidance by instating a corrected TPC as the arm approached the target. The approach to such a new TPC would take more time, on the average, than the final approach to the previously tracked TPC, thereby causing greater velocity profile asymmetry. In our simulation results, velocity profiles become more symmetric as movement

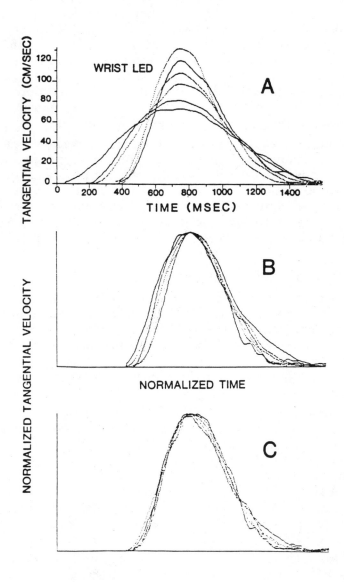

Figure 13.7. Velocity profiles from movements of similar duration are approximately superimposable following velocity and time axis rescaling. Reprinted with permission from Atkeson and Hollerbach (1985).

speed increases and eventually exhibit a symmetry reversal even in the absence of newly instated TPC's. Thus the greater symmetry of velocity profiles at higher speeds may be due to the combined effects of PPC updating properties as the GO signal is parametrically increased, and to the consequent elimination of corrective TPC's as the target is rapidly approached. In support of this analysis, Jeannerod (1984, p.252) noted that "the low velocity phase is still observed in the absence of visual feedback, and even in the no-vision situation. This finding, however, does not preclude that visual feedback, when present, will be incorporated ... In the present study, movement duration and low-velocity phase duration were found to be increased in the visual feedback situation."

In summary, our explanation of these data shows how a circuit capable of flexibly binding muscle groups into synchronous synergies automatically implies the trends observed in data on velocity profile asymmetry. Thus we suggest an explanation of movement invariants, such as duration invariance and synchrony, using a control circuit which never computes an explicit trajectory and whose outputs exhibit a type of speed-dependent asymmetry which other models have not been able to explain.

13.13. Vector Cells in Motor Cortex

Before quantitatively developing our model, it remains to indicate how the present position command (PPC) is gradually updated until it matches a fixed target position command (TPC). Sections 13.15–13.18 motivate this mechanism through an analysis of the types of information that can be used by a developing system to learn TPC's. The summary here is merely descriptive and is made to link these introductory remarks to supportive neural data.

When a new TPC is switched on, its relationship to the current PPC can be arbitrary. Any realizable pair of positions can be coded by the TPC and the PPC. In order to track the TPC, the PPC needs to change in a *direction* determined by the difference between the TPC and the PPC. In addition, the *amount* of required change is also determined by this difference. An array which measures both the direction and the distance between a pair of arrays TPC and PPC is called a *difference vector*, or DV. At any given time, the DV between the TPC and the PPC—namely, $DV = TPC - PPC$—is computed at a match interface (Figure 13.8).

How does such a DV (difference vector) update the current PPC? Clearly the PPC must be updated in the direction specified by the DV. Hence we assume that the PPC cumulatively adds, or *integrates*, through time all the DV's which arise at the match interface. Due to this arrangement, the PPC gradually approaches the TPC. At a time when the PPC equals the TPC, the DV equals zero; hence, although the PPC may continue to integrate DV's, it will not further change until either the switching on of a new TPC creates a non-zero DV, or the PPC is updated by inflow information during a passive movement (Section 13.30). To summarize these relations, we call our model the Vector-Integration-To-Endpoint (VITE) Model.

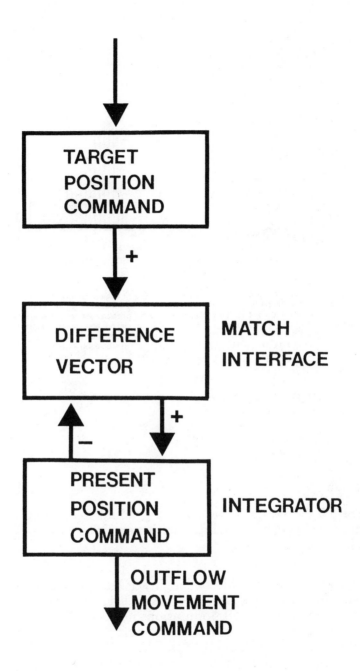

Figure 13.8. A match interface within the motor command channel continuously computes the difference between the target position and present position, and adds the difference to the present position command.

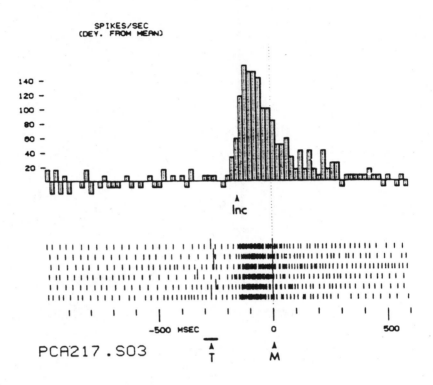

Figure 13.9. Quick buildup and gradual decline of activity in motor-cortical vector cells. Reprinted with permission from Georgopoulos *et al.* (1982).

Georgopoulos and his colleagues (Georgopoulos, Kalaska, Caminiti, and Massey, 1982; Georgopoulos, Kalaska, Crutcher, Caminiti, and Massey, 1984) have found cell populations in the motor cortex whose collective properties mirror those of the vector-computing nodes at the match interface of our model (Figure 13.8). The activity of each such node models the average potential of a population of neural cells with similar receptive field properties. Figure 13.9 shows a histogram of the average number of spikes per unit time recorded from a single such neuron. This temporal behavior closely matches that of a DV cell population in the model (Figure 13.18). The vector cells in motor cortex, just like the DV cell populations in the model, are very broadly tuned to direction (Figure 13.10a); that is, there exists a broad range of directions in which a given component of the model DV is positive.

Figure 13.11 further explicates these properties. Figure 13.11a clarifies why cells at the DV stage may be called vector cells at all. For simple movements, at increasing times $t_o < t_1 < t_2 < \ldots$, the relative sizes of the activities across the DV populations do not change. Hence these populations code a vector direction, even though their individual absolute activities sweep out an approximately bell-shaped curve through time. Figure 13.11b ilustrates that, as movement direction is parametrically changed, the relative activations of an agonist-antagonist pair of DV populations change systematically in such a way that individual populations may remain active over a broad range of directions, as in Figure 13.10a. Figure 13.11b also schematizes the fact that different agonist muscles may remain active over different ranges of direction, depending upon the movement in question. Although Figure 13.11a schematizes a formal DV, this DV may have many components because it controls many muscle groups. In contrast, the 3-dimensional vector which represents the direction of the arm's movement in Euclidean space has only three components. One of the major outstanding problems in arm movement control is to relate the geometry of the high dimensional muscle space with the geometry of Euclidean space.

Due to the importance of explaining why each DV population is sensitive to a broad range of directions, we further comment on this property below. The PPC outflow channels must control several different muscle groups at each joint, and several different joints in each arm. Because of the opponent organization of the muscles (Figure 13.11b), up to one half of the cellular components composing the DV stage will have positive activities during a given movement.

Each initial positive-valued component $DV_i(0) = TPC_i(0) - PPC_i(0) > 0$ of the difference vector DV corresponds to an expected change in length of one of the many muscle groups whose shortening contributes a motion component to the overall limb movement. If there were only one active agonist-antagonist muscle pair driving the movement, the movement would always tend to follow a preferred direction. Where more than one agonist-antagonist pair guides the movement, however, a muscle can facilitate motion along directions other than its preferred direction. In this case, the net direction of limb motion depends upon the relative sizes $DV_i(0) > 0$ of the cooperating agonists, so that each DV_i population can be active across a broad range of movement directions, as in Figure 13.11b. Since the net movement direction shifts continuously with the relative sizes $DV_i(0)$ of the cooperating agonists, it should be possible to predict the direction of a forthcoming limb movement.

Both of these conclusions have been supported by Georgopoulos, Kalaska, Crutcher, Caminiti, and Massey (1984) and Georgopoulos, Schwartz, and Kettner (1986). Figure 13.10a illustrates that vector cells in motor cortex are, indeed, broadly tuned to direction. Figure 13.10b illustrates that the aggregate activity of a large sample of active vector cells [read,

Bullock and Grossberg

(A)

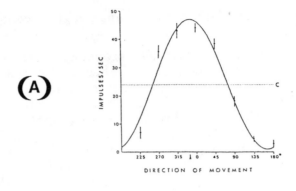

(B)

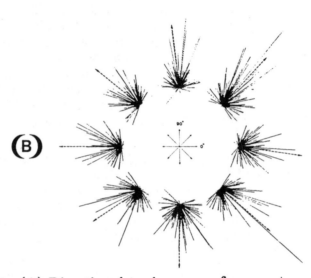

Figure 13.10. (A) Directional tuning curve for a motor-cortical cell exhibiting peak activity during a 0° (center-to-right) arm movement. Dotted line indicates control period discharge rate. Thus this cell is inhibited when movement direction falls outside the 180° hemisphere of movements to which it can contribute a positive motion component. Reprinted with permission from Kalaska *et al.* (1983). (B) Each dotted arrow in the central graphic indicates the direction of a radial (center-out) movement, and points to a representation of the cellular activites observed during that movement. In each plot of cellular activites, the *direction* of each solid black line corresponds to the direction of movement for which a given cell fired maximally, whereas the *length* of each solid black line corresponds to the firing rate of the same cell during the indicated movement. The single dashed line with arrowhead in each plot represents the vector sum of all the neural vectors (solid block lines) generated during the indicated movement. Note the correspondence between the direction of the vector sum (dashed line with arrowhead) and the direction of the actual movement (indicated by the dotted arrow in the central graphic). All cells were related to muscle groups acting at the shoulder, a ball-and-socket joint. Figures reprinted with permission from Georgopoulos *et al.* (1984).

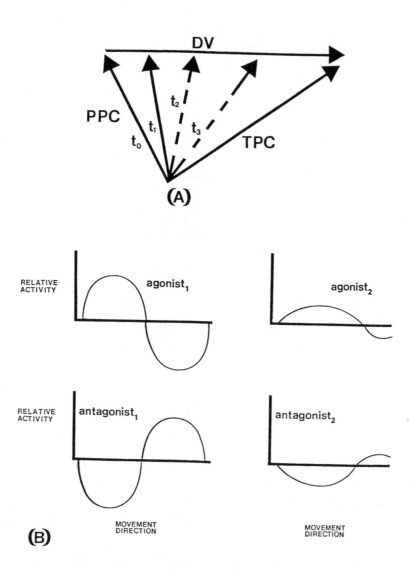

Figure 13.11. (A) As the movement unfolds through times $t_o, t_1, t_2, \ldots$ the present position command (PPC) approaches the target position command (TPC) in such a way that the difference vector (DV) does not change direction as its length approaches zero. (B) Over a full range of movement directions, DV cells associated with opposing muscles (AG_1 $vs.$ $ANTAG_1$ or AG_2 $vs.$ $ANTAG_2$) show reciprocal patterns of activation and inhibition. The zero-crossings can occur at different points along the direction scale for different opponent pairs (AG_1 - $ANTAG_1$ $vs.$ AG_2 - $ANTAG_2$).

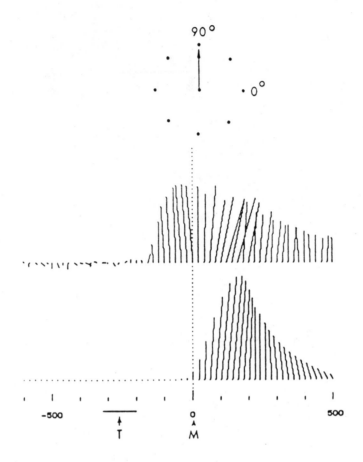

Figure 13.12. (A): A comparison of the population vector of 241 directionally tuned cells (upper figure) with the velocity vector of the hand (lower figure), each measured at 20 msec. intervals during the reaction time and during movement. Note the asymmetry (longer right tail) in both. Reprinted with permission from Georgopoulos *et al.* (1984).

cells from different DV_i populations] can be used to accurately predict the direction of the forthcoming movement.

Figure 13.12 plots data from a vector cell population *in vivo* alongside the velocity profile of the corresponding movement. Note that the asymmetry in the velocity profile is in the same direction as the asymmetry in the vector cell population profile. This correspondence suggests that the velocity asymmetry is related to the neural control circuit, as our model also suggests.

Georgopoulos *et al.* (1984, p.510) also noted that: "No obvious invariance in cell discharge was observed when the final position was the same ... these results show that, at the level of motor cortex, it is the direction of movement and not its endpoint that is the principle determinant of cell discharge during the initiation and execution of movement. Therefore, if the hypothesis be true that the endpoint of the movement is the controlled spatial variable (Polit and Bizzi, 1979) then the motor cortex seems to be distal to that end-point specifying process." In other words, if one accepts the STE Model, these data suggest that the TPC cells occur closer to the periphery than the DV cells. On the other hand, if one accepts our model, these data imply that the PPC cells occur closer to the periphery than the DV cells, but that the TPC cells occur more central than the DV cells. A combination of anatonomical and physiological experiments can be used to test this prediction. It should also be noted, however, that the STE Model on which the conclusion of Georgopoulos *et al.* (1984) is based is inconsistent with the very existence of vector cells, because the spring-like properties of the muscles themselves, rather than a neural computation of vectors, determines the direction and length of movement in the STE Model.

Several further properties of cells in precentral motor cortex, documented by Evarts and Tanji (1974; Tanji and Evarts, 1976), lend support to identifying them with the vector cells in our model. In their experiments, monkeys were trained to either push or pull a lever. During each trial (schematized in Figure 13.13a) animals first held the lever in a medial position for 2-4 sec. Then either a green or a red *priming* signal was illuminated. If green, the forthcoming movement required for reward was a push; if red, a pull. Finally, .6–1.2 seconds after the priming signal, the *release* signal occurred. This release signal took the form of an externally imposed push or pull on the lever held by the monkey. It both cued movement onset and perturbed the position of the lever so as to increase or decrease its initial distance from target.

Figure 13.13b summarizes operating characteristics of two cells. The first cell increased its activity after a "push" priming signal, but was inhibited by a "pull" priming signal; the second cell showed the opposite response. From these data alone, it would not be clear whether these cells' activities code DV's or TPC's. However, their further characteristics confirm their status as DV cells. The second bracket for each cell in Figure 13.13b indicates that their activities decline as movement proceeds in their preferred direction. This decline rules out the TPC interpretation. In the model, it occurs because the movement progressively cancels the difference with which DV cell activity is correlated.

The third bracket for each cell indicates that the initial position perturbations also have the effect they must have if the DV interpretation is correct: perturbations that make the starting point closer to target subtract from activity levels, whereas contrary perturbations add to activity levels. This occurs automatically in the model because PPC's, and thus the corresponding DV's, are updated by sensory feedback during passive movements (Section 13.30).

Though the foregoing considerations argue strongly for the existence of DV cells in precentral motor cortex, it might be argued that the DV's

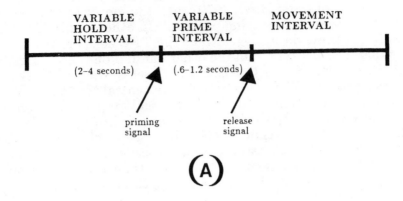

(A)

CELL 1 OPERATING CHARACTERISTICS

⇑ priming signal	produced	↑ activity
⇓ priming signal	produced	↓ activity

⇑ movement	produced	↓ activity

⇑ prime + ⇓ perturbation	produced	greater ↑ activity
⇑ prime + ⇑ perturbation	produced	less ↑ activity

CELL 2 OPERATING CHARACTERISTICS

⇓ priming signal	produced	↑ activity
⇑ priming signal	produced	↓ activity

⇓ movement	produced	↓ activity

⇓ prime + ⇑ perturbation	produced	greater ↑ activity
⇓ prime + ⇓ perturbation	produced	less ↑ activity

(B)

Figure 13.13. (A): The time course of each trial in the push-or-pull task used by Evarts and Tanji (1974). (B): Operating characteristics of two motor-cortical cells. Solid arrows indicate increases (upward arrow) or decreases (downward arrow) in cell discharge rates. Hollow arrows indicate a push-(upward arrow) or pull-(downward arrow) related event: either the push/pull priming signal, a push/pull movement, or the push/pull perturbation that also served as the release signal.

could be measuring force rather than positional values. Indeed, Evarts interpreted his early experimental data (Evarts, 1968) as suggestive of force coding. However, the data of Schmidt, Jost and Davis (1975) appear to rule out this alternative interpretation. After varying position and force independently, they concluded that "motor cortex cell firing patterns appear to be unrelated to the large values of rate of change of force seen in this experiment" (p.213).

The data summarized in Sections 13.7–13.13 weigh heavily against the STE Model and models based upon optimization principles. So too do the formal shortcomings of these models noted in Sections 13.7 and 13.12. We now show that the Vector-Integration-to-Endpoint (VITE) Model overcomes these formal shortcomings and provides a parsimonious quantitative explanation of all the behavioral and neural data summarized above and in the subsequent sections.

13.14. Learning Constraints Mold Arm Control Circuits

Rejecting the Spring-To-Endpoint (STE) Model does not entail rejecting all dependence upon endpoint commands. An analysis of sensory-motor learning during eye-hand coordination enables us to identify processes which supplement endpoint, or target position, commands to overcome the shortcomings of the STE Model (Grossberg, 1978a). The central role of learning constraints in the design of sensory-motor systems has elsewhere been developed for the case of the saccadic eye movement system (Grossberg and Kuperstein, 1986).

We focus our discussion of learning within the arm movement system upon the basic problem of how, when an observer looks at an object, the observer's hand knows where to move in order to touch the object. We discuss this issue from the perspective of eye-hand coordination in a mammal, but the issues that are raised, as well as the conclusions that are drawn, generalize to many other species and sensory-motor systems. Why learning processes are needed to solve this problem is illustrated by the following example.

The movement command which guides the hand to a visual target at a fixed position relative to the body is not invariant under growth. If a young arm, with relatively short limb segments, and an old arm with relatively long limb segments, react to the same command—that is, assume equal angles at analogous joints—then the tips of the two arm's fingers will be at different loci with respect to the body frame. In short, any animal that grows over an extended period will need to adaptively modify movement commands even if its only ambition is to perform the same act earlier and later in its life cycle. Put the other way, that animals do remain able to reach desired targets throughout periods of limb growth implies plasticity in their sensory-motor commands. Because such growth is slow relative to the rate of learning, failures of sensory-motor coordination are rarely noticeable. In humans, exceptions occur during the first few months of life, prior to experiential tuning of the infant's initially coarse sensory-motor mapping (Fetters and Todd, 1987; von Hofsten, 1979, 1982).

13.15. Comparing Target Position with Present Position to Gate Intermodality Learning

Thus, as the arm grows, the motor commands which move it to a fixed position in space with respect to the body must also change through learning. Many arm movements are activated in response to visually seen objects that the individual wishes to grasp. We therefore formulate this learning process as follows: How is a transformation learned and adaptively modified between the parameters of the eye-head system and the hand-arm system so that an observer can touch a visually fixated object?

Following Piaget's (1963) analysis of *circular reactions*, let us imagine that an infant's hand makes a series of unconditional movements, which the infant's eyes unconditionally follow. As the hand occupies a variety of positions that the eye fixates, a transformation is learned from the parameters of the hand-arm system to the parameters of the eye-head system. A reverse transformation is also learned from parameters of the eye-head system to parameters of the hand-arm system. This reverse transformation enables an observer to intentionally move its hand to a visually fixated position.

How do these two sensory-motor systems know what parameters are the correct ones to map upon each other? This question raises the fundamental problem that many neural signals, although large, are unsuitable for being incorporated into behavioral maps and commands. They are "functional noise" to the motor learning process. The learning process needs to be actively modulated, or gated, against learning during inappropriate circumstances.

In the present instance, not all positions that the eye-head system or the hand-arm system assume are the correct positions to associate through learning. For example, suppose that the hand briefly remains at a given position and that the eye moves to foveate the hand. An infinite number of positions are assumed by the eye as it moves to foveate the hand. Only the final, intended, or expected position of the eye-head system is a correct position to associate with the position of the hand-arm system.

Learning of an intermodal motor map must thus be prevented except when the eye-head system and the hand-arm system are near their intended positions. Otherwise, all possible positions of the two systems could be associated with each other, which would lead to behaviorally chaotic consequences. Several important conclusions follow from this observation (Grossberg, 1978a; Grossberg and Kuperstein, 1986).

(1) All such adaptive sensory-motor systems compute a representation of target position (also called expected position, or intended position). Thus the importance of endpoint computations is confirmed. This representation is the TPC (target position command). In addition:

(2) All such adaptive sensory-motor systems also compute a representation of present position. This representation is the PPC (present position command).

(3) During movement, target position is matched against present po-

sition. Intermodal map learning is prevented except when target position approximately matches present position (Figure 13.14). A *gating*, or modulator, signal is thus controlled by the network at which target position is matched with present position. This gating signal enables learning to occur when a good match occurs and prevents learning from occurring when a bad match occurs. This matching process takes place at the match interface that was described in Section 13.13. The DV (difference vector) controls the gating signal.

(4) In order to compare target positions with present positions, both types of data must be computed in the same coordinate system. Present eye position is computed with respect to head coordinates. Thus there is an evolutionary pressure to encode target position in head coordinates.

13.16. Trajectory Formation using DV's: Automatic Compensation for Present Position

The above discussion of how *intermodality* sensory-motor transformations are learned also sheds light upon how *intramodality* movement trajectories are formed. Intermodality transformations associate TPC's because only such transformations can avoid the multiple confusions that could arise through associating arbitrary positions along a movement trajectory. TPC's are not, however, sufficient to generate intramodality movement trajectories. In response to the same TPC, an eye, arm, or leg must move different distances and directions depending upon its present position when the target position is registered.

PPC's can be used to convert a single TPC into many different movement trajectories. Computation of the difference between target position and present position at the match interface in Figure 13.8 generates a difference vector, or DV, that can be used to automatically compensate for present position. Such automatic compensation accomplishes a tremendous reduction in the memory load that is placed upon an adaptive sensory-motor system. Instead of having to learn whole movement trajectories, the system only has to learn intermodality maps between TPC's. As shall be shown below, the DV's which are computed from target positions and present positions at the match interface can be used to automatically and continuously update the PPC movement commands from which the trajectory is formed. In summary, consideration of the types of information that can be used to learn intermodality commands during motor development leads to general conclusions about the quantities from which intramodality movement trajectories are formed, and thus about the way in which other neural systems, such as sensory, cognitive, and motivational systems, can influence the planning of such trajectories.

Computation of TPC's, PPC's, and DV's is a qualitatively different approach to generating a trajectory than are traditional computations based upon a Newtonian analysis of movement kinematics. In a Newtonian analysis, every position within the trajectory is assumed to be explicitly controlled (Atkeson and Hollerbach, 1985; Brody and Paul, 1984; Hogan, 1984; Hollerbach, 1984). Such computations lead to a combinatorial ex-

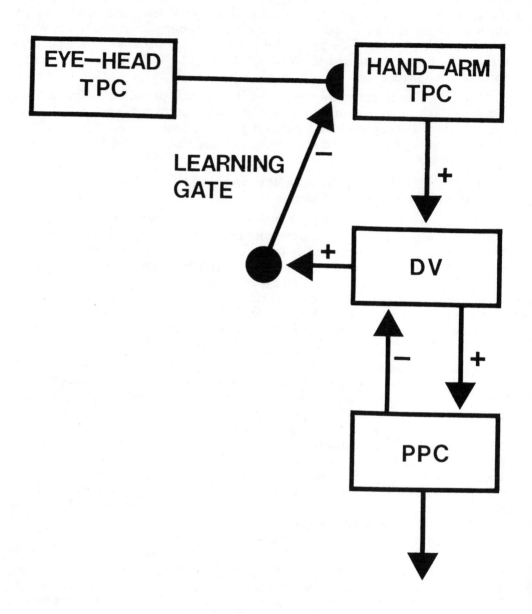

Figure 13.14. Learning in sensory-motor pathways is gated by a DV process which matches TPC with PPC to prevent incorrect associations from forming between eye-head TPC's and hand-arm TPC's.

plosion which is hard to reconcile with the rapidity of biological movement generation in real-time. In a vector computation, the entire trajectory is never explicitly planned. Instead, a TPC is computed which determines where the movement expects, or intends, to terminate. The subtraction of the PPC is an automatic process which compensates for the variability of the starting position. The DV which is hereby computed can be used to generate an accurate movement without ever explicitly computing a planned sequence of trajectory positions for the whole movement. In arm movements, a continuous comparison is made between a fixed TPC and all the PPC's that are computed during the movement. All of these compensations for changes in present position are automatically registered, and therefore place no further burden upon the computation of planned movement parameters. In addition, such automatic compensations for present position spontaneously generate the major invariants of arm movements that have been discovered to date (Sections 13.22–13.29). Thus the general problem of how DV's are computed is a central one for the understanding of trajectory formation in several movement systems.

13.17. Matching and Vector Integration during Trajectory Formation

We now specify in greater detail a model of how TPC's, PPC's, and DV's interact with each other through time to synthesize a movement trajectory. Each PPC generates a pattern of outflow movement signals to arm system muscles (Figure 13.8). Each such outflow pattern acts to move the arm system towards the present position which it encodes. Thus, were only a single PPC to be activated, the arm system would come to rest at a single physical position. A complete movement trajectory can be generated in the form of a temporal succession of PPC's. Such a movement trajectory can be generated in response to a single TPC that remains active throughout the movement. Although a TPC explicitly encodes only the endpoint of the movement, the process whereby present positions are automatically and continuously updated possesses properties that are much more powerful than those of an STE Model.

This process of continuous updating proceeds as follows. At every moment, a DV is computed from the fixed TPC and the PPC (Figure 13.8). This DV encodes the difference between the TPC and the PPC. In particular, the DV is computed by subtracting the PPC from the TPC at the match interface.

Because a DV computes the difference between the TPC and the PPC, the PPC equals the TPC only when all components of the DV equal zero. Thus, if the arm system's commands are calibrated so that the arm attains the physical position in space that is coded by its PPC, then the arm system will approach the desired target position in space as the DV's computed during its trajectory approach zero. This is accomplished as follows.

At each time, the DV computes the direction and amplitude which must still be moved to match the PPC with the TPC. Thus the DV computes an error signal of a very special kind. These error signals are used to continuously update the PPC in such a way that the changing PPC approaches the fixed TPC by progressively reducing the vector error to zero. In particular, the match interface at which DV's are computed sends excitatory signals to the stage where PPC's are computed. This stage integrates, or adds up, these vector signals through time. The PPC is thus a cumulative record of all past DV's, and each DV brings the PPC a little closer to the target position command.

In so doing, the DV is itself updated due to negative feedback from the new PPC to the match interface (Figure 13.8). This process of updating present positions through vector integration and negative feedback continues continuously until the PPC equals the TPC. Several important conclusions follow from this analysis of the trajectory formation process.

Two processes within the arm control system do double duty: A PPC generates feedforward, or outflow, movement signals *and* negative feedback signals which are used to compute a DV. A DV is used to update intramodality trajectory information *and* to gate intermodality learning of associative transformations between TPC's. Thus the match interface continuously updates the PPC when the arm is moving *and* disinhibits the intermodality map learning process when the arm comes to rest.

Within the circuit depicted in Figure 13.8, "position" and "direction" information are separately coded. Positional information is coded within the PPC and directional information is coded by the DV at the match interface. On the other hand, the computations which give rise to positional and directional information are not independent, since DV's are integrated to compute PPC's, and PPC's are subtracted from TPC's to compute DV's.

In Figure 13.8, the PPC is computed using outflow information, but not inflow information. This property emphasizes the need to mechanize concepts about how present position is computed. Using an outflow-based PPC clarifies how targets can be reached when sources of inflow information are eliminated (Polit and Bizzi, 1978) without being forced into the erroneous conclusion that no information about present position is needed to form a trajectory. In addition, although the PPC integrates outflow DV signals during active movements, inflow signals are used to update the PPC during passive movements (Section 13.30), thereby clarifying the data of Polit and Bizzi (1978) concerning failure of monkeys to compensate for passive shifts of their initial upper arm position in the deafferented state. The PPC feedback shown in Figure 13.8 is an "efference copy" of a "premotor" command (von Holst and Mittelsteadt, 1950). The VITE model's use of efferent feedback distinguishes it from an alternative class of models, which propose that present position information is derived from afferent feedback from sensory receptors in the limb. In particular, the far reaching consequences of its use of efferent, as opposed to afferent, feedback make the VITE model fundamentally different from the classical closed-loop servo recommended by Adams (1971, 1977) as a model of human motor performance. Further differences are introduced by the VITE model's use of the time-varying multiplicative GO signal introduced in Section 13.11 and elaborated below.

13.18. Intentionality and the GO Signal: Motor Priming without Movement

The circuit depicted in Figure 13.8 embodies the concept of intention, or expectation, through its computation of a TPC. The complete movement circuit embodies intentionality in yet another sense, which leads to a circuit capable of variable speed control. The need for such an additional process can also be motivated through a consideration of eye-hand coordination (Grossberg, 1978a, 1982a).

When a human looks at a nearby object, several movement options for touching the object are available. The object could be grasped with the left hand or the right hand. The object could even be touched with one's nose or one's toes! We assume that the eye-head system can simultaneously activate TPC's in several motor systems via the intermodality associative transformations that are learned to these systems. An additional "act of will," or GO signal, is required to convert one or more of these TPC's into overt movement trajectories within only the selected motor systems.

There is only one way to implement such a GO signal within the circuit depicted in Figure 13.8. This implementation is described in Figure 13.15. The GO signal must act at a stage intermediate between the stages which compute DV's and PPC's: The GO signal must act after the match interface so that it does not disrupt the process whereby DV's become zero as PPC's approach the TPC. The GO signal must act before the stage which computes PPC's so that changes in the GO signal cannot cause further movement after the PPC matches the TPC. Thus, although the GO signal changes the outputs from the match interface before they reach the present position stage, the very existence of such processing stages for continuous formation of a trajectory enables the GO signal to act without destroying the accuracy of the trajectory.

The detailed computational properties of the GO signal are derived from two further constraints. First, the absence of a GO signal must prevent the movement from occurring. This constraint suggests that the GO signal multiplies, or *shunts*, each output pathway from the match interface. A zero GO signal multiplies every output to zero, and hence prevents the PPC from being updated. Second, the GO signal must not change the direction of movement that is encoded by a DV. The direction of movement is encoded by the *relative* sizes of all the output signals generated by the vector. This constraint reaffirms that the GO signal *multiplies* vector outputs. It also implies that the GO signal is *nonspecific*: The *same* GO signal multiplies each output signal from the matching interface so as not to change the direction encoded by the vector.

In summary, the GO signal takes a particularly simple form. When it equals zero, the present position signal is not updated. Hence no overt movement is generated. On the other hand, a zero GO signal does not prevent a TPC from being activated, or a DV from being computed. Thus

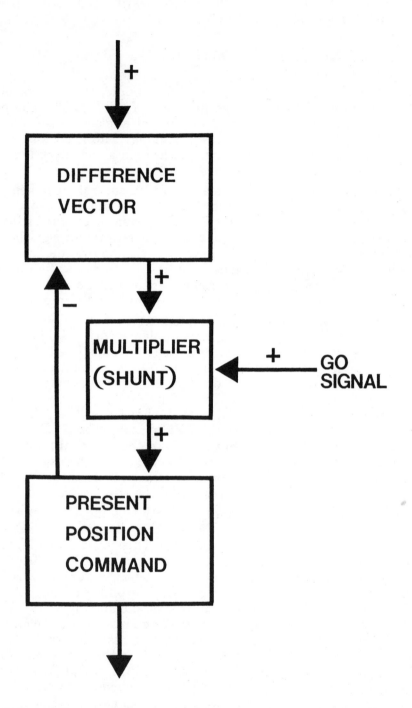

Figure 13.15. A GO signal gates execution of a primed movement vector and regulates the rate at which the movement vector updates the present position command.

a motor system can become ready, or primed, for movement before its GO signal turns on. When the GO signal does turn on, the movement can be rapidly initiated. The size of the GO signal regulates overall movement speed. Larger GO signals cause faster movements, other things being equal, by speeding up the process whereby directional information from the match interface is integrated into new PPC's. In models of cognitive processing, the functional analog of the GO signal is an attentional gain control signal (Carpenter and Grossberg, 1987a, 1988a; Grossberg, 1987b, 1987c; Grossberg and Stone, 1986a).

Georgopoulos, Schwartz, and Kettner (1986) have reported data consistent with this scheme. In their experiment, a monkey is trained to withhold movement for 0.5 to 3 seconds until a lighted target dims. They reported that cells with properties akin to DV cells computed a direction congruent with that of the upcoming movement during the waiting period. These data support the prediction that the neural stage where the GO signal is registered lies between the DV stage and the PPC stage.

13.19. Synchrony, Variable Speed Control, and Fast Freeze

The circuit in Figure 13.15 is now easily seen to possess qualitative properties of synchronous synergetic movement, variable speed control, and fast freeze-and-abort. We apply the circuit properties that each muscle synergist's motor command is updated at a rate that is proportional both to the synergist's distance from its target position and to a variable-magnitude GO signal, which is broadcast to all members of the synergy to initiate and sustain the parallel updating process.

To fix ideas, consider a simple numerical example. Suppose that, prior to movement initiation, muscle synergist A is 4 distance units from its target position and muscle synergist B is 2 distance units from its target position. In that case, if the mean rates at which PPC's are updated for the two synergists are in the same proportion as the distance (i.e., 2:1), then the updating of synergist A will take 4/2 time units while the updating of synergist B will take 2/1 time units. Thus both processes will consume approximately 2 time units. Although the PPC updating process occurs at different rates for different synergists, it consumes equal times for all synergists. The result is a synchronous movement despite large rate variations among the component motions.

Changing the magnitude of the GO signal governs variable speed control. Because both of the updating rates in the example (2 and 1) are multiplied by the same GO signal, the component motions will remain synchronous, though of shorter or longer duration, depending on whether the GO signal multiplier is made larger or smaller, respectively. In general, the GO signal's magnitude varies inversely with duration and directly with speed. Finally, if the value of the GO signal remains at zero, no updating and no motion will occur. Thus very rapid freezing can be achieved by completely inhibiting the GO signal at any point in the trajectory. The fact that target position may be very different from present position when the GO signal is withdrawn does not interfere with freezing, as it would using a STE Model, because the arm position closely tracks the PPC, which stops changing as soon as the signal shuts off.

Grossberg (1978a, Section 54; reprinted in Grossberg, 1982a) suggested an alternative scheme whereby actively moving muscles could be opposed by properly scaled antagonist co-contractions in response to a sudden unexpected event. In this scheme, agonist-antagonist motor commands are organized as gated dipole opponent processes and the unexpected event triggers a burst of nonspecific arousal to all the command sources. Each gated dipole opponent process reacts to such a nonspecific arousal burst by causing an antagonistic rebound whose size is scaled to that of the dipole's prior on-response. The rate of antagonist contraction generated by such a scheme is thus matched to the size of the just-previous rate of agonist contraction. Both types of mechanism—inhibition of GO signal and onset of arousal burst to opponent motor controls—are worthy of further neurophysiological testing. Another role for the opponent organization of motor commands is summarized in the next section.

13.20. Opponent Processing of Movement Commands

Mammalian motor systems are organized into pairs of agonist and antagonist muscles. We now note a new functional role for such an opponent organization: An opponent organization is needed to convert DV's into PPC's which can eventually match an arbitrary TPC. Figure 13.16 depicts how opponent organization is joined to the system's other processing constraints.

The need for opponent signals can be seen from the following examples. If a target position signal is larger than the corresponding present position signal, then a positive output signal is generated by the corresponding component of the DV. Such positive output signals increase the present position signal until it matches the target position signal. Increasing the present position signal causes the target muscle group to contract. The opponent muscle group must also simultaneously relax. Inhibitory signals to the present position node of the opponent muscle instate this latter property. When these inhibitory signals are integrated by the present position node of the opponent muscle, the output signal to the opponent muscle decreases, thereby relaxing the muscle.

The need for opponent processing can also be seen by considering the case in which the target position signal is smaller than the present position signal. Then the corresponding component of the DV is negative. Since only nonnegative activities can generate output signals, no output signal is generated by this component of the DV to its corresponding present position node. How, then, is this present position signal decreased until it matches the target position signal? The answer is now obvious, since we have just considered the same problem from a slightly different perspective: If a negative vector component corresponds to an antagonist muscle group, a positive vector component corresponds to its opponent agonist muscle group. This positive vector component generates inhibitory signals to the present position command of the antagonist muscle, thereby

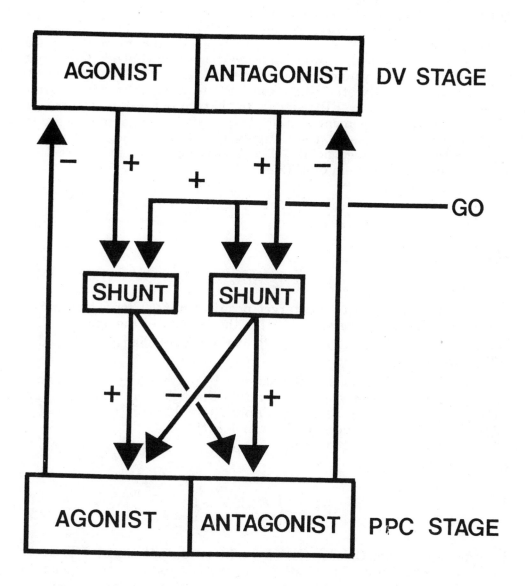

Figure 13.16. Opponent interactions among channels controlling agonists and their antagonists enable coordinated, automatic updating of their present position commands (PPCs). DV = difference vector.

relaxing the antagonist muscle until its PPC equals its TPC.

13.21. System Equations

A quantitative analysis of movement invariants requires the development of a rigorous real-time mathematical model of the constraints summarized in the preceding sections. Qualitative algebraic analysis is insufficient because the trajectory is an emergent property of a nonlinear integration and feedback process under variable gain control. Our model defines the simplest system that is consistent with these constraints. To fix ideas, we explicitly study how the TPC to an agonist muscle group generates a trajectory of PPC signals to that muscle group. Generalizations to synergetic movement of multiple agonist-antagonist muscle groups follow directly from this analysis. Figure 13.17 locates the mathematical variables that are defined below. The network depicted in Figure 13.17 obeys the following system of differential equations:

$$\frac{dV}{dt} = \alpha(-V + T - P) \tag{13.2}$$

and

$$\frac{dP}{dt} = G[V]^+. \tag{13.3}$$

In (13.2) and (13.3), $T(t)$ is a target position input, $V(t)$ is the activity of the agonist's DV population, $P(t)$ is the activity of the agonist's PPC population, $G(t)$ is the GO signal, $\frac{dV}{dt}$ is the rate of change of V, and $\frac{dP}{dt}$ is the rate of change of P.

Equation (13.2) says that the activity $V(t)$ averages the difference of the input signals $T(t)$ and $P(t)$ at a rate α through time. The TPC input $T(t)$ excites $V(t)$, whereas the PPC input $P(t)$ inhibits $V(t)$ as part of the negative feedback loop between $V(t)$ and $P(t)$.

Equation (13.3) says that $P(t)$ cumulatively adds, or integrates, the product $G[V]^+$, where

$$[V]^+ = \begin{cases} V & \text{if } V > 0 \\ 0 & \text{if } V \leq 0. \end{cases} \tag{13.4}$$

In other words, the DV population elicits an output signal $[V]^+$ to the PPC population only if the activity V exceeds the output threshold 0. The output signal is a linear function of V at suprathreshold values. The output signal $[V]^+$ is multiplied, or gated, by the GO signal $G(t)$ on its way to the PPC stage. The activity $P(t)$ at the PPC stage integrates the gated signal through time.

In particular, $G(t) = 0$ implies $\frac{dP}{dt}(t) = 0$. In other words, if the GO signal is shut off within a given time interval, the $P(t)$ is constant throughout that time interval. Fast-freeze can hereby be rapidly obtained

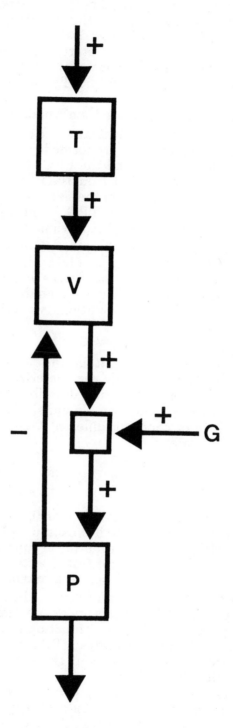

Figure 13.17. Network variables employed in computer simulations. See text equations (13.2) and (13.3).

by simply switching $G(t)$ quickly to zero no matter how far $P(t)$ may be from $T(t)$ at that time. In addition, this circuit generates compensatory, or "error correcting," trajectories, as described in Section 13.10. For example, suppose that the GO signal starts out larger than usual or that there is a slight delay in instatement of the TPC relative to onset of the GO signal. In either case, $P(t)$ can initially increase faster than usual. As a result, $T - P(t)$ can rapidly become smaller than usual. Consequently, updating of $P(t)$ terminates earlier than usual.

This compensatory process illustrates two critical features of the VITE Model: (1) Trajectories are not pre-formed. (2) Because the GO signal feeds in between the DV stage and the PPC stage and because the DV is continuously inhibited by feedback from the PPC stage, accuracy is largely insulated from random variations in the size or onset time of the GO signal, variations in the onset time of the TPC, or momentary perturbations of the PPC due to internal noise or inflow signals.

The system of equations (13.2)–(13.4) is explicitly solved for a particular choice of GO signal in Appendix 1. In Sections 13.22–13.29, we display the results of computer simulations which demonstrate that this simple model provides a quantitative explanation of all the data thus far summarized. In most of these simulations, we write the GO signal in the form

$$G(t) = G_0 g(t). \tag{13.5}$$

Constant G_0 is called the GO *amplitude* and function $g(t)$ is called the GO *onset function*. The GO amplitude parameterizes how large the GO signal can become. The GO onset function describes the transient build-up of the GO signal after it is switched on. In our simulations, we systematically studied the influence of choosing different GO amplitudes G_0 and onset functions from the family

$$g(t) = \begin{cases} \frac{t_n}{\beta_n + \gamma t_n} & \text{if } t \geq 0 \\ 0 & \text{if } t < 0. \end{cases} \tag{13.6}$$

In (13.6), we chose β and γ equal to 1 or 0. If $\beta = 0$ and $\gamma = 1$, then $g(t)$ is a step function which switches from 0 to 1 at time $t = 0$. If $\beta = 1$ and $\gamma = 1$, then $g(t)$ is a slower-than-linear function of time if $n = 1$ and a sigmoid, or S-shaped, function of time if $n > 1$. In both of these cases, function $g(t)$ increases from $g(0) = 0$ to a maximum of 1, and attains the value $\frac{1}{2}$ at time $t = \beta$. If $\beta = 1$ and $\gamma = 0$, then $g(t)$ is a linear function of time if $n = 1$ and a faster-than-linear function of time if $n > 1$. We will demonstrate below that an onset function which is a faster-than-linear or sigmoid function of time generates a PPC profile through time that is in quantitative accord with data about the arm's velocity profile through time. On the other hand, if muscle and arm properties attenuate the increase in velocity at the beginning of a movement, then linear or even slower-than-linear onset functions could also quantitatively fit the data. Direct physiological measurements of the GO signal and PPC updating processes would enable a more definitive selection of the onset function to be made.

13.22. Computer Simulation of Movement Synchrony and Duration Invariance

In simulations of synchronous contraction, the same GO signal $G(t)$ is switched on at time $t = 0$ across all VITE circuit channels. We consider only agonist channels whose muscles contract to perform the synergy. Antagonist channels are controlled by opponent signals as described in Section 13.20. We assume that all agonist channels start out at equilibrium before their TPC's are switched to new, sustained target values at time $t = 0$. In all agonist muscles, $T(0) > P(0)$. Consequently, $V(t)$ in (13.2) increases, thereby increasing $P(t)$ in (13.3) and causing the target muscle to contract. Different muscles may be commanded to contract by different amounts. Then the size of $T(0) - P(0)$ will differ across the VITE channels inputting to different muscles. Thus, equations (13.2)–(13.4) describe a generic component of a TPC $(T_1, T_2, \ldots, T_n)$, a DV $(V_1, V_2, \ldots, V_n)$, and a PPC $(P_1, P_2, \ldots, P_n)$. Rather than introduce subscripts $1, 2, \ldots, n$ needlessly, we merely note that our mathematical task is to show how the VITE circuit (13.2)–(13.4) behaves in response to a single GO function $G(t)$ if the initial value $T(0) - P(0)$ is varied. The variation of $T(0) - P(0)$ can be interpreted as the choice of a different setting for each of the components $T_i(0) - P_i(0), i = 1, 2, \ldots, n$. Alternatively it can be interpreted as the reaction of the same component to different target and initial position values on successive performance trials.

Figure 13.18 depicts a typical response to a faster-than-linear $G(t)$ when $T(0) > P(0)$. Although $T(t)$ is switched on suddenly to a new value T, $V(t)$ gradually increases-then-decreases, while $P(t)$ gradually approaches its new equilibrium value, which equals T. The rate of change $\frac{dP}{dt}$ of P provides a measure of the velocity with which the muscle group that quickly tracks $P(t)$ will contract. Note that $\frac{dP}{dt}$ also gradually increases-then-decreases with a bell-shaped curve whose decelerative portion $(\frac{d_2 P}{dt_2} <$ 0) is slightly longer than its accelerative portion $(\frac{d_2 P}{dt_2} > 0)$, as in the data described in Sections 13.8, 13.9, 13.12, and 13.13.

Figure 13.19 demonstrates movement synchrony and duration invariance. This figure shows that the V curves and the $\frac{dP}{dt}$ curves generated by widely different $T(0) - P(0)$ values and the same GO signal $G(t)$ are perfectly synchronous through time. This property is proved mathematically in Appendix 2. The simulated curves mirror the data summarized in Sections 13.12 and 13.13. These results demonstrate that the PPC output vector $(P_1(t), P_2(t), \ldots, P_n(t))$ from a VITE circuit dynamically defines a synergy which controls a synchronous trajectory in response to any fixed choice $(T_1, T_2, \ldots, T_n)$ of TPC, any initial positions $(P, (0), P_2(0), \ldots, P_n(0))$, and any GO signal $G(t)$.

13.23. Computer Simulation of Changing Velocity Profile Asymmetry at Higher Movement Speeds

The next simulations reproduce the data reviewed in Section 13.12

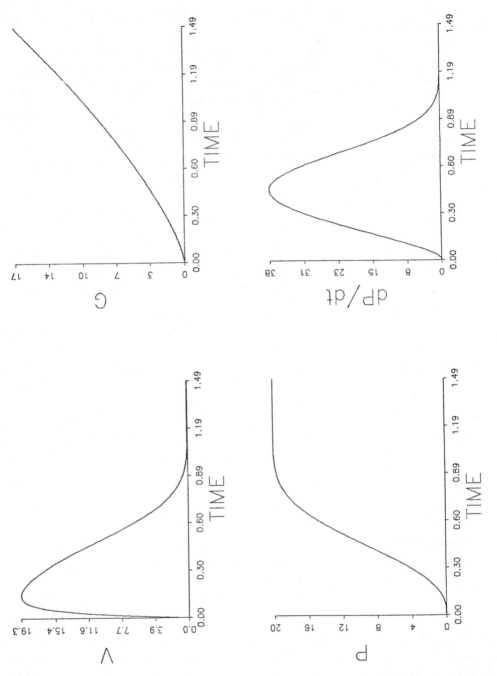

Figure 13.18. The simulated time course of the neural network activities V, G, and P during an 1100 msec. movement. The variable T (not plotted) had value 0 at $t < 0$, and value 20 thereafter. The derivative of P is also plotted to allow comparison with experimental velocity profiles. Parameters for equations (13.2), (13.3), (13.6): $\alpha = 30$, $n = 1.4$, $\beta = 1$, $\gamma = 0$.

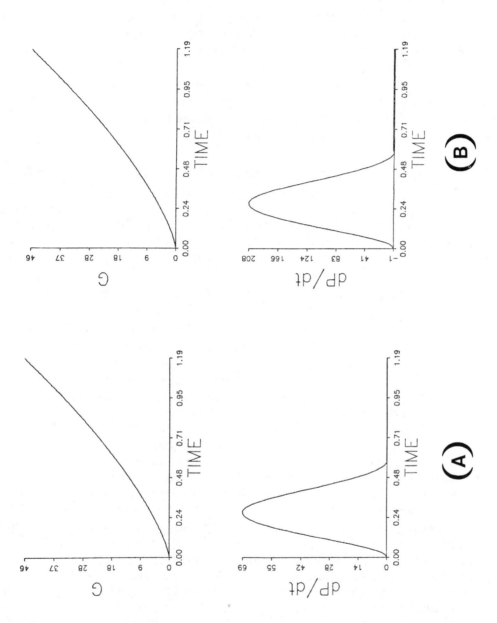

Figure 13.19. With equal GO signals, movements of different size have equal durations and perfectly superimposable velocity profiles after velocity axis rescaling. (A, B): GO signals and velocity profiles for 20 and 60 unit movements lasting 560 msec. (See Figure 13.18 caption for parameters.)

Bullock and Grossberg

concerning the greater symmetry of velocity profiles at higher movement velocities. In these simulations, the initial difference $T(0) - P(0)$ between TPC and PPC was held fixed and the GO amplitude G_0 was increased. Figure 13.20a–c shows that the profile of $\frac{dP}{dt}$ becomes more symmetric as G_0 is increased. At still larger G_0 values, the direction of asymmetry reversed; that is, the symmetry ratio exceeded .5, as in the data of Zelaznik, Schmidt, and Gielen (in press). Figure 13.20d shows that if both the time axis t and the velocity axis $\frac{dP}{dt}$ are rescaled, then curves corresponding to movements of the same size at different speeds can approximately be superimposed, except for the mismatch of their decelerative portions, as in the data summarized in Section 13.12.

13.24. Why Faster-than-Linear or Sigmoid Onset Functions?

The parametric analysis of velocity profiles in response to different values of $T(0) - P(0)$ and G_0 led to the choice of a faster-than-linear or sigmoid onset function $g(t)$. In fact, the faster-than-linear onset function should be interpreted as the portion of a sigmoid onset function whose slower-than-linear part occurs at times after $P(t)$ has already come very close to T.

Figure 13.21 shows what happens when a slower-than-linear $g(t) = t(\beta + t)^{-1}$ or a linear $g(t) = t$ is used. At slow velocities (small G_0), the velocity profile $\frac{dP}{dt}$ becomes increasingly asymmetric when a slower-than-linear $g(t)$ is used. At a fixed slow velocity, the degree of asymmetry increases as the slower-than-linear $g(t)$ is chosen to more closely approximate a step function. A linear $g(t)$ leads to an intermediate degree of asymmetry. A faster-than-linear, or sigmoid, $g(t)$ leads to slight asymmetry at small values of G_0 as well as greater symmetry at large values of G_0. A sigmoid $g(t)$ can be generated from a sudden onset of GO signal if at least two cell stages average the GO signal before it gates $[V]^+$ in (13.3). A sigmoid $g(t)$ contains a faster-than-linear part at small values of t, and an approximately linear part at intermediate values of t. Thus a sigmoid $g(t)$ can generate different degrees of asymmetry depending upon how much of the total movement time occurs within each of these ranges.

We have also simulated a VITE circuit using sigmoid GO signals whose rate of growth increases with the size of the GO amplitude. Such covariation of growth rate with amplitude is a basic property of neurons which obey membrane, or shunting, equations (Grossberg, 1970, 1973, 1982a; Sperling and Sondhi, 1968). Such a sigmoid GO signal $G(t)$ can be simply defined as the output of the second neuron population in a chain of shunting equations perturbed by a step function input with amplitude G_0. Thus, let

$$G_0(t) = \begin{cases} G_0 & \text{if } t \geq 0 \\ 0 & \text{if } t < 0 \end{cases} \tag{13.7}$$

$$\frac{d}{dt}G_1 = -AG_1 + (B - G_1)G_0 \tag{13.8}$$

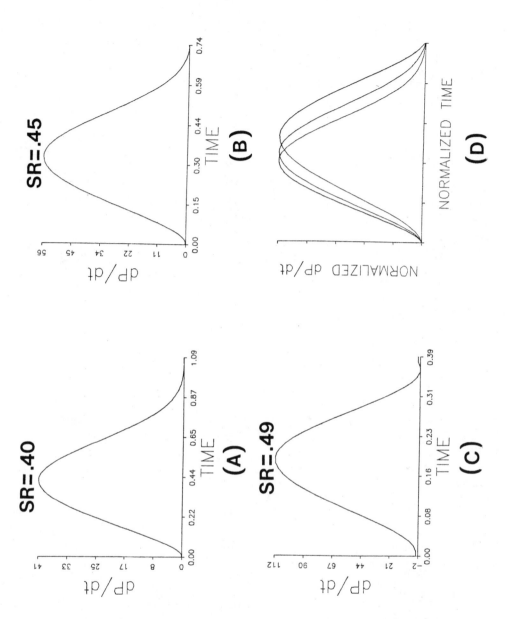

Figure 13.20. (A, B, C): Velocity profiles associated with a slow, medium, and fast performance of a 20 unit movement. Each SR value gives the trajectory's *symmetry ratio*; that is, the time taken to move half the distance, $.5(T(0) - P(0))$, divided by the total movement duration, MT. These ratios indicate progressive symmetrization at higher speeds. (D): The velocity profiles shown in (A), (B), and (C) are not perfectly superimposable. (See Figure 13.18 for parameters.)

Bullock and Grossberg

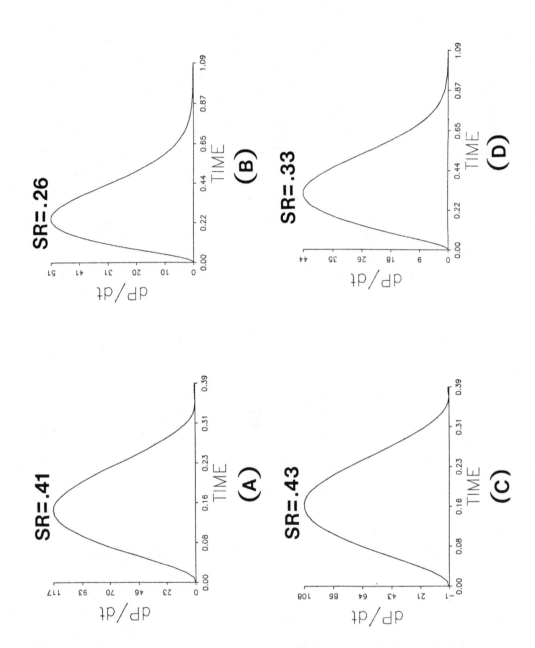

Figure 13.21. (A, B): Velocity profiles for a slow and a fast movement with a slower-than-linear $g(t)$: $\alpha = 30$, $n = 1$, $\beta = 1$, $\gamma = 1$. (C, D): Velocity profiles for a slow and a fast movement with a linear $g(t)$: $\alpha = 30$, $n = 1$, $\beta = 1$, $\gamma = 0$. (SR = symmetry ratio.)

and

$$\frac{d}{dt}G_2 = -AG_2 + (B - G_2)G_1. \qquad (13.9)$$

Then $G_2(t)$ is a sigmoid function of the desired shape. The GO signal $G(t)$ can be set equal to $G_2(t)$, as we did, or even to a sigmoid signal $f(G_2(t))$ of $G_2(t)$. A typical result is shown in Figure 13.22. In the series of simulations exemplified by Figure 13.22, the range of symmetry ratios, namely .44–.50 was similar to that found in Figure 13.19 using a faster-than-linear signal function. Final choice of a best-fitting $G(t)$ awaits a more direct experimental determination of the PPC profile through time.

13.25. Computer Simulation of Velocity Amplification during Target Switching

Velocity amplification by up to a factor of three can be obtained by switching to a new value of T while a previously activated GO signal is still on. Figure 13.23 demonstrates this effect by comparing two computer simulations. In the first simulation, onset of $T(t)$ and $g(t)$ were both synchronous at time $t = 0$ (Figure 13.23a). In the second simulation, onset of $g(t)$ preceded onset of $T(t)$ by a time equivalent to about 300 msec (Figure 13.23b). Note the much higher peak velocity (235 versus 102) attained in Figure 13.23b. This effect, which matches the "anomalous" velocity multiplication observed in the target-switching experiments of Georgopoulos et al. (1981), is due to the prior build-up of the GO signal during response execution.

In the ensuing sections, computer simulations will be compared with a variety of data which were not reviewed in the preceding sections.

13.26. Reconciling Staggered Onset Times with Synchronous Termination Times

Within the context of a target-switching experiment, velocity amplification may appear to be a paradoxical property. On the other hand, such a property has an adaptive function in the many situations where a hand will fail to reach a moving target unless it both changes direction and speeds up. In addition, we now show that the same mechanism can generate synchronous termination times of synergetic muscle components which may individually start to move at staggered onset times.

The need for this latter property has recently been emphasized by a study of Hollerbach, Moore, and Atkeson (1986), who showed that nearly straight movement paths can result from muscle coordinate planning if the onset times of muscles acting at different joints are appropriately staggered *and* if all the muscles reach their final positions synchronously. Their study did not, however, explain how a neural mechanism could generate synchronous muscle offsets despite staggered muscle onsets.

We now show that the posited interaction of a growing GO signal with components of a DV that may be switched on at different times automatically generates synchronous offsets as an emergent property of

Bullock and Grossberg

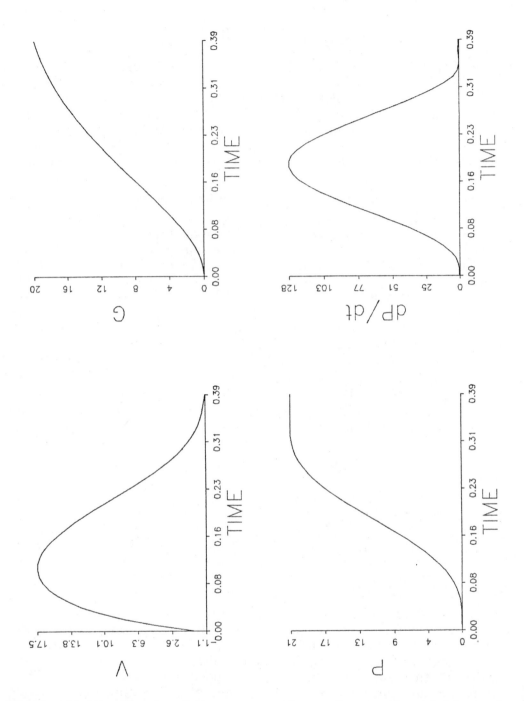

Figure 13.22. Simulated time course of neural network activities and $\frac{dP}{dt}$ for a 350 msec movement. Note the S-shaped growth in G (sigmoid GO signal). Parameter values for equations (13.2), (13.3), (13.8), (13.9): $\alpha = 25$, $A = 1$, $B = 25$.

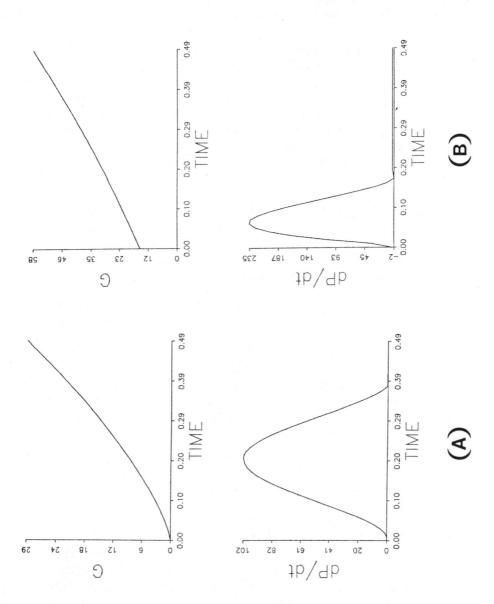

Figure 13.23. A much higher peak velocity is predicted by the model whenever a target is activated after the GO signal has already had time to grow. (A): The control condition, in which T and the GO signal growth process are activated synchronously. (B): Same T as in (A), but here T was activated after $G(t)$ had been growing for 300 msec. (See Figure 13.18 for parameters.)

the VITE circuit. Thus the interaction of a GO signal with a DV both helps to linearize the paths generated by individual TPC's and, as in the target-switching experiments, enables the hand to efficiently track a moving target by quickly reacting to read-out of an updated TPC.

Figure 13.24 depicts the results of four blocks, labelled I, II, III, and IV, of computer simulations. Each block represents the onset time, offset time, and duration of three simulations. In the leftmost simulations of each block, onset of a DV component and a GO signal were synchronous. In the other two simulations of each block, a different DV component was read-out at successively longer delays with respect to the onset time of the GO signal. Due to duration invariance (Appendix 2), the results are independent of the initial sizes of the $T(0) - P(0)$ values of these components.

The four blocks (I, II, III, IV) correspond to four increasing values of the GO amplitude G_0 $(10, 20, 40, 80)$. The approximate invariance of termination times across components with different onset delays is indicated by the nearly equal *heights* reached by all the bars within the block. The different *lengths* of bars within each block show that less time is needed to update those components whose onset times are most delayed. Thus, in block I, all the components terminate almost synchronously even though their onset times are staggered by as much as 26% of the total movement time. In block II, almost synchronous terminations occur even though onset times are staggered by as much as 39% of the total movement time. At very large choices of G_0 (blocks III and IV), synchrony begins to gently break down because the earliest components have executed over 50% of their trajectories before later components even begin to move. These and other results in the article suggest the critical importance of experimentally testing the existence and predicted properties of GO–DV interactions, notably the predicted correlations between the temporal evolution of the GO signal and the DV.

13.27. Computer Simulation of the Inverse Relation between Duration and Peak Velocity

Each curve depicted in Figure 13.25a summarizes a series of simulations in which $T(0) - P(0)$ was held constant while G_0 was varied . In this way, a series of velocity profiles were generated whose peak velocities differed even though their trajectories traversed the same distance. The duration of each movement was computed by measuring the interval between velocity profile zero crossings. The different curves in Figure 13.25a used different values of the distance parameter $T(0) - P(0)$.

These curves mirror the data of Lestienne (1979) summarized in Figure 13.25b. Figure 13.25b plots agonist burst duration against peak velocity. The overall shapes of the plots of simulated durations (Figure 13.25a) and agonist burst durations (Figure 13.25b) as a function of peak velocity are similar. This similarity reinforces the postulate that the VITE circuit operates in agonist-antagonist muscle coordinates (Sections 13.3 and 13.20). It also suggests that the relationship between VITE circuit outputs, mo-

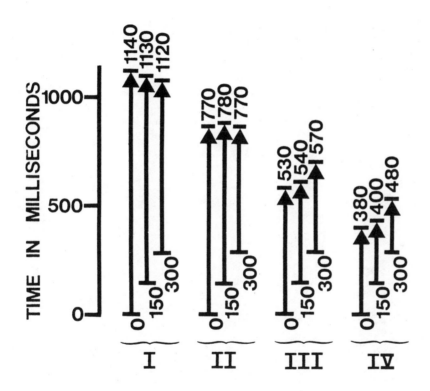

Figure 13.24. Simulation results showing automatic VITE circuit compensation for contraction-onset-time staggering across components of a synergy. Each block (I, II, III, IV) shows results for a different value (10, 20, 40, and 80, respectively) of the GO signal scalar, G_0. (See Figure 13.18 for parameters.)

Bullock and Grossberg

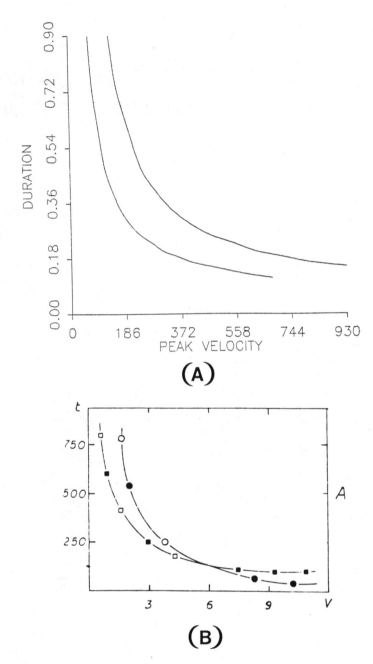

Figure 13.25. (A): Simulation of movement duration (sec) as a function of peak velocity (deg/sec) for a 30° (lower curve) and a 60° (upper curve) movement. (See Figure 13.18 for parameters.) (B): Data on agonist burst duration (squares) and antagonist burst onset-time (dots) as a function of peak velocity (rad/sec) for a 60° movement. Reprinted with permission from Lestienne (1979).

toneuron inputs, and actual muscle activities might be relatively simple (Bullock and Grossberg, 1988b).

Nevertheless, two caveats deserve mention. First, were Figure 13.25a a plot of movement duration (MT) against *mean* velocity $(\overline{V})$, it would necessarily have the shape shown, since by definition,

$$MT = \frac{D}{\overline{V}}, \tag{13.10}$$

where D denotes the distance. Multiplying by different values of D generates a family of curves similar in shape to those shown in Figure 13.25a. The VITE model generates the curve in Figure 13.25a because mean velocity and peak velocity are strongly correlated in these VITE trajectories due to the duration invariance described in Section 13.22.

The second caveat acknowledges that the VITE circuit cooperates with several other circuits to generate a controllable trajectory in response to unexpected loads and to variable velocities (Bullock and Grossberg, 1988b). For example, during medium and high speed movement, the duration of the initial agonist burst may be only one fourth the duration of the corresponding movement. If we assume that the PPC updating process consumes most of the movement time, then these short duration EMG bursts are further evidence that the PPC stage must not be identified with—and must be higher in the outflow channel than—the spinal motorneurons whose suprathreshold activities are directly reflected in the EMG bursts.

This conclusion is consonant with available data on the genesis of EMG burst patterns. In vivo, EMG activites are often sculpted into multiphasic burst patterns by several subnetworks that converge on and embed the spinal motorneurons. In particular, during high-speed movements, muscle changes lag behind neural changes early in response development. This leads to registration of "lag errors" at model regulatory circuits (Bullock and Grossberg, 1988b; Feldman, 1986; Ghez and Martin, 1982; Grossberg and Kuperstein, 1986), including the stretch reflex and cerebellar circuits, which translate these error signals into large agonist activations and antagonist inhibitions. If the large agonist activations accelerate the limb so much that it begins to overshoot the intended position, this overshoot is registered as an error opposite in sign to the initial lag error, and the result is a large antagonist braking activity in concert with agonist inhibition. Such braking may slow the movement enough that a smaller lag-error is once again registered. Though this results in a second agonist burst, and transient antagonist inhibition, this last phasic modulation fades quickly and gives way to the tonic EMG pattern required to hold the arm at the final postural position. A similar analysis may be given for isometric contractions.

TABLE 13.1

FOR FIXED DURATION (MT), ERROR
GROWS IN PROPORTION TO DISTANCE

MT	DISTANCE	ERROR
.56	10	.084
.56	20	.170
.56	40	.349
.56	80	.700

13.28. Speed-Accuracy Trade-off: Woodworth's Law and Fitts' Law

The VITE Model circuit predicts a speed-accuracy trade-off which quantitatively fits the classical laws of Woodworth (1899) and of Fitts (1954). The existence of a speed-accuracy trade-off *per se* can be understood by considering the role of the rate parameter α in equation (13.1). The case of an overshoot error is considered for definiteness.

Given *any* finite value of the averaging rate α in equation (13.2), $V(t)$ takes some time to react to changes in $P(t)$. In particular, even if $P(t) = T$ at a given time $t = t_0$, $V(t)$ will typically require some extra time after $t = t_0$ to decrease to the value 0, and by (13.3) $P(t)$ will continue to increase during this extra time. If α is very large, $V(t)$ can approach 0 quickly. Consequently, by (13.3), $V(t)$ will not allow $P(t)$ to overshoot the target value T by a large amount. On the other hand, given *any* choice of α, the *relative* amount whereby $P(t)$ overshoots the target T depends upon the size of the GO amplitude G_0. This is true because a larger value of G_0 causes $P(t)$ to increase faster, due to (13.3), and thus $P(t)$ can approach T faster. In contrast, $V(t)$ can only respond to the rapidly changing values of $T - P(t)$ at the constant rate α. As a result, $V(t)$ tends to be larger at a time $t = t_0$ when $P(t_0) = T$ if G_0 is large than if G_0 is small. It therefore takes $V(t)$ longer to equal 0 after $t = t_0$ if G_0 is large. Thus $P(t)$ overshoots T more if G_0 is large. This covariation of amount of overshoot with overall movement velocity is a speed-accuracy trade-off.

Fitts' Law, as described in equation (13.1), relates movement time (MT), distance (D), and target width (W). The target width may be thought of as setting the criterion for what counts as an error. The law may be given two complementary readings. The first notes that for a fixed movement time, error grows in proportion to amplitude. This component of the law was discovered by Woodworth (1899). Table 13.1 presents simulation results based on the same parameter choices used in Figure 13.18. The results show that, in a parameter range where model overshoot errors occur, the model's error also grows in proportion to amplitude. In these simulations, G_0 was held fixed and $T(0) - P(0)$ was varied.

The second way of reading the law notes that in order to maintain

TABLE 13.2
FOR FIXED ERROR LEVEL, DURATION (MT)
GROWS LINEARLY WITH DISTANCE DOUBLING

ERROR	DISTANCE	MT
.059	2	.39
.057	4	.49
.058	8	.59
.059	16	.70
.057	32	.80
.059	64	.91

a fixed absolute error size, or to fall within a target zone of fixed width, while increasing movement distance, it is necessary to allow more time for completing the movement. In particular, every doubling of distance will add a constant amount, b, to the time needed to perform the movement with the same level of accuracy. Allowing less than b more time for a movement of twice the distance will lead to a less accurate movement.

Table 13.2 presents the results of a simulation (parameters as in Figure 13.18) in which the rate parameter α was small enough that modest error resulted even at the smallest distance, or initial value of $T(0) - P(0)$, that was tested, namely a distance of 2 units. Then the distance $T(0) - P(0)$ was repeatedly doubled, and the value of G_0 progressively decreased, such that the error level was held approximately constant. As can be seen, movement time increased approximately linearly with each doubling of distance, as required by a logarithmic relation between MT and D. It should be noted that the "errors" shown in Tables 13.1 and 13.2 are defined relative to a mathematical point, that is a target having zero width along the direction of motion. If subjects adjust their GO signal so that expected error is no greater than the width of a physical target, then by choosing a TPC corresponding to the near side of the target, they can produce the "errorless" movements required in the Fitts task. The model's striking replication of the laws of Woodworth and Fitts, together with its other successes in experimental results, increases our confidence that the VITE Model captures some of the basic neural design principles that underly trajectory generation *in vivo*.

Woodworth's Law is a consequence of duration invariance in the model. This can be seen from the mathematical analysis provided in Appendix 2. There it is proved that the PPC value $P(t)$ can be written in the form

$$P(t) = P(0) + (T(0) - P(0)q(t)) \qquad (13.11)$$

given *any* continuous GO signal $G(t)$. In (13.11), $T(0) - P(0)$ represents the amount of contraction, or "distance" to be moved, that is mandated by the TPC value $T(0)$ and the initial PPC value $P(0)$. Function $q(t)$

is independent of $P(0)$ and $T(0)$. By (13.11), $P(t)$ approaches $T(0)$ as $q(t)$ approaches 1, and $P(t)$ overshoots or undershoots if $q(t)$ approaches a value greater or less than 1, respectively. Since $q(t)$ is multiplied by $T(0) - P(0)$, the amount of error (undershoot or overshoot), is proportional to distance, as in Woodworth's Law.

Whereas the proof of Woodworth's Law is a general consequence of duration invariance in the model, Fitts' Law has been mathematically proved in only one case as of the present time (Appendix 1), although our computer simulations demonstrate that it occurs with greater generality. In this case, the GO signal $G(t)$ switches on from value 0 at times $t < 0$ to the constant value $G_0 > 0$ at times $t \geq 0$. In addition, G_0 is chosen sufficiently large to generate overshoot errors. In particular, when $4G_0 > \alpha$,

$$MT = \frac{2}{\alpha} \log\left(\frac{T(0) - P(0)}{E}\right) \tag{13.12}$$

where E is the amount of overshoot error in the VITE command.

These instances of Woodworth's Law and Fitts' Law are generated by the VITE circuit itself, without the intervention of visual feedback. A number of authors have commented upon the applicability of these laws when visual feedback is inoperative. For example, Keele (1982, pp.152–153) has written: "What is the underlying nature of the movement system that yields Fitts' Law? ... One factor is the intrinsic accuracy of the motor control system when visual feedback is unavailable. When the eyes are closed during a movement (or the lights are turned off), an average movement will miss target by about 7% of the total distance moved." Schmidt (1982, pp.253–254) summarized error functions for sighted and blind movements across various movement times from studies of Keele and Posner (1968) and Zelaznik, Hawkins, and Kisselburgh (1983). A clear speed-accuracy trade-off was observed. Meyer, Smith, and Wright (1982, p.450) have reviewed data comparing the initial impulse phase of a movement, where visual feedback is unimportant, with the subsequent current-control phase, where visual feedback may be used to improve accuracy. They noted that "the initial-impulse phase was found to contribute directly to the speed-accuracy trade-off. Even when subjects had to perform with their eyes closed and relied on just this phase to execute their movements, they still produced a trade-off ... models that attempt to account for the speed-accuracy trade-off ... must include mechanisms that modulate the trade-off during the initial-impulse phase, not just during the current-control phase." The VITE circuit's ability to reproduce both Woodworth's Law and Fitts' Law as emergent properties of the PPC updating process satisfies this requirement.

It should be emphasized that the VITE circuit is also capable of generating a PPC that approaches the TPC without error in some parameter ranges (Appendix 1). In these parameter ranges, an undershoot error will occur if the GO signal is prematurely terminated or if the effects of small DV signals get lost in ambient cellular noise. A range effect has also been reported (Georgopoulos, 1986, p.151) such that "subjects tended to overshoot the target in small movements (2.5 cm) and to undershoot in large movements (40 cm)." A number of factors may influence this result. For example, during high speed small movements, auxiliary circuits for controlling the arm's inertial effects may not have a sufficient opportunity to act (Grossberg and Kuperstein, 1986, Chapters 3 and 5). During large movements, the distance to be moved may be visually underestimated, thereby leading to instatement of an incorrect TPC. The choice of GO signal amplitude as a function of target distance may contribute to the range effect. The relative importance of such factors will be easier to assess as new experiments and the theory are progressively elaborated with the aid of the quantitative VITE circuit analysis that is provided herein.

Even the definition of what constitutes a movement "error" during ecologically useful motor behavior deserves further commentary. For example, Carlton (1979) asked subjects to keep their movement errors below 5 percent. Subjects typically chose a two-part movement strategy whose first velocity component undershot the target, and whose second velocity component made the final approach to the target at a much lower speed. Such results suggest that subjects found it easier to achieve greater accuracy by breaking up the movement into parts than by launching the movement ballistically over the full distance. The first movement part, albeit strictly speaking an "undershoot error", provides the occasion for updating TPCs and choosing small GO signals during the final part of the movement, thereby achieving high accuracy without too great an increase in total movement duration. Because GO signal adjustments may also be necessary during the final components of such composite movements, these components may also obey a speed-accuracy tradeoff, as Carlton (1979) found.

13.29. Computer Simulation of Peak Acceleration Data

Bizzi *et al.* (1984) measured the peak accelerations of medium-speed forearm movements by monkeys. They considered movements around the elbow that swept out 20° and 60°. A computer simulation is compared with their data in Table 13.3. In order to make this comparison, we scaled 1 time unit in our simulation to equal 10 msec. We then chose two values of the GO amplitude parameter G_0 which generated trajectories of duration approximately equal to 554 msec. and 692 msec., respectively. Due to duration invariance (Section 13.22), the same durations obtain given these choices of G_0 over a wide range of choices of the distance measure $T(0) - P(0)$. The fact that movements were 20° or 60° was translated into the constraint that the $T(0) - P(0)$ value corresponding to the smaller choice of G_0 must be chosen three times larger than the $T(0) - P(0)$ value corresponding to the larger choice of G_0. Then we searched for values of $T(0) - P(0)$ that gave the best fit to the peak acceleration data subject to this constraint.

The result is compared in Table 13.3 with the data, and with the fit of the Minimum-Jerk Model of Hogan (1984). The VITE Model fit these data substantially better than the Minimum-Jerk Model. The values associated with the VITE[+] model indicate that a perfect fit can be

TABLE 13.3
A COMPARISON OF THREE MODELS' ABILITIES
TO PREDICT DATA ON PEAK ACCELERATION ($\ddot{P}$)

DISTANCE	MT	PEAK $\ddot{P}$	PEAK $\ddot{P}$ SOURCE
20°	.554	$397°/sec^2$	Bizzi *et al.* (1984)
60°	.692	$1130°/sec^2$	(experimental data)
20°	.554	$376°/sec^2$	Minimum-jerk model
60°	.692	$722°/sec^2$	(simulation)
20°	.554	$394°/sec^2$	VITE model
60°	.692	$854°/sec^2$	(simulation)
20°	.554	$396°/sec^2$	VITE$^+$ model
60°	.692	$1127°/sec^2$	(simulation)

obtained (with Figure 13.18 parameters) if DV readout to the shunting stage, rather than being instantaneous, occurs over a brief interval whose length is proportional to the size of the DV.

As noted in Section 13.12, the Minimum-Jerk Model also erroneously predicts a symmetric velocity profile, at least at the level of the central controller. Moreover, it is hard to see how this model could explain the velocity amplification that occurs during target switching (Section 13.11). Finally, the Minimum-Jerk Model does not contain any representation that may be compared with the existence of vector cells or with the manner in which vector cell activities are integrated into outflow movement commands (Section 13.13). We therefore believe that the VITE Model provides a better foundation for developing a quantitative neurally-based theory of arm movements than does the Minimum-Jerk Model. The VITE model, in addition to the model circuits developed in Grossberg and Kuperstein (1986), also provides a mechanistic neural explanation of some of the types of invariant behaviors for whose analysis the task dynamics approach to motor control was developed (Saltzman and Kelso, 1983).

13.30. Updating the PPC using Inflow Signals during Passive Movements

Despite these successes, the VITE Model as described above is far from complete. In this section, a solution of one additional design problem is outlined. Bullock and Grossberg (1988b) suggest solutions of a number of the other design problems whereby a VITE circuit can effectively move an arm of variable mass subjected to unexpected perturbations at variable velocities through a Newtonian world.

In Section 13.6, we noted that inflow signals are needed to update the PPC during a passive movement. For example, Gellman, Gibson, and Houk (1985) have described cells in the cat inferior olive that are sensitive to passive body displacement but not to active movement, and Clark, Burgess, Chapin, and Lipscomb (1985) have analysed muscle proprioceptive contributions to position sense during passive finger movements in humans. Two basic problems motivate our model of PPC updating by inflow signals. First, the process of updating the PPC during passive movements must continue until the PPC registers the position coded by the inflow signals. Thus a difference vector of inflow signals minus PPC outflow signals updates the PPC during passive movements. We denote this difference vector by DV_p to distinguish it from the DV which compares TPC's with PPC's. At times when $DV_p = 0$, the PPC is fully updated. Although the DV_p is not the same as the DV which compares a TPC with a PPC, the PPC is a source of inhibitory signals, as will be seen below, in computing both difference vectors.

Second, PPC outflow signals and inflow signals may, in principle, be calibrated quite differently. We will show how corollary discharges of the PPC outflow signals are adaptively recalibrated until they are computed in the same numerical scale as the inflow signals to which they are compared. We also show that this adaptive recalibration mechanism automatically computes a DV_p which updates the PPC by just the correct amount.

Figure 13.26 schematizes a model circuit for adaptively computing this DV_p. We call this circuit the *passive update of position (PUP) model*. In Figure 13.26, the PPC sends inhibitory corollary discharge signals towards the outflow-inflow match stage where the inflow signals are registered. It is assumed that this stage is inhibited except when the movement command circuit is inactive. A simple way to achieve this property is to assume that the GO signal in the movement command circuit inhibits the outflow-inflow match stage, as in Figure 13.25. Thus the mismatches of outflow and inflow signals that occur during every active movement do not erroneously update the outflow-inflow match stage. In addition, the GO signal is assumed to inhibit learning at the LTM traces which multiply the PPC signals on their way to the outflow-inflow match stage.

This assumption is consistent with arm movement results of Evarts and Fromm (1978) which showed greater modulation of vector cells in precentral motor cortex by inflow signals during small slow movements than during posture, and strongly attenuated modulation during large fast movements. In the model, the amount of attenuation increases with the size of the GO signal. The gating signal which attenuates the inflow process may be a nonlinear (e.g., sigmoid) function of the GO signal. Parametric analysis of the degree of inflow attenuation as a function of overall active movement speed would provide valuable information about the form of this hypothesized gating signal.

After a movement is over, both the outflow-inflow match stage and the LTM traces are released from inhibition. Typically, the PPC represents the same position as the inflow signals, but perhaps in a different numerical

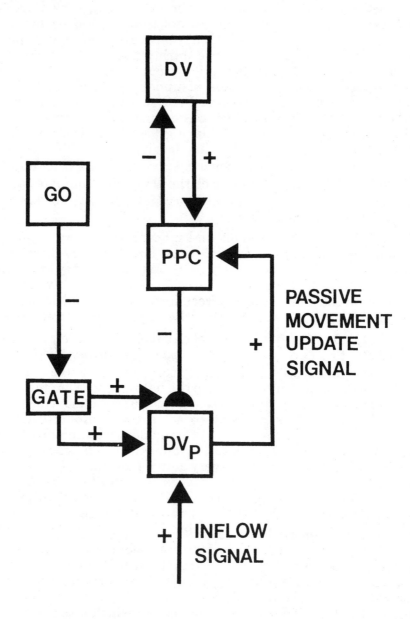

Figure 13.26. A passive update of position (PUP) circuit. An adaptive pathway $PPC \rightarrow DV_P$ calibrates PPC-outflow signals in the same scale as inflow signals during intervals of posture. During passive movements, output from DV equals zero. Hence the passive difference vector DV_P updates the PPC until it equals the new position caused by any passive movements that may occur due to the application of external forces.

scale. The learning laws described in Appendix 3 define LTM traces which change until the PPC *times* the LTM trace equals the inflow signal. After a number of such learning trials during stable posture, $DV_p = 0$ and the PPC signals are rescaled by the LTM traces to correctly match the inflow signals.

During a passive movement, the PPC does not change, but the inflow signal may change. If the DV_p becomes positive, it causes an increase in the PPC until the DV_p decreases to 0 and the PPC is correctly updated by the inflow signals. If the DV_p becomes negative, then the DV_p of the opponent muscle can decrease the PPC until a match again occurs.

13.31. Concluding Remarks

The present article introduces a circuit for automatically translating a target position command into a complete movement trajectory via a mechanism of continuous vector updating and integration. A wide variety of behavioral and neural data can be quantitatively explained by this mechanism. The model also provides a foundation for clarifying some of the outstanding classical issues in the motor control literature, highlights the relevance of learning constraints upon the design of neural circuitry, and may be viewed as a specialized version of a more general architecture for movement control.

The VITE circuit and the PUP circuit do not, however, exhaust the total neural machinery that is needed for the control of arm movements. Mechanisms for properly timed sequential read-out of TPC's in a serial motor plan, such as during reaching and grasping or during a dance (Grossberg and Kuperstein, 1986, Chapter 9), for adaptive linearization of a non-linear muscle plant (Grossberg and Kuperstein, 1986, Chapter 5), and for automatically or predictively adapting to the inertial properties generated by variable loads and velocities (Bullock and Grossberg, 1988b) also form essential parts of the arm control system. When all of these systems are joined together, however, one can begin to understand quantitatively how the arm system achieves its remarkable flexibility and versatility, and can begin to build a new type of biologically inspired adaptive robot whose design is qualitatively different from the algorithms offered by traditional approaches to artificial intelligence.

APPENDIX 1

Bell-Shaped Velocity Profile, Fitts' Law, and Staggered Onset Times

This Appendix solves the system of equations

$$\frac{d}{dt}V = \alpha(-V + T - P) \tag{A1}$$

$$\frac{d}{dt}P = G[V]^+ \tag{A2}$$

under the simplifying assumption that the GO signal G is a step function. Then the system can easily be integrated to demonstrate some basic properties.

In many situations, the system starts out in an equilibrium state such that the PPC equals the TPC. Then a new TPC is switched on and the system approaches a new equilibrium. Before the new TPC is switched on, $P = T$ in (A1). Since the system is at equilibrium, $\frac{d}{dt}V = 0$. Thus, by (A1), it also follows that $V = 0$ under these circumstances.

Suppose that a new TPC value is switched on at time $t = 0$. If the system represents an agonist muscle, then $T(0) > P(0)$ so that the PPC increases when $T(0)$ turns on, thereby causing more contraction of its target muscle group. Thus by (A1),

$$V(0) = 0, \tag{A3}$$

and

$$\frac{d}{dt}V(0) = \alpha(T(0) - P(0)) > 0. \tag{A4}$$

Consequently $V(t) \geq 0$ for all times t such that $0 \leq t \leq S$, where S is the first positive time, possibly infinite, at which $V(S) = 0$. While $V(t) \geq 0$ it follows by (A2) that

$$\frac{d}{dt}P = GV \tag{A5}$$

To solve equations (A1) and (A5), differentiate (A1) at times when $V(t) \geq 0$. Then

$$\frac{d^2}{dt^2}V = \alpha(-\frac{dV}{dt} - \frac{dP}{dt}), \tag{A6}$$

because T is constant. Substituting (A5) into (A6) yields the equation

$$\frac{d^2}{dt^2}V + \alpha\frac{d}{dt}V + \alpha GV = 0 \tag{A7}$$

subject to the initial data (A3) and (A4).

This equation can be solved by standard methods. The solution takes the form

$$V(t) = (T(0) - P(0))f(t), \qquad (A8)$$

where $f(t)$ is independent of $T(0)$ and $P(0)$. Thus $V(t)$ equals the initial difference between the new TPC and the initial PPC multiplied by a function $f(t)$ which is independent of the new TPC and the initial PPC. By (A2),

$$\frac{d}{dt}P = (T(0) - P(0))g(t), \qquad (A9)$$

where $g(t) = Gf(t)$. Integration of (A9) yields

$$P(t) = P(0) + (T(0) - P(0)) \int_0^t g(v)dv. \qquad (A10)$$

Since $\frac{d}{dt}P$ provides an estimate of the arm's velocity profile, (A9) illustrates the property of duration invariance in the special case that $G(t)$ is constant. Duration invariance is proved using a general $G(t)$ in Appendix 2. Equation (A9) also illustrates how the velocity profile can respond to a sudden switch in the TPC with a gradual increase-then-decrease in its shape, although $g(t)$ assumes a different form if $\alpha > 4G$, $\alpha = 4G$, or $\alpha < 4G$. When $\alpha > 4G$,

$$g(t) = \frac{\alpha G}{\sqrt{\alpha^2 - 4\alpha G}} e^{-\frac{\alpha}{2}t} \left[e^{\frac{t}{2}\sqrt{\alpha^2 - 4\alpha G}} - e^{-\frac{t}{2}\sqrt{\alpha^2 - 4\alpha G}} \right]. \qquad (A11)$$

Term $[\exp(\frac{t}{2}\sqrt{\alpha^2 - 4\alpha G})] - [\exp(-\frac{t}{2}\sqrt{\alpha^2 - 4\alpha G})]$ in (A11) increases exponentially from the value 0 at $t = 0$, whereas term $\exp[-\frac{\alpha}{2}t]$ decreases exponentially towards the value 0 at a faster rate. The net effect is a velocity function that increases-then-decreases with an approximately bell-shaped profile. In addition, $g(t) \geq 0$ and

$$\int_0^\infty g(t)dt = 1. \qquad (A12)$$

By (A10) and (A12), $P(t)$ increases towards T as t increases. Thus $P(t)$ either approaches $T(0)$ with an arbitrarily small error, or an undershoot error occurs if the GO signal is switched off prematurely.

If $\alpha = 4G$, then

$$g(t) = \alpha Gte^{-\frac{\alpha}{2}t}. \qquad (A13)$$

Again the velocity profile gradually increases-then-decreases, but starts to increase linearly before it decreases exponentially. The function in (A13) also satisfies (A12), so that accurate movement or undershoot occur, depending upon the duration of the GO signal.

Bullock and Grossberg

The case of $\alpha < 4G$ deserves special attention. In this case, the rate G with which P is updated in equation (A2) exceeds the ability of the rate α in equation (A1) to keep up. As a result, an overshoot error can occur. In particular,

$$g(t) = \frac{2\alpha G}{\sqrt{4\alpha G - \alpha^2}} e^{-\frac{\alpha}{2}t} \sin\left(\frac{\sqrt{4\alpha G - \alpha^2}}{2}t\right) \qquad (A14)$$

if $0 \leq t \leq \dfrac{2\pi}{\sqrt{4\alpha G - \alpha^2}}$. When t exceeds $\dfrac{2\pi}{\sqrt{4\alpha G - \alpha^2}}$, function $g(t)$, and thus $V(t)$, becomes negative. By (A2), $[V(t)]^+ = 0$ when t exceeds $\dfrac{2\pi}{\sqrt{4\alpha G - \alpha^2}}$, so that, by (A2), $P(t)$ stops moving at this time. The movement time in this case thus satisfies

$$MT = \frac{2\pi}{\sqrt{4\alpha G - \alpha^2}}. \qquad (A15)$$

Within this time frame, the velocity profile is the symmetric function $\sin\left(\dfrac{\sqrt{4\alpha G - \alpha^2}}{2}t\right)$ multiplied by the decaying, hence asymmetric, function $e^{-\frac{\alpha}{2}t}$. Greater overall symmetry of $g(t)$ is achieved if the rate $\dfrac{\sqrt{4\alpha G - \alpha^2}}{2}$ with which the sine function changes is rapid relative to the rate $\dfrac{\alpha}{2}$ with which the exponential function changes; viz., if $2G \gg \alpha$.

Since $P(t)$ stops changing at time $t = \dfrac{2\pi}{\sqrt{4\alpha G - \alpha^2}}$, the final PPC value found from equation (A10) is

$$P\left(\frac{2\pi}{\sqrt{4\alpha G - \alpha^2}}\right) = P(0) + (T(0) - P(0))(1 + e^{-(\alpha\pi/\sqrt{4\alpha G - \alpha^2})}). \qquad (A16)$$

Thus an overshoot error occurs of size

$$E = (T(0) - P(0))e^{-(\alpha\pi/\sqrt{4\alpha G - \alpha^2})}. \qquad (A17)$$

In accordance with Woodworth's Law, the error is proportional to the distance $(T(0) - P(0))$. Fitts' Law can be derived by holding E constant in (A17) and varying $(T(0) - P(0))$ to test the effect on the MT in (A15). Substituting (A15) into (A17) shows that

$$E = (T(0) - P(0))e^{-\frac{\alpha MT}{2}} \qquad (A18)$$

which implies Fitts' Law

$$MT = \frac{2}{\alpha} \log\Big(\frac{T(0) - P(0)}{E}\Big). \qquad (A19)$$

The initial condition $V(0) = 0$ in (A3) obtains if the system has actively tracked a constant TPC until its PPC attains this TPC value. Under other circumstances, $V(0)$ may be negative. When this occurs, $\frac{d}{dt}P$ in (A2) may remain 0 during an initial interval while $V(t)$ increases to nonnegative values. Thus P begins to change only after a staggered onset time. Some properties of staggered onset times are derived below.

A negative initial value of $V(0)$ may obtain if a particular muscle group has been passively moved to a new position either by an external force or by the prior active contraction of other muscle groups. In such a situation, $P(t)$ may be changed by the PUP circuit (Section 13.30) even if $T(t) = 0$, and $V(t)$ may track $P(t)$ via equation (A1) until a new equilibrium is reached. Under these circumstances, (A1) implies that

$$0 = \frac{d}{dt}V = \alpha(-V + 0 - P). \qquad (A20)$$

If we assume that this equilibrium value obtains at time $t = 0$, then

$$V(0) = -P(0) < 0, \qquad (A21)$$

and equation (A2) implies that

$$\frac{d}{dt}P = G[V]^+ = 0. \qquad (A22)$$

Thus P remains constant until V becomes positive. If a new TPC is switched on at time $t = 0$ to an agonist muscle which satisfies (A21), then $T(0) > P(0)$. By (A1), V increases according to the equation

$$\frac{d}{dt}V + \alpha V = \alpha(T(0) - P(0)), \qquad (A23)$$

where $\alpha(T(0) - P(0))$ is a positive constant, until the time $t = t_1$ at which $V(t_1) = 0$. Thereafter $[V]^+ = V > 0$ so that V and P mutually influence each other through equations (A1) and (A5).

Time t_1 is computed by integrating equation (A10). We find

$$V(t) = V(0)e^{-\alpha t} + (T(0) - P(0))(1 - e^{-\alpha t}) \qquad (A24)$$

for $0 \le t \le t_1$. By (A21),

$$V(t) = -P(0) + T(0)(1 - e^{-\alpha t}). \qquad (A25)$$

Thus

$$t_1 = \frac{1}{\alpha} \, ln \, \left[1 - \left(\frac{P(0)}{T(0)}\right)\right]^{-1}. \tag{A26}$$

By (A26), t_1 is a function of the ratio of the initial PPC value to the new TPC value.

For times $t \geq t_1$, equations (A1) and (A5) can be integrated just as they were in the preceding case. Indeed,

$$V(t_1) = 0 \tag{A27}$$

by the definition of t_1, and

$$\frac{d}{dt}V(t_1) = \alpha(T(0) - P(0)) \tag{A28}$$

by (A23) and (A28). The initial data (A27) and (A28) are the same as the initial data (A3) and (A4) except for a shift of t_1 time units. Consequently if the GO signal onset time is also shifted by t_1 time units, then it follows from (A8) that at times $t \geq t_1$,

$$V(t) = (T(0) - P(0))f(t - t_1). \tag{A29}$$

An estimate of such a velocity profile is found by piecing together (A24) and (A29). Thus

$$\frac{d}{dt}P = \begin{cases} 0 & \text{for } 0 \leq t < t_1 \\ G(T(0) - P(0))f(t - t_1) & \text{for } t_1 \leq t \end{cases}. \tag{A30}$$

Equation (A30) illustrates how a velocity profile with a staggered onset time can occur if $V(0) < 0$. As shown in Section 13.26, the VITE command to a muscle group can compensate for a staggered onset time if its DV is multiplied by the same GO signal as other muscles in the synergy. In this case, the GO signal onset time is not shifted to match the onset time of each component of the VITE command.

APPENDIX 2

Synchrony and Duration Invariance

Consider equations (A1) and (A2) under the influence of an arbitrary nonnegative and continuous GO function $G(t)$. As in Appendix 1, let

$$V(0) = 0 \qquad (A3)$$

and $P = T$ before T is switched to a new value. Suppose for definiteness that $T(t)$ switches from the value T_0 to T_1 at time $t = 0$, and that

$$T_1 > T_0 = P(0). \qquad (A31)$$

Consequently, equations

$$\frac{d}{dt}V = \alpha(-V + T - P) \qquad (A1)$$

and

$$\frac{d}{dt}P = GV \qquad (A5)$$

hold for an interval of values $t \geq 0$. Define the new PPC variable

$$Q(t) = P(t) - T_0 \qquad (A32)$$

and the new target position constant

$$T_2 = T_1 - T_0. \qquad (A33)$$

Then (A1) and (A5) can be replaced by equations

$$\frac{d}{dt}V = \alpha(-V + T_2 - Q) \qquad (A34)$$

and

$$\frac{d}{dt}Q = GV. \qquad (A35)$$

By (A31),

$$Q(0) = 0. \qquad (A36)$$

Thus by (A3) and (A36), both V and Q start out with 0 values at $t = 0$.
Now define new variables

$$v(t) = \frac{V(t)}{T_2} \qquad (A37)$$

and

$$q(t) = \frac{Q(t)}{T_2}. \tag{A38}$$

By (A34) and (A35), these variables obey the equations

$$\frac{d}{dt}v = \alpha(-v + 1 - q) \tag{A39}$$

and

$$\frac{d}{dt}q = Gv. \tag{A40}$$

In addition,

$$v(0) = q(0) = 0 \tag{A41}$$

by (A3) and (A36). It is obvious that a unique solution of (A39)–(A41) obtains no matter how T_2 and T_1 are chosen, if $T_2 > T_1$.

By combining (A31), (A32), (A33), and (A38), we find that

$$P(t) = P(0) + (T_1 - P(0))q(t), \tag{A42}$$

where $q(t)$ is independent of T_1 and $P(0)$. Equation (A42) proves duration invariance given a general GO function $G(t)$. Indeed, differentiating (A42) yields

$$\frac{d}{dt}P = (T_1 - P(0))\frac{d}{dt}q(t) \tag{A43}$$

which shows that function $\frac{d}{dt}q$ generalizes function $g(t)$ in equation (A9).

APPENDIX 3

Passive Update of Position

Mathematical equations for a PUP circuit are described below. As in our description of a VITE circuit, equations for the control of a single muscle group will be described. Opponent interactions between agonist and antagonist muscles also exist and can easily be added once the main ideas are understood.

The PUP circuit supplements the equation

$$\frac{d}{dt}P = G[V]^+ \tag{A2}$$

whereby the PPC integrates DV's through time. A PUP circuit obeys equations

Present Position Command

$$\frac{d}{dt}P = G[V]^+ + G_p[M]^+, \tag{A44}$$

Outflow-Inflow Interface

$$\frac{d}{dt}M = -\beta M + \gamma I - zP, \tag{A45}$$

Adaptive Gain Control

$$\frac{d}{dt}z = \delta G_p(-\epsilon z + [M]^+). \tag{A46}$$

The match function M in (A45) rapidly computes a time-average of the difference between inflow (γI) and gated outflow (zP) signals. Thus

$$M \simeq \frac{1}{\beta}(\gamma I - zP). \tag{A47}$$

If the inflow signal γI exceeds the gated outflow signal zP, then $[M]^+ > 0$ in (A47). Otherwise $[M]^+ = 0$. The *passive gating function* G_p in (A44) is positive only when the muscle is in a passive, or postural, state. In particular, $G_p > 0$ only when the GO signal $G(t) \simeq 0$ in the VITE circuit. Figure 13.26 assumes that a signal $f(G(t))$ inhibits a tonically active source of the gating signal G_p. Thus G_p is the output from a "pauser" cell, which is a tonically active cell whose output is attenuated during an active movement. Such cells are well-known to occur in saccadic eye movement circuits (Grossberg and Kuperstein, 1986; Luschei and Fuchs, 1972; Raybourn and Keller, 1977). If both G_p and $[M]^+$ are positive in (A44), then $\frac{d}{dt}P > 0$. Consequently, P increases until $M = 0$; that is, until the gated outflow signal zP equals the inflow signal zI. At such a time, the PPC is updated to match the position attained by the muscle during a passive movement. To see why this is true, we need to consider the role of function z in (A45) and (A46).

Function z is a long term memory (LTM) trace, or associative weight, which adaptively recalibrates the scale, or gain, of inflow signals until they are in the same scale as outflow signals. Using this mechanism, a match between inflow and outflow signals accurately encodes a correctly updated PPC. Adaptive recalibration proceeds as follows.

In equation (A46), the learning rate parameter δ is chosen to be a small constant to assure that z changes much more slowly than M or P. The passive gating function G_p also modulates learning, since z can change only at times when $G_p > 0$. At such times, term $-\epsilon z$ describes a very slow forgetting process which prevents z from getting stuck in mistakes. The forgetting process is much slower than the process whereby z grows when $[M]^+ > 0$. Since function M reacts quickly to its inputs γI and $-zP$, as in (A47), term $[M]^+ > 0$ only if

$$\gamma I > zP. \tag{A48}$$

The outflow signal P is multiplied, or gated, by z on its way to the match interface where M is computed (Figure 13.26).

Because z changes only when the muscle is in a postural, or a passive state, terms γI and P typically represent the same position, or state of contraction, of the muscle group. Then inequality (A48) says that the scale γI for measuring position I using inflow signals is larger than the scale zP for measuring the same position using outflow signals. When this happens, z increases until $M = 0$; viz., until outflow and inflow measurement scales are equal.

On an occasion when the arm is passively moved by an external force, the inflow signal γI may momentarily be greater than the outflow signal zP. Due to past learning, however, the inflow signal satisfies

$$\gamma I = zP^*, \tag{A49}$$

where P^* is the outflow command that is typically associated with I. Thus by (A47),

$$M \simeq \frac{z}{\beta}(P^* - P). \tag{A50}$$

By (A44) and (A50), P quickly increases until it equals P^*. Thus, after learning occurs, P approaches P^*, and M approaches 0 very quickly, so quickly that any spurious new learning which might have occurred due to the momentary mismatch created by the onset of the passive movement has little opportunity to occur, since z changes slowly through time. What small deviations may occur tend to average out due to the combined action of the slow forgetting term $-\epsilon z$ in (A46) and opponent interactions.

Equations (A45) and (A46) use the same formal mechanisms as the *head-muscle interface* (HMI) described by Grossberg and Kuperstein (1986). The HMI adaptively recodes a visually activated target position coded in head coordinates into the same target position coded in agonist-antagonist muscle coordinates. Such a mechanism for adaptive matching of two measurement scales may be used quite widely in the nervous system. We therefore call all such systems Adaptive Vector Encoders.

CHAPTER 14

A COMPARATIVE ANALYSIS
OF NEURAL MECHANISMS, RECENT DATA,
AND ALTERNATIVE MODELS

Stephen Grossberg

14.1. Comparative Analysis of Neural Models

The previous chapters illustrate how contemporary neural network models provide insights into some of the organizational principles that govern biological sensory-motor systems, and offer a level of computational precision that enables sharp comparisons and contrasts to be made between different sensory-motor systems. The capacity of these models to clarify, integrate, and predict behavioral and neural data is predicated upon the coordinated use of theoretical, mathematical, computational and empirical tools in a manner that reveals many more constraints on brain design than empirical tools alone. No single experimental paradigm in the behavioral and brain sciences provides sufficiently many data to uniquely characterize a neural system. Interdisciplinary theoretical and empirical approaches that can coordinate and discover both top-down and bottom-up constraints at multiple levels of behavioral and neural organization provide a much greater level of guidance towards characterizing brain designs.

Where insufficient guidance to derive a unique model is provided by all the available top-down and bottom-up theoretical and data constraints, it is advisable to develop fully the major model types that are consistent with all known constraints. Such a comparative approach to model development was followed, for example, in Chapters 3, 5, 6, 10, and 11. By rendering explicit the theoretical relationships among each model's parts, a relatively small number of new experiments can efficiently rule out many otherwise plausible solutions to a prescribed neural problem. A comparative approach to neural modelling is also advisable to cope with the facts of evolutionary variation. One model realization of a fundamental neural design may exist in some species, whereas a different realization may have evolved in other species. One helpful way to understand the invariant properties of a neural design is to carefully articulate its major design variations. Last but not least, a comparative analysis also provides neural network technologists with several ways to implement a desired functional competence.

The present chapter carries out a comparative analysis in two different senses. First it compares variations on an important neural design that is realized differently within the eye and arm movement systems, as well as at different processing stages of the same system. This type of comparative analysis helps to sharpen our understanding of each system by clarifying why it is computationally different from other systems that share

share some of its design properties. Then comparisons of our models are made with subsequent models and data of other investigators. This type of comparative analysis may help the reader to form a more unified understanding of the complex and often fragmented literature on adaptive sensory-motor control.

14.2. Comparative Analysis of Movement Vectors in Eye and Arm Movements

The design principle of vector encoding has been described in both the control of saccadic eye movements by the superior colliculus (Mays and Sparks, 1980, 1981; Sparks, 1978; Sparks and Jay, 1987; Sparks and Mays, 1981) and the control of arm movements by the motor cortex (Evarts and Tanji, 1974; Georgopoulos, 1986; Georgopoulos, Kalaska, Caminiti, and Massey, 1982; Georgopoulos, Kalaska, Crutcher, Caminiti, and Massey, 1984; Georgopoulos, Kettner, and Schwartz, 1988; Georgopoulos, Schwartz, and Kettner, 1986; Kettner, Schwartz, and Georgopoulos, 1988; Schwartz, Kettner, and Georgopoulos, 1988; Tanji and Evarts, 1976).

Although neural vectors are encoded in both of these systems, they are encoded differently in each system. Why do both systems employ a neural code which, in its broad outline, seems similar, but in its computational realization is grossly different? Models of saccadic eye movements (Chapter 4) and of arm movements (Chapter 13) have been developed in which these distinct types of vector coding are utilized. The models suggest that the design constraints which force these differences concern different problems of learning and coordinate transformation that are solved by the eye and arm movement systems. These constraints were necessarily scattered across several of the previous chapters in order to develop each of them technically. The present discussion summarizes and compares these constraints in a single place, and suggests additional experiments that may be used to further test the models.

14.3. Map Vectors and Difference Vectors

Because different types of vectors seem to exist, we need simple but evocative names to clearly distinguish them. The experiments of Sparks and his colleagues on the deeper layers of monkey superior colliculus have revealed a type of vector coding that may conveniently be called a *vector map code* (see pp.307–308). In such a vector representation, each location in a spatially organized map encodes a different vector, hence, a different combination of movement length and direction. The most eccentric locations tend to code the longest movements. Changing the polar angle of a location tends to change movement direction. Exciting cells at a prescribed location in the map tends to cause a saccadic eye movement of corresponding length and direction. Populations of cells are activated under normal behavioral conditions. The eye movement triggered by such a population has a length and direction that corresponds to the average length and direction coded by all of the cells in the population.

The experiments of Georgopoulos and his colleagues on monkey motor cortex have revealed a type of vector encoding that may conveniently be called a *vector difference code* (see p. 316). In such a vector representation, each cell tends to generate a broad unimodal tuning curve of direction preference that may include 180° of movement directions. Coding of movement amplitude tends to covary with the firing rate of cells in their direction of maximal sensitivity. Moreover, changes in the initial position of the arm covary with changes in the baseline level of cell activity. Thus a vector difference code does not encode amplitude and direction via different locations in a spatial map.

The computation and design significance of these map vectors and difference vectors are clarified from the viewpoint of the system's total behavioral competence.

14.4. Vector Integration to Endpoint and GO Signal Modulation in Arm Movement Control

Difference vectors are found in the model of arm trajectory control, called the Vector Integration to Endpoint (VITE) model, that was described in Chapter 13. This model predicts how read-out of a target position command, or TPC, that specifies a desired target position, or motor expectation, is translated into a present position command, or PPC, that causes a synergy of arm muscles to contract and relax synchronously until the PPC equals the TPC. Figure 13.1 reviews the main variables that are computed by the VITE circuit.

Figure 13.1 shows that a TPC is subtracted from a PPC at a network stage at which a difference vector (DV) is computed. As discussed in Chapter 13, model DV properties are remarkably similar to data properties reported by Georgopoulos and his colleagues. In particular, a large DV may be active without causing an overt movement. Such DV activation, called *motor priming*, has been reported by Georgopoulos, Schwartz, and Kettner (1986). The next stage of the model (Figure 13.1) computes the product of a DV and a GO signal, or gain control signal, that controls read-out of the movement command. The product DV × GO is integrated through time by the subsequent PPC stage. Due to this circuit design, the PPC stage generates a continuous trajectory of synchronous outflow movement commands that gradually causes the PPC to approach the TPC at a speed that is regulated by the amplitude of the GO signal.

Since the completion of Chapter 13, a still larger body of behavioral and neural data about arm and speech articulator movements has been analysed by comparison with emergent properties of the VITE model (Bullock and Grossberg, 1988a; Cohen, Grossberg, and Stork, 1989). Here I summarize some neural data that support the existence of a GO signal, some predictions to further test the circuit's overall design, and a learning problem from which the circuit was derived to prepare the ground for comparative analysis with the vector map concept.

14.5. GO Signal Generator in Globus Pallidus

Additional physiological support for the VITE model comes from recent experiments involving lesions and electrical stimulation of the basal ganglia. Data from a set of experiments by Horak and Anderson (1984a, 1984b) are consistent with the interpretation that the internal segment of the globus pallidus is an *in vivo* analogue of the VITE model's GO-signal generator.

An *in vivo* candidate for a GO-signal generator must pass three tests. First, stimulation at some site in the proposed pathway must have an effect on the *rate* of muscle contractions. Second, it must have this effect without affecting the *amplitude* of the contractions. Thus stimulation should have no effect on movement accuracy. Third, this rate-modulating effect should be *nonspecific*: it should affect all muscles that are typically synergists for the movement in question.

The studies conducted by Horak and Anderson (1984a, 1984b) addressed these issues. Horak and Anderson (1984a) showed that "when neurons in the globus pallidus were destroyed by injections of kainic acid (KA) during task execution, contralateral arm movement times (MT) were increased significantly, with little or no change in reaction times (p.290)." This satisfies the rate criterion. Moreover, the rate of motor recruitment was depressed "in all the contralateral muscles studied at the wrist, elbow, shoulder, and back, but there were no changes in the sequential activation of the muscles (p.20)." This satisfies the non-specificity criterion. Finally, the authors also noted that "animals displayed no obvious difficulty in aiming accurately ... they did not miss the 1.5-cm target more often following KA injections, and there was no noticeable dysmetria around the target (p.300)." This satisfies the accuracy criterion.

Horak and Anderson (1984b) used an electrical stimulation paradigm instead of a lesion paradigm. They found that "stimulation in the ventrolateral internal segment of the globus pallidus (GP_i) or in the ansa lenticularis reduced movement time, whereas stimulation at many sites in the external pallidal segment (GP_e), dorsal (GP_i), and putamen increased movement times for the contralateral arm (p.305)." Once again, these effects were non-specific: "no somatotopic effects of stimulation were evident. If stimulation at a site produced slowing, it produced a depression of activity in all the muscles studied. Even stimulus currents as low as 25 μA affected proximal as well as distal muscles, flexor as well as extensor muscles, and early- as well as late-occurring activity (p.309)."

In the VITE model, activation of the GO-signal pathway produces movement only if instatement of a TPC different from the current PPC leads to the computation of a non-zero DV. In agreement with this property, Horak and Anderson (1984b) observed that "stimulation at sites that speeded movements did not induce involuntary muscle activation in resting animals nor did it change background EMG activity prior to self-generated activity during task performance (p.313)." In Chapter 13, it was noted that "very rapid freezing can be achieved by completely inhibiting the GO signal at any point in the trajectory". This property of the model has also been shown to be a property of the GP system. In particular, Horak and Anderson reported that "stimulation with 50 or 100 μA at ... sites ventral and medial to typical GP_i neuronal activity completely and immediately halted the monkey's performance in the task (p.315)." Taken together, their experiments led Horak and Anderson (1984b) to conclude that "the basal ganglia ... determine the speed of the movement" (p.321).

14.6. Factorization of Position and Velocity Control

The striking correspondence between the experimental results of Georgopoulos *et al.* and of Horak and Anderson and the theoretical predictions of the VITE model regarding separate DV and GO-signal processes is important because it supports the hypothesis that motor systems, like sensory systems, implement a factorization of pattern and energy (Grossberg, 1970, 1978a, 1982a). In the motor system, this factorization means that a movement's velocity ("energy") can be scaled up or down over a wide range without disrupting the movement's direction or terminal position ("pattern"). Moreover, by using a GO-signal that grows gradually during the movement time, as in Figures 13.18 and 13.22, all synergists will complete their contractions at approximately the same time even if movement onset times of different synergists are staggered by a large amount (Bullock and Grossberg, 1988a, 1988b). These properties of the model, together with the growing evidence for separate DV and GO-signal pathways *in vivo*, provide a basis for understanding how primates can achieve space-time equifinality—all synergists reaching their length targets at equal times—yet retain separate control of velocity and position (Figure 13.24). Note that rate-control models relying on *static* stiffness adjustments (e.g., Cooke, 1980) lack the critical temporal-equifinality property.

14.7. Amplification of Peak Velocity and a GO Signal Test

Chapter 13 noted that in addition to compensating for muscles that begin to contract at staggered onset times, the VITE circuit automatically compensates for changes of target position during the movement time. In particular, it was shown that the model generates the amplification of peak velocity (Figure 13.23) that occurs during target-switching experiments (Georgopoulos, Kalaska, and Massey, 1981). Such a velocity amplification facilitates reaching the target after an incorrect initial TPC is replaced by an updated TPC. This speed-up occurs "on-the-fly." It is not preprogrammed, but is rather an automatic emergent property of VITE circuit interactions. It is caused as follows.

First there is a rapid change in the TPC and thus in the DV. Then a more gradual change occurs in the DV and the PPC as the PPC integrates the DV through time. The velocity amplification is predicted to be caused by interaction of the new DV with the GO signal that was activated by the previous movement command. This prediction can be physiologically tested using an experiment that would also provide another opportunity to test if the Horak-Anderson cells in globus pallidus generate GO signals. Such a test would directly stimulate, at increasing levels of intensity,

Horak-Anderson cells during a target switching task. Observed changes in movement velocity could then be used to calibrate the amount of change in GO signal amplitude caused by each level of stimulation.

14.8. Prediction and Test of Cells that Multiplex a Code for Local Velocity

The property of motor priming in motor cortex supports the VITE circuit prediction that there exists a stage subsequent to the DV stage at which an overt movement command is activated. The data of Horak and Anderson (1984a, 1984b) support the prediction that such activation may be partially controlled by a GO signal from the globus pallidus.

The VITE model may be further tested by recording from cells at the stage to which the motor cortex vector cells of Georgopoulos project. The cells at this subsequent stage should compute a measure of local movement velocity. This can be seen as follows.

These cells are predicted to compute (Figure 14.1) the product of rectified difference vector $[V]^+ = \max(V, 0)$ and GO signal G, namely

$$[V]^+ G. \tag{14.1}$$

The subsequent PPC stage computes a present position command P that performs a time integral of $[V]^+ G$, namely

$$P(t) = \int^t [V]^+ G \, dt. \tag{14.2}$$

Differentiating (14.2) shows that

$$\frac{dP}{dt} = [V]^+ G. \tag{14.3}$$

If subsequent network mechanisms cause the arm to follow closely the outflow movement command $P(t)$, then $\frac{dP}{dt}$ in (14.3) provides a good estimate of local movement velocity.

Equation (14.3) is of great interest from a conceptual point of view. It shows that the quantity $[V]^+ G$, which itself does not explicitly compute a velocity signal, *becomes* a velocity signal because of the manner in which it is transformed at subsequent network stages, in particular because it is integrated through time at the PPC stage.

The definition of this local velocity signal also depends upon the existence of a feedback loop between successive network stages (Figure 14.1). This feedback loop is needed to generate movements that are goal-oriented. This feedback loop is defined as follows. Quantity V in (14.3) computes a time-average of the difference between P and T, as in

$$\frac{d}{dt} V = \alpha(-V + T - P). \tag{14.4}$$

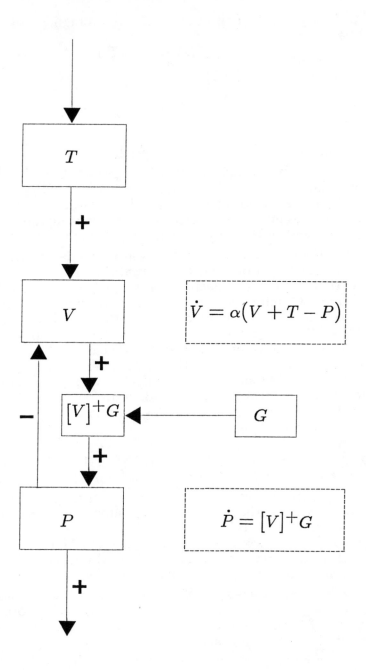

Figure 14.1. Main variables of the VITE circuit: T = target position command, V = difference vector, G = GO signal, P = present position command. The circuit does not include the opponent interactions that exist between the VG and P stages of agonist and antagonist muscle commands.

For simplicity, consider the case when the averaging rate α is large. Then, by (14.4),

$$V \cong T - P. \tag{14.5}$$

Hence, by (14.3) and (14.5),

$$\frac{d}{dt}P \cong [T - P]^{+}G, \tag{14.6}$$

which summarizes the action of the feedback loop.

The approximate equation (14.6) shows that the local velocity signal is an emergent property of the entire network. It multiplexes quantities T, P, and G that are computed at three different network stages. It converts these quantities into a local velocity signal by using the feedback loop that exists between the DV stage and the PPC stage.

Given the motor cortical vector cells as an anatomical marker, it seems to be an experiment of great conceptual importance to test the existence of cells that code local velocity at one of their target nuclei. If the stage coding local velocity is found, then a retrograde marker applied at this stage may identify a location in, or near, the global pallidus. Then a direct neurophysiological test of the existence of a GO signal may be made to supplement the data of Horak and Anderson (1984a, 1984b). If globus pallidus cells are not marked, then this experiment may discover the true location of the GO signal generator. An anterograde marker applied at the local velocity stage may be used to discover the location of the PPC stage. Then a direct neurophysiological test can determine its ability to time-integrate local velocity signals.

14.9. Learning an Associate Map between Target Position Maps of the Eye-Head and Hand-Arm Movement Systems

Our theory suggests that the VITE circuit plays two distinct roles. One role, reviewed above, concerns trajectory formation within a sensory-motor system. This role may be called *intramodal trajectory formation*. The second role concerns *intermodal learning of target position maps* (Figure 13.14). The remarkable fact is that the same TPC, DV, and PPC stages are predicted to accomplish both roles.

The learning process transforms stored representations of a target position coded with respect to the eye-head system into a target position command of the hand-arm system for moving the arm, via VITE dynamics, to that position in space.

As pointed out in Section 13.14, not all positions that the eye-head system or the hand-arm system assume are the correct positions to associate through learning. For example, suppose that the hand briefly remains at a given position and that the eye moves to foveate the hand. An infinite number of positions are assumed by the eye as it moves to foveate the hand. Only the final, intended, or expected position of the eye-head system is a correct position to associate with the position of the hand-arm system.

Learning of an intermodal motor map must thus be prevented except when the eye-head system and the hand-arm system are near their intended positions. Otherwise, all possible positions of the two systems could be associated with each other, which would lead to behaviorally chaotic consequences. Several important conclusions follow from this observation:

(1) All such adaptive sensory-motor systems compute a representation of target position. This representation is the TPC.

(2) All such adaptive sensory-motor systems also compute a representation of present position. This representation is the PPC.

(3) During movement, target position is matched against present position. Intermodal map learning is prevented except when target position approximately matches present position, that is, except when the DV is small (Figure 13.14). A *learning gate*, or modulator, signal is thus controlled by the DV. This gating signal enables learning to occur when a good match occurs and prevents learning from occurring when a bad match occurs.

In summary, we trace the existence of vector difference codes to two fundamental computational problems: intermodal learning of target position transformations, and intramodal performance of synchronous trajectories within dynamically determined motor synergies.

14.10. Visually Reactive Movements and the Vector Map Code within Superior Colliculus

The type of vector map code described by Sparks and his colleagues may be analysed as part of a circuit design that realizes a different type of learning process. This learning process enables the *visually reactive movement system* to generate accurate reactive eye movements in response to flashing or moving lights on the retina (Chapters 2, 3, and 11). The role of map vectors in the visually reactive movement system has been analysed in several previous chapters as part of a developmental sequence during which reactive eye movements to flashing or moving lights on the retina are supplemented by attentionally mediated movements towards motivationally interesting sensory cues. These movements are supplemented once again by predictive eye movements that form part of planned sequences of complex movement synergies capable of ignoring the sensory substrate on which they are built. Each of these categories of eye movement requires one or more types of learning in order to achieve high accuracy. The movement systems wherein attention and intention play an increasingly important role base their adaptive success upon the prior learning of the more primitive, visually reactive types of movement.

14.11. Three Interacting Coordinate Systems: Retinotopic, Motor Sector, and Map Vector

The visually reactive movement system uses learning based upon visual error signals to improve the accuracy of its movements. It is assumed that a target light is chosen and stored in short term memory (STM) before a movement starts (Figure 2.4). This stored representation activates a movement along an unconditioned movement pathway. The movement amplitude and direction, before learning, are controlled by a transformation of the retinal location of the stored representation into a motor representation in which the most eccentric positions generate the largest movement signals. This is accomplished by decomposing the motor representation into hemifields (Figure 2.1), and assuming that the gradient of connections to the corresponding pairs of agonist and antagonist muscles increases with eccentricity (Edwards, 1980; Gisbergen, Robinson, and Gielen, 1981).

The target light is stored in STM so that it can benefit from a visual error signal after the movement terminates. The stored representation samples this visual error signal along a conditioned movement pathway (Figure 2.4) whose output summates with that of the unconditioned pathway to generate the total movement signal. Thus learning within this system controls a feedforward adaptive gain that is changed by visual error signals.

How these visual error signals are coded clarifies one aspect of why a vector map exists in the deeper layers of superior colliculus. As illustrated by Figure 2.4, each light plays two roles: it acts as a movement signal for the next movement, and an error signal for the last movement. Thus the retinal location of each light must be remapped into a type of motor coordinates that can correct the full range of typical movement errors. The theory suggests that this is accomplished as follows.

14.12. Automatic Gain Control of Movement Commands by Visual Error Signals: Cerebellar Learning

The theory predicts how each movement command pathway can individually benefit from visual error signals to generate a more accurate movement in the future. Its analysis leads to a model of learning by the cerebellum which extends earlier models of cerebellar learning (Chapter 3). I emphasize two key properties of this model herein for purposes of comparative analysis: (i) the dual action of each light; and (ii) the learning of a motor synergy. The previous section summarized the network anatomy that subserves the dual action property.

14.13. Learning a Motor Synergy: Opponent Processing of Error Signals

The second key property of the AG stage concerns its ability to convert visual error signals, which individually activate only a *single* retinal position, into correct and synchronous movement commands to *all* muscles which move the eye. Learning of a motor synergy takes place in the Adaptive Gain Stage, or AG stage. The AG stage is identified with the cerebellar vermis, based upon data which show that this brain region controls modification of a saccade's *pulse gain* (Optican and Robinson, 1980). The conditioned movement pathway generates sampling signals which pass through the AG stage and add or subtract a conditionable movement signal to the total movement command. An error signal acts to change the size, or gain, of the conditionable movement signal. Thus the AG stage is a region where automatic gain control of the total movement command takes place.

In order to learn a motor synergy, the system preprocesses the error signals before they can be sampled by the conditioned movement pathway. Two processing constraints conceptualize these preprocessing stages: (a) the Opponent Processing constraint, and (b) the Equal Access constraint. The need for Opponent Processing—which is a new feature of our model—can be seen as follows.

Each eye is moved by three pairs of agonist and antagonist muscles. One pair moves the eye horizontally. The other two pairs move the eye obliquely, and together can generate vertical movements (Figure 1.2). The model assumes that a learned *increase* in the gain of an agonist muscle command must generate a *decrease* in the gain of the corresponding antagonist muscle command, and conversely. In other words, each visual error signal has antagonistic, or opponent, effects on the conditionable gains of the muscle commands which it changes.

In order to realize this Opponent Processing constraint, suppose that the retina is topographically transformed from retinotopic coordinates into a motor map containing six sectors (Figure 2.2). This motor sector map is an idealization that may be compared to the data of Sparks and his colleagues. Each pair of agonist-antagonist muscles—(α^+, α^-), (β^+, β^-), (γ^+, γ^-)—is represented by opposite sectors in the sector map. A visual error signal which falls within a prescribed sector increases the conditioned gain of the corresponding muscle and decreases the conditioned gain of the antagonistic muscle. As shown in Figure 3.5 and the surrounding discussion, this type of retinal-to-motor transformation can be used to correct undershoot, overshoot, and skewed movement errors.

14.14. The Equal Access Constraint

In response to a light to a fixed retinal position, the system cannot *a priori* predict which type of error will occur as a result of its inadequately tuned parameters. In order to correct any possible error, each position must be able to activate a conditioned movement pathway that is capable of sampling error signals delivered to *any* of the motor sectors. This is the Equal Access constraint, which was first articulated in a formal model of cerebellar learning by Grossberg (1964, 1969a).

In order to realize the Equal Access constraint, we have assumed that the motor sectors are mapped, via a complex logarithmic map (Schwartz, 1980), into motor strips (Figure 3.9). Then a single conditioned movement pathway can sample gain changes due to error signals which activate any motor strip. Figure 3.6 describes two variants of this design. Each variant realizes both the Opponent Processing constraint and the Equal Access constraint.

The by now classical cerebellar interpretation of this anatomy (Figures 3.8 and 3.10) is that the sampling signals are carried by parallel fibers through the dendrites of Purkinje cells, whereas the error signals are carried by climbing fibers to the Purkinje cell dendrites (Albus, 1971; Grossberg, 1964, 1969a, 1972a; Ito, 1974; Marr, 1969).

In summary, visual error signals are mapped from retinotopic coordinates into motor sector coordinates and then into motor strip coordinates. Then any visual error signal can be sampled by any stored movement command within pathways organized to learn and read-out the correct conditioned gain signals to all the target muscles. Such a transformation provides a simple explanation of the type of vector map described by Sparks: An increase in map eccentricity increases movement length and a change in map polar angle changes movement direction because such a representation enables visual error signals to be mapped into motor commands that are capable of correcting undershoot, overshoot, and skewed errors in visually reactive movements.

14.15. The Vector-to-Sector Transform: Dimensional Consistency of Planned Vectors and Reactive Retinotopic Commands

It remains to discuss why the deeper layers of superior colliculus code movement *vectors*, rather than merely motorically transformed retinotopic commands. An analysis of this problem is spread over several chapters of this volume, namely Chapters 3, 4, 6, 10, 11. Here I outline some of the main design themes.

Perhaps the most salient issue concerns the apparent absurdity of using vector encoding when the problem is considered from a common-sense point of view. In order to compute a vector, the retinotopic location R of a light must be combined with the initial position E of the eye in the head to generate a target position T of the light in head coordinates. Let us symbolically represent this transformation by

$$T = R + E. \tag{14.7}$$

Then a vector V is computed by subtracting E from T:

$$V = T - E. \tag{14.8}$$

On the other hand, the eye moves in the head. Thus, all motor commands M must be recoded into head-coordinates again before activating the saccade generator that moves the eye:

$$M = V + E. \tag{14.9}$$

A comparison of equations (14.7)–(14.9) seems to suggest much ado about nothing, because (14.7) implies that

$$R = T - E, \tag{14.10}$$

so that M could have been derived directly from T without computing V at all!

The functional significance of these transformations is clarified by noting that vector coordinates V are consistent with retinotopic coordinates R, but head coordinates, T and M, are not. Visual error signals within the visually reactive movement system are retinotopically coded before being remapped into a retinally consistent motor sector map. In order for head-centered, attentive, planned movement commands T to benefit from the movement accuracy that is learned using visual error signals, they must be transformed into a retinally consistent coordinate system. Comparison of (14.8) and (14.9) illustrates that movement vectors V are consistent with retinal and motor sector coordinates.

Such vectors V are suggested in Sections 4.6–4.8 to be difference vectors, rather than the map vectors studied by Sparks and his colleagues. Thus both difference vectors and map vectors are suggested to exist as part of the eye movement control system. As with the difference vectors described by Georgopoulos and his colleagues for the control of arm movements, the difference vectors used in eye movement control are suggested to be computed in cerebral cortex (Sections 11.10 and 11.11).

In summary, the head commands T are transformed into vectors V so that the vectors V can be transformed into a motor sector code. In this way, attentive, planned movements can achieve the learned accuracy of visually reactive movements. This vector-to-sector transformation converts the motor sector map into a vector map.

14.16. Movement Gating, Intermodal Mapping, and Competition between Planned and Reactive Movements

The vector-to-sector transform is a learned transformation. Our model of how this learning process occurs (Sections 11.2 and 11.3) clarifies how vectors V can learn to control the movement pathways activated by a retinal position R during visually reactive movements when the vector V is generated by R, and thus $V = R$. The model also predicts how, after learning is over, a visually reactive movement to position R can be suppressed via a spatially organized competitive interaction when an intended movement command V is activated such that $V \neq R$. Despite this suppression, the model explains how the movement controlled by V achieves the accuracy derived from the cerebellar gains learned by visually reactive error signals. The same analysis also suggests how auditory signals (Section 11.4) and planned movement sequences (Chapter 9 and Sections 11.11 and 11.12) can activate accurate saccadic eye movements, and how inhibitory gating of superior colliculus by substantia nigra enables planned attentive movement commands to successfully compete with more rapidly processed reactive movement commands (see pages 131 and 286).

In summary, this comparative analysis clarifies the functional role played by two types of vector codes—vector map codes and vector difference codes—in the control of saccadic eye movements by the superior colliculus and the control of planned arm movements by the motor cortex, respectively. Vector difference codes form part of the Vector Integration to Endpoint (VITE) Model that converts a target position command into a series of continuously integrated present position commands which are capable of generating a synchronous arm movement trajectory. The difference vectors are converted into overt movement commands by a gain control signal, called the GO signal, whose generator may be in globus pallidus. The VITE circuit is also predicted to play a role in modulating the learning of transformations from parietal target position representations of the eye-head system to target position commands of the hand-arm system.

The vector map codes are suggested to arise due to the interaction of several subsystems of the saccadic eye movement system. A visually reactive movement system uses visual error signals to correct motor synergies that are activated by visual signals. To accomplish this visual-to-motor learning process, the visual error signals are recoded into a motor sector map. An analysis of how movement errors are corrected by this system suggests a refined model of cerebellar learning, notably learning in the cerebellar vermis.

In order for the planned and attentive saccadic eye movement subsystems to benefit from visually reactive learning, they code their movement commands into vectors which are dimensionally compatible with the motor sector code, and then transform the vectors into the motor sector code. This vector-to-sector transformation converts the motor sector code into the type of vector map found in the deeper layers of superior colliculus. The properties of this transformation clarify how auditory signals and planned, attentive movement sequences may benefit from learning within the visually reactive movement system, and how gating of superior colliculus by substantia nigra enables the competition between these several movement systems to be successfully completed.

14.17. Data and Models of Posterior Parietal Target Positions Coded in Head-Centered Coordinates

The remainder of this chapter compares our theory with some of the relevant data and models that have appeared subsequent to the completion of the first edition of this book in 1985. When work on the book first began, few individuals were actively exploring self-organizing mechanisms of neural sensory-motor control. Now this literature is expanding rapidly. Thus the discussion herein does not aim for completeness. Rather its goal is to form some conceptual linkages that may be used by the reader to better understand the connections between our own results and those described by other investigators.

One area of great current interest concerns the existence and structure of a target position map coded in head-centered coordinates within the posterior parietal cortex. The need for such a map was impressed upon us by our discovery of system-level constraints concerning the manner in which visual targets coded in retinotopic coordinates could generate eye-movement commands coded in head coordinates. It hereby became clear that combinations of visual signals and eye position signals would need to be combined in a distributed fashion in order to generate a head-centered target position map, or TPM. Chapter 10 described three related models in which invariant, but distributed, TPMs could be synthesized from combinations of non-invariant visual and eye position data. In the self-organizing model of this process (Sections 10.3–10.8), the initial position of the light on the retina and the initial position of the eye in the head are stored in short term memory before an eye movement begins. Early in the learning process, the eye movement is triggered by a visually reactive eye movement system. This system is sensitive to rapid changes in lights registered on the retina. After a movement is completed, a teaching vector $(I_1, I_2, \ldots, I_m)$ is derived from an outflow signal that characterizes the final position of the eye. However, the task of this TPM-learning system is to learn a correct *target* position, not just any final eye position of a movement.

Such accuracy is derived from the fact that the visually reactive movement system is sensitive to visual error signals that compute whether or not the eye movement enabled the eye to foveate the target light (Chapter 3). These error signals are used to trigger a learning process that enables visually reactive movements to become accurate. When these movements become accurate, the final eye position generates an internal representation of target position that is used as a teaching vector to learn an invariant TPM.

Our theory assumes that learning of an invariant TPM takes place while the system is making visually reactive movements. Thus an invariant TPM can be learned because the visually reactive movement system can correct its movement errors.

As reviewed in Section 14.15, target position commands within this TPM are transformed into vectors so that they can be associated, in a dimensionally consistent way, with retinotopically coded movement pathways within the visually reactive system.

14.18. Parallel Maps of Eye Position: An Application of Competitive Learning to Gaussian and Linear Teaching Vectors

In order to learn such an invariant TPM, two distinct representations of eye position information need to be computed in parallel and stored at different times during the eye movement cycle. The first eye position representation, which is denoted by EPM_I for *initial eye position map*, stores the position of the eye before the movement begins. This map is called EPM_1 in Chapter 10. A retinotopic map, which is denoted by RM, stores the retinotopic position of the target light before the movement starts. The second eye position representation, which is denoted by EPM_T for *target eye position map*, reads-out the eye position after the movement terminates. This map is called EPM_2 in Chapter 10. Both the RM and the EPM_I send sampling signals to the EPM_T. The EPM_T is the recipient of the teaching vector $(I_1, I_2, \ldots, I_m)$ after a movement terminates. Thus the model describes how an EPM_T can be adaptively transformed into an invariant TPM, by building upon the learning of the (non-invariant) visually reactive movement system.

The theory assumes that both EPMs are derived from outflow signals that define the present position of the eye-in-the-head. These outflow signals are computed in motor coordinates that calibrate how much each of the six muscles that hold each eye in the head is contracted. Such a six-dimensional motor vector is transformed into an EPM via the mechanism of competitive learning (Sections 6.4–6.5). The most extreme form of competitive learning compresses a multidimensional vector into the choice of a single node, or cell population, in the EPM. Different nodes represent different motor vectors in such a map. A less extreme form of competitive learning converts a motor vector into a unimodal Gaussian activity profile within the TPM. Such a unimodal teaching vector for the EPM$_T$ is used in one of the simulated models. See equation (10.49).

At the other extreme, the competitive learning mechanism does not distort the read-out of the motor vector. In effect, the motor vector is itself the teaching vector for the EPM$_T$. In this case, the teaching vector components I_k are (approximately) a linear function of eye position. This is a consequence of adaptive linearization (Chapter 5), which enables the muscles to respond linearly to motor commands, so that corollary discharges, in the form of EPM$_T$ signals, can be used as an accurate teaching vector. This linear teacher defines the second model that was simulated. See equation (10.30). Also see equation (10.29), which assumes that the teacher is derived from an agonist-antagonist organization of eye position commands.

While the first edition of the book was being completed, Anderson, Essick, and Seigel (1984) presented some of their neurophysiological data about cells in posterior parietal cortex, and while the book was in press, Anderson, Essick, and Siegel (1985) published an article whose details supported the model's main predictions: that a distributed representation of target position in head-centered coordinates is implicitly generated by interacting combinations of visual and eye position signals, and that the receptive fields of the cells exhibit combinations of Gaussian and linear (or "planar") properties.

14.19. Back Propagation Model of Target Position: Comparison with Competitive Learning

Zipser and Anderson (1988) recently described a back propagation model of target position formation which built upon the data of Anderson, Essick, and Seigel (1985). This model assumes that RM, EPM$_I$, and EPM$_T$ maps exist with Gaussian and linear receptive fields. It also assumes the existence of an extra intermediate level of "hidden units," or interneurons, between these maps in order to provide enough degrees of freedom for the steepest-descent curve-fitting mechanism of the algorithm to converge.

I do not believe that back propagation, at least in its present form, is a viable model of any brain process. This conclusion does not imply that the algorithm may not be very useful in technological applications. The results of Zipser and Anderson (1988) illustrate my concerns about its use as a biological model.

First, there is a metatheoretical concern. With what probability will a model that was not derived to explain a particular set of physical or biological phenomena succeed in explaining it? For example, who would expect a theory of electrons to work if it was not derived from an analysis of data about electrons? At best, such a theory might capture the model-independent properties of electrons or, said in another way, the properties that have little to do with electrons.

Then there are a series of fundamental technical issues which too many proponents of back propagation, as a biological model, have heretofore either ignored or misrepresented. Sometimes this seems to have been the case because the practitioners do not understand how the model actually works. I have talked with scientists who have made use of convenient software tools to apply the model even though they do not know how it is defined.

This remarkable state of affairs has been justified by the claim that it does not matter how the model works. It is claimed that the model will generate the same "optimal" solution that a more biological model would also generate. Significantly, a similar type of claim was made about Artificial Intelligence models of brain processes when people worried that von Neumann computer architectures are different from biological brains. We now all realize that that claim was spurious.

The present claim as yet has no scientific justification. In fact, many properties of the algorithm strongly suggest that the claim is false and that back propagation will generate both quantitatively different results and qualitatively different heuristics than biologically motivated learning models.

For example, back propagation is, at bottom, a device for adaptive data compression. The number of hidden units is a key parameter in determining how compressed the data will become. This is, however, false in biological models such as competitive learning. There, as illustrated in Chapters 2, 6, and 10, an arbitrarily large number of hidden units may coexist with an arbitrary degree of data compression. The degree of compression is determined by how sharply the lateral inhibition, or competition, is tuned, not by how many hidden units exist.

This difference between the models leads to a second key difference. In back propagation, a single, teacher-determined, global error signal is broadcast throughout the network as a basis for changing its adaptive weights, or LTM traces. In competitive learning, there is no teacher, and all LTM weight changes are localized to the set of synapses that are contiguous to nodes that win the competition.

Perhaps the most unbiological feature of back-propagation is its use of a non-local transport of adaptive weights, or LTM traces, from its bottom-up filter to its top-down error signal (Figure 14.2). This computation lies at the heart of the algorithm. By this scheme, the numerical values of

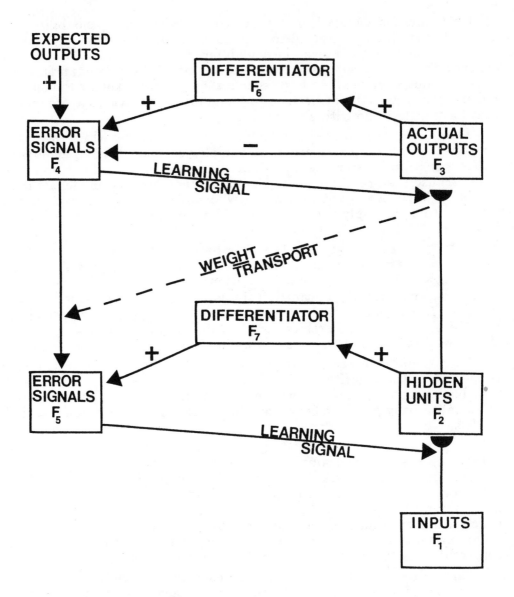

Figure 14.2. Circuit diagram of the back propagation model: In addition
to processing levels F_1, F_2, F_3, there are also levels F_4, F_5, F_6, and F_7
to carry out the computations which control the learning process. The
transport of learned weights from the $F_2 \to F_3$ pathways to the $F_4 \to F_5$
pathways shows that this algorithm cannot represent a learning process
in the brain.

LTM traces that are computed within the $F_2 \to F_3$ pathway must be transported, with great precision, to distinct pathways $F_4 \to F_5$ elsewhere in the network. Such a non-local event has no support in neural data.

It is sometimes claimed that this weight transport operation somehow captures the familiar fact that reciprocal top-down pathways exist in all thalamo-cortical and cortico-cortical interactions. This claim is at best misleading. The top-down signals $F_4 \to F_5$ in Figure 14.2 do not directly influence the fast information processing at level F_2. Rather, they only have a slow and indirect effect on learning by the LTM traces in the $F_1 \to F_2$ pathways. Top-down, locally defined interactions which do influence fast information processing, as in Adaptive Resonance Theory, give rise to qualitatively different computational properties (Carpenter and Grossberg, 1987b, 1988b; Grossberg, 1987d). It is also well-known that the back-propagation algorithm may become seriously unstable when arbitrarily many inputs perturb it in real-time, when input statistics are nonstationary, or when learning rates are sped up to biologically plausible levels. Such problems do not occur, for example, in Adaptive Resonance Theory.

To sidestep these obstacles, some scientists point to the good fit of back propagation simulations to biological data. Unfortunately, no criteria of good fit are offered. One is invited to inspect a series of experimental receptive field properties and a series of simulated receptive fields which are acknowledged to contain significant discrepancies. In all examples that I have studied to date, even the qualitative fits are poor and typically worse than the fits achieved by alternative models in the literature.

In comparing the model of Zipser and Anderson (1988) with the models in Chapter 10, note in particular that the Zipser-Anderson model needs a level of hidden units, whereas the model of Chapter 10 does not; the Zipser-Anderson model uses non-local weight transport, whereas the model of Chapter 10 uses only local operations; the Zipser-Anderson model assumes Gaussian and linear receptive fields, whereas the model of Chapter 10 predicted such receptive fields. Further developments of such models should continue comparative analyses along these lines.

Perhaps the most unfortunate side effect of back propagation is that it seems to act as a mental soporific. At first, it seems to be so easy to use. As with all general curve-fitting techniques, one can always eventually manage to reduce the error by assuming enough degrees of freedom. Which degrees of freedom might be relevant to biological processing do not, however, seem to be suggested by the algorithm. As one who has always worked hard to find the kernel of truth in any work and then to run with it, I am still looking for signs that this technique can be used to generate new and nontrivial insights into neural representation.

14.20. Comparison of Mammalian and Anuran Head and Vector Representations

Cross-species comparisons and contrasts are of great importance for discovering computational invariants of the evolutionary process. A notable homology exists between the mammalian superior colliculus and the anuran tectum. Grobstein and his colleagues have made significant experimental advances and probing theoretical commentaries in their search for evolutionary invariants by using the frog tectum and related structures as an experimental model.

In their analysis of frog prey capture behavior, this group early noted the need for a target position representation coded in body-centered co-ordinates. In particular, Grobstein, Comer, and Kostyk (1981, p. 344) wrote that:

> "while a given retinal and tectal region corresponds to a single direction in an eye-centered co-ordinate frame, they in fact correspond to a set of directions in a body-centered or movement co-ordinate frame. Conversely, a given point in a movement co-ordinate frame in fact corresponds to a set of points in an eye-centered co-ordinate frame such as the retina or the tectum. We are intrigued by the possibility that between the tectum and the pattern generating circuitry there may be an intermediate level of circuitry into which space is represented in a body-centered or movement co-ordinate frame. Because of the many to one and one to many character of the transformation in going from an eye-centered to a body-center or movement co-ordinate frame, disturbances of circuitry involved in this transformation might be expected to result not in disconnection of particular tectal regions from pattern generating circuitry but rather in an alteration in the particular output associated with activation of given tectal regions."

More recent work has led Grobstein (1987) to posit the concept of an *activity gated divergence* as a path structure to link the retinotectal map with pattern generating circuitry. This concept embraces the several processing steps whereby a retinally coded visual input is transformed into a head-centered target position representation before being transformed once again into a vector map representation in the deep layers of the superior colliculus (see Sections 14.15–14.18). Using this interpretive bridge, one can make a link from the present book to Grobstein's data and his sophisticated commentary about other recent experimental and theoretical contributions.

14.21. The Transformation from Head-Centered Eye Movement Maps to Body-Centered Arm Movement Maps: Neck Corollary Discharges as a Map Teaching Signal

Chapter 10 described models of how retinally coded visual cues could be transformed into a target position map (TPM) in head-centered coordinates. Chapter 11 explained how this TPM could be used to generate saccadic eye movements towards a visual target, or towards a remembered target. Chapter 13 suggested how the same TPM could be used to generate visually-guided arm movements (Figure 13.14).

In order to carry out the transformation from an eye-head TPM to a hand-arm TPM, head-centered coordinates need to be transformed into body-centered coordinates by taking into account the position of the head in the body. Such a transformation can be learned by using convergent head-coordinate signals from the eye-head TPM and corollary discharges from the neck musculature to learn a representation of hand-arm target position with respect to the body. The model in Chapter 10 can be used to learn this transformation, just as it was used to learn the transformation from retinal to head-centered coordinates. Corollary discharges of arm position would replace the corollary discharges of eye position that were used as a teaching vector in Chapter 10.

In all, these considerations suggest that the same TPM that controls saccadic eye movements can be used to control arm movements in response to both momentary visual signals and remembered visual signals.

Nemire and Bridgeman (1987) have generated data which support this concept. Their studies confirm an earlier investigation by Gielen, van den Heuvel, and van Gisbergen (1984). In their experiments, forty large saccadic eye movements in darkness resulted in significant ocular undershoot of a remembered eccentric target position. Let us assume that this remembered target position was stored in short-term memory within the head-centered TPM. They also found a comparable amount of undershoot with manual pointing of the arm to the same remembered targets. Saccadic and arm movement measures were also highly correlated within sessions as well as between sessions. Because arm pointing could be changed by manipulating only saccades, the authors concluded that both systems share a single map of space.

14.22. Transformation from Auditory Maps to Visually-Activated Eye Movement Maps

The previous section discussed one type of intermodality transformation; namely, between the eye-head TPM and the hand-arm TPM. Both of these TPMs develop in response to visual cues. Sections 1.15 and 11.4–11.6 analysed how auditory cues can trigger saccadic eye movements. There it was noted that an incorrect eye movement in response to an auditory source does not generate an auditory error signal. In order to achieve accurate eye movements in response to auditory cues, it was predicted (pp. 22–23) that "Intermodality sharing of retinally activated saccadic command pathways can be achieved if there exists a processing stage at which signals generated by auditory cues feed into visually calibrated saccadic command pathways. Then auditory cues can use the visually learned saccadic parameters by activating these visually calibrated commands ... a learned mapping of auditory signals onto a visually derived head coordinate map would achieve the most parsimonious solution of this problem." This analysis thus led to the prediction that visual signals guide the learned adjustment of the map for auditory localization. See Figure 11.12.

Data from the laboratories of Knudsen and Konishi concerning the existence of a head-centered auditory map in barn owls were cited (p. 22), but evidence was lacking concerning the main prediction that vision guides the adjustment of auditory localization.

While the first edition of this book was in press, experiments on barn owls that more directly supported this prediction were published (Knudsen, 1985; Knudsen and Knudsen, 1985). In these experiments, it was shown that barn owls raised with one ear plugged made systematic errors in auditory localization after the earplug was removed. These localization errors then corrected themselves within a few weeks in young owls, but not in adult owls, thus demonstrating a critical period of developmental plasticity. However, even young animals did not correct their auditory localization errors when deprived of vision. Moreover, when prisms were placed in front of their eyes, they adjusted their auditory localization to match the visual error induced by the prisms. Thus the visual system provides the spatial organization to which auditory localization is tuned.

14.23. A Related Model of Auditory-to-Visual Transformation: Neuronal Group Selection

Pearson, Sullivan, Gelfand, and Peterson (1987) responded to these Knudsen data by describing a model wherein auditory signals that are initially broadly distributed become more focused due to associative learning from the auditory map to the visual map. The model which they used is a variant of the competitive learning model that was used in this book for the same purpose.

However, instead of explicitly representing the competitive interaction in the network geometry, and the gating effects of the competition on associative learning, these authors used a lumped version of the competitive learning model. In this lumped model, the effects of the competition are directly built into thresholds for weakening or strengthening the auditory-to-visual LTM traces. This lumped competitive learning model is often called *neuronal group selection* in the writings of Edelman (1987).

14.24. Predictive Saccades and Saccade Sequences: The LTM Invariance Principle

Section 1.16, Chapter 9, and Sections 11.8–11.13 modelled a separate subsystem for storing predictive saccadic commands and sequences of commands in TPMs, for automatically reading-out these command sequences, and for adaptively calibrating the accuracy of predictive movements by using the visually reactive movement system as a source of accurate movement parameters.

Bronstein and Kennard (1987) have since reported additional data supporting the concept that the predictive saccadic movement and visually reactive movement systems are different.

Zingale and Kowler (1987) have reported parametric properties of predictive sequences of saccades. They noted that the latency of the first saccade in a sequence and the duration of intervals between subsequent saccades increased with sequence length, and varied with ordinal position in the sequence. Our model (Section 9.4) for storing predictive saccadic commands in short term memory has all of these properties. It was derived to explain data about storing temporal order information in short term, or working, memory in a variety of perceptual, cognitive, and motor paradigms. The use of a similar circuit for all of these storage tasks was derived from the fact that all of these tasks face a common computational challenge: to store temporal order information in a way that permits its stable encoding into sequence codes, or chunks, in long-term memory. The design principle that constrains all such circuits is called the *LTM Invariance Principle* (Grossberg, 1978a, 1978c).

Zingale and Kowler (1987) noted the similarity of their data to data about typing, speech, and related motor tasks. The LTM Invariance Principle was used to explain such data in Grossberg (1986b).

14.25. Comparison of Saccade Generator Models

Sections 14.10–14.16 reviewed our theory of how a vector map code is generated in the deeper layers of the superior colliculus. The present section discusses recent modelling results relevant to our model of how vector commands from the superior colliculus input to the saccade generator (SG) to cause a saccadic eye movement. Section 2.5 and Chapter 7 develop this model.

Scudder (1988) has published a new model of the saccade generator. This model is an attempt to avoid the hypothesis of the Robinson (1975) model that a representation of target position is the input to the burst generator of the SG. Subsequent data, such as those of Mays and Sparks (1980) and Bruce and Goldberg (1985), have suggested that the superior colliculus and frontal eye fields generate inputs to the SG in the form of discrete vectors that do not change during the saccade. Scudder (1980, p. 1458) also makes this assumption; namely, that "the position of the eye relative to the target is evaluated once, the colliculus issues a command specifying the size and direction of the appropriate saccade, and the burst generator then executes it." Scudder contrasts his model with that of Keller (1979, 1980), in which the superior colliculus computes a motor error that continuously diminishes as the saccade progresses, a property that has not been supported by subsequent experiments.

In order to make a dimensionally consistent model, Scudder subtracts a vector specifying how much the eye has moved from the discrete vector that generates the SG movement command. This is accomplished by assuming that a type of inhibitory feedback neuron (IFN) exists in the SG that has not yet been experimentally discovered. The model also does not produce microsaccadic oscillations or saccade staircases.

Our own SG model shares a key property with the Scudder (1988) model; namely, we also assume that the superior colliculus generates inputs in the form of discrete vectors to the superior colliculus. On the other hand, our model does explain microsaccadic oscillations and saccade staircases, as well as such finer data features as antagonistic bursts near the end of a saccade, isometric coactivation during perpendicular saccades, and saccadic undershoot during a fatigued state (Chapter 7). Our model achieves this greater explanatory range, moreover, without positing the existence of an IFN.

Instead, our model includes a postulate that partially supports the basic intuition behind the Robinson (1975) model, but also explains why a target position input to the SG has not been discovered. This is the postulate that an eye position representation, or EPM, adds to the vector representation, or RM, that is derived from the superior colliculus at the SG (Section 7.4). Both the RM and the EPM are switched on once and for all before the movement starts. The EPM is, however, normally cancelled by inhibitory feedback from the tonic cells (Figure 7.4). Thus its effects are not normally visible in the cell profiles of the SG. However, during the abnormal experimental conditions that generate saccade staircases, the EPM signal is not cancelled, and a saccade staircase is generated by the action of an Eye Position Update Network, or EPUN (Section 7.6). This prediction of our model may be used to differentiate it from the Scudder (1980) model by repeating the experiment of Schiller and Stryker (1972) to produce saccade staircases, while also recording from SG burst cells.

14.26. Applications of the Model's Circular Reaction to Eye-Hand Coordination by an Adaptive Robot

Kuperstein (1987, 1988a, 1988b) has used the models developed in this book to define a complete system for eye-hand coordination that he has implemented in a working robot. His system builds upon the concept of circular reaction (Section 1.3) and of the concepts developed in this book to computationally model such a sensory-motor cycle. Kuperstein also extends the models developed herein by defining representations of binocular eye position and binocular visual disparity and showing how to use these representations to generate accurate reaching movements to an object located in three-dimensional space.

Although Kuperstein has not yet incorporated all the models developed herein into his robot, his work provides an important existence proof that these models provide the foundation for "a novel approach to adaptive control of multijoint positioning which is at the boundary of both engineering and neuroscience. It is based on a new adaptive network control theory ... which allows a control system to learn a 'sense of space' by its own experience" (Kuperstein, 1987).

REFERENCES

Abend, W., Bizzi, E., and Morasso, P. (1982). Human arm trajectory formation. *Brain*, **105**, 331–348.

Adams, J.A. (1971). A closed-loop theory of motor learning. *Journal of Motor Behavior*, **3**, 111–149.

Adams, J.A. (1977). Feedback theory of how joint receptors regulate the timing and positioning of a limb. *Psychological Review*, **84**, 504–523.

Albus, J.S. (1971). A theory of cerebellar function. *Mathematical Biosciences*, **10**, 25–61.

Andersen, R.A., Essick, G.K., and Siegel, R.M. (1984). The role of eye position on the visual response of neurons in area 7A. *Society for Neuroscience Abstracts*, **10**, 274.11.

Anderson, R.A, Essick, G.K., and Siegel, R.M. (1985). Enclosing of spatial location by posterior parietal neurons. *Science*, **230**, 456–458.

Armstrong, D.M. and Drew, T. (1980). Responses in the posterior lobe of the rat cerebellum to electrical stimulation of cutaneous afferents to the snout. *Journal of Physiology (London)*, **309**, 357–374.

Atkeson, C.G. and Hollerbach, J.M. (1985). Kinematic features of unrestrained vertical arm movements. *Journal of Neuroscience*, **5**(9), 2318–2330.

Bahill, A.T. and Stark, L. (1979). The trajectories of saccadic eye movements. *Scientific American*, **240**, 108–117.

Baker, R. and Berthoz, A. (1977). **Control of gaze by brain stem neurons: Developmments in neuroscience**, Vol. 1. Amsterdam: North-Holland.

Beggs, W.D.A. and Howarth, C.I. (1972). The movement of the hand towards a target. *Quarterly Journal of Experimental Psychology*, **24**, 448–453.

Bell, C.C. (1981). An efference copy which is modified by reafferent input. *Science*, **214**, 450–453.

Bernstein, N.A. (1967). **The coordination and regulation of movements**. London: Pergamon Press.

Bizzi, E. (1968). Discharge of frontal eye field neurons during saccadic and following eye movements in unanesthetized monkeys. *Experimental Brain Research*, **6**, 69–80.

Bizzi, E. (1980). Central and peripheral mechanisms in motor control. In G.E. Stelmach and J. Requin (Eds.), **Tutorials in motor control**. Amsterdam: North-Holland.

Bizzi, E., Accornero, N., Chapple, W., and Hogan, N. (1982). Arm trajectory formation in monkeys. *Experimental Brain Research*, **46**, 139–143.

Bizzi, E., Accornero, N., Chapple, W., and Hogan, N. (1984). Posture control and trajectory formation during arm movement. *Journal of Neuroscience*, **4**(11), 2738–2744.

Bizzi, E. and Schiller, P.H. (1970). Single unit activity in the frontal eye fields of unanesthetized monkeys during head and eye movement. *Experimental Brain Research*, **10**, 151–158.

Blakemore, C., Carpenter, R.H., and Georgeson, M.A. (1970). Lateral inhibition between orientation detectors in the human visual system. *Nature*, **228**, 37–39.

Bloedel, J.R., Ebner, T.J., and Yu, Q.-X. (1983). Increased responsiveness of Purkinje cells associated with climbing fiber inputs to neighboring neurons. *Journal of Neurophysiology*, **50**, 220–239.

Bloedel, J.R. and Roberts, W.J. (1971). Action of climbing fibers in cerebellar cortex of the cat. *Journal of Neurophysiology*, **34**, 17–31.

Bower, J.M. and Woolston, D.C. (1983). Congruence of spatial organization of tectile projections to granule cell and Purkinje cell layers of cerebellar hemispheres of the albino rat: Vertical organization of cerebellar cortex. *Journal of Neurophysiology*, **49**, 745–766.

Brindley, G.S. (1964). The use made by the cerebellum of the information that it receives from sense organs. *International Brain Research Organizational Bulletin*, **3**, 80.

Brody, M. and Paul, R. (Eds.) (1984). **Robotics research: The first international symposium.** Cambridge, MA: MIT Press.

Bronstein, A.M. and Kennard, C. (1987). Predictive eye saccades are different from visually triggered saccades. *Vision Research*, **27**, 517–520.

Brooks, V.B. (1979). Motor programs revisited. In R.E. Talbott and D.R. Humphrey (Eds.), **Posture and movement: Perspective for integrating sensory and motor research on the mammalian nervous system.** New York: Raven Press, pp.13–49.

Brooks, V.B. (1986). **The neural basis of motor control.** New York: Oxford University Press.

Bruce, C.J. and Goldberg, M.E. (1984). Physiology of the frontal eye fields. *Trends in Neurosciences*, **7**, 436–441.

Bruce, C.J. and Goldberg, M.E. (1985). Primate frontal eye fields, I: Single neurons discharging before saccades. *Journal of Neurophysiology*, **53**, 603–635.

Buchanan, T.S., Almdale, D.P.J., Lewis, J.L., and Rymer, W.Z. (1986). Characteristics of synergic relations during isometric contractions of human elbow muscles. *Journal of Neurophysiology*, **56**, 1225–1241.

Buchtel, H.A. and Guitton, D. (1980). Saccadic eye movements in patients with discrete unilateral frontal-lobe removals. *Society for Neuroscience Abstracts*, **6**, 316.

Bullock, D. and Grossberg, S. (1986). Neural dynamics of planned arm movements: Synergies, invariants, and trajectory formation. Paper presented at the Symposium on Neural Models of Sensory-Motor Control at the annual meeting of the Society for Mathematical Psychology, Cambridge, MA, August 20.

Bullock, D. and Grossberg, S. (1988a). The VITE model: A neural command circuit for generating arm and articulator trajectories. In J.A.S. Kelso, A.J. Mandell, and M.F. Shlesinger (Eds.), **Dynamic patterns in complex systems**. Singapore: World Scientific Press, 305–326.

Bullock, D. and Grossberg, S. (1988b). Neuromuscular realization of planned arm movement trajectories. *Neural Networks*, **Supplement 1**, 329.

Carlton, L.G. (1979). Control processes in the production of discrete aiming responses. *Journal of Human Movement Studies*, **5**, 115–124.

Carpenter, G.A. (1979). Bursting phenomena in excitable membranes. *SIAM Journal on Applied Mathematics*, **36**, 334–372.

Carpenter, G.A. (1981). Normal and abnormal signal patterns in nerve cells. In S. Grossberg (Ed.), **Mathematical psychology and psychophysiology**. SIAM–AMS Proceedings, **13**, 49–90.

Carpenter, G.A. and Grossberg, S. (1983). A neural theory of circadian rhythms: The gated pacemaker. *Biological Cybernetics*, **48**, 35–59.

Carpenter, G.A. and Grossberg, S. (1984). A neural theory of circadian rhythms: Aschoff's rule in diurnal and nocturnal mammals. *American Journal of Physiology*, **247**, R067–R1082.

Carpenter, G.A. and Grossberg, S. (1985a). A neural theory of circadian rhythms: Split rhythms, after-effects, and motivational interactions. *Journal of Theoretical Biology*, **113**, 163–223.

Carpenter, G.A. and Grossberg, S. (1985b). Category learning and adaptive pattern recognition: A neural network model. *Proceedings of the Third Army Conference on Applied Mathematics and Computing*, **ARO 86-1**, 37–56.

Carpenter, G.A. and Grossberg, S. (1987a). A massively parallel architecture for a self-organizing neural pattern recognition machine. *Computer Vision, Graphics, and Image Processing*, **37**, 54–115.

Carpenter, G.A. and Grossberg, S. (1987b). Associative learning, adaptive pattern recognition, and competitive decision making by neural networks. In H. Szu (Ed.), **Optical and hybrid computing**. SPIE, **634**, 218–247.

Carpenter, G.A. and Grossberg, S. (1988a). Neural dynamics of category learning and recognition: Attention, memory consolidation, and amnesia. In J. Davis, R. Newburgh, and E. Wegman (Eds.), **Brain structure, learning, and memory**. Boulder, CO: Westview Press, 233–290.

Carpenter, G.A. and Grossberg, S. (1988b). The ART of adaptive pattern recognition by a self-organizing neural network. *Computer*, **21**, 77–88.

Clark, F.J., Burgess, R.C., Chapin, J.W., and Lipscomb, W.T. (1985). Role of intramuscular receptors in the awareness of limb position. *Journal of Neurophysiology*, **54**, 1529–1540.

Cody, F.W.J. and Richardson, H.C. (1979). Mossy and climbing fibre mediated responses evoked in the cerebellar cortex of the cat by trigeminal

Grossberg and Kuperstein

afferent stimulation. *Journal of Physiology (London)*, **287**, 1–14.

Coffey, G.L., Godwin-Austen, R.B.., MacGillivray, B.B., and Sears, T.A. (1971). The form and distribution of the surface evoked responses in cerebellar cortex from intercostal nerves in the cat. *Journal of Physiology (London)*, **212**, 129–147.

Cohen, M.A. and Grossberg, S. (1983). Absolute stability of global pattern formation and parallel memory storage by competitive neural networks. *Transactions IEEE on Systems, Man, and Cybernetics*, **SMC-13**, 815–826.

Cohen, M.A. and Grossberg, S. (1984a). Some global properties of binocular resonances: Disparity matching, filling-in, and figure-ground synthesis. In P. Dodwell and T. Caelli (Eds.), **Figural synthesis**. Hillsdale, NJ: Erlbaum.

Cohen, M.A. and Grossberg, S. (1984b). Neural dynamics of brightness perception: Features, boundaries, diffusion, and resonance. *Perception and Psychophysics*, **36**, 428–456.

Cohen, M.A. and Grossberg, S. (1986). Neural dynamics of language coding: Developmental programs, perceptual grouping, and competition for short term memory. *Human Neurobiology*, **5**, 1–22.

Cohen, M.A., Grossberg, S., and Stork, D. (1988). Speech perception and production by a self-organizing neural network. In Y.C. Lee (Ed.), **Evolution, learning, cognition, and advanced architectures**. Hong Kong: World Scientific Publishers.

Cooke, J.D. (1980). The organization of simple, skilled movements. In G.E. Stelmach and J. Requin (Eds.), **Tutorials in motor behavior**. Amsterdam: Elsevier/North-Holland, 199–212.

Cubeddu, L.X., Hoffmann, I.S., and James, M.K. (1983). Frequency-dependent effects of neuronal uptake inhibitors on the autoreceptor-mediated modulation of dopamine and acetylcholine release from the rabbit striatum. *Journal of Pharmacology and Experimental Therapeutics*, **226**, 88– 94.

Dubocovich, M.L. and Weiner, N. (1982). Modulation of the stimulation-evoked release of 3H-dopamine through activation of dopamine autoreceptors of the D-2 subtype in the isolated rabbit retina. In M. Kohsaka *et al.* (Eds.), **Advances in the biosciences, Vol. 37: Advances in dopamine research**. New York: Pergamon Press.

Ebner, T.J. and Bloedel, J.R. (1981). Correlation between activity of Purkinje cells and its modification by natural peripheral stimuli. *Journal of Neurophysiology*, **45**, 948–961.

Ebner, T.J., Yu, Q.-X., and Bloedel, J.R. (1983). Increase in Purkinje cell gain associated with naturally activated climbing fiber input. *Journal of Neurophysiology*, **50**, 205–219.

Eccles, J.C. (1953). **The neurophysiological basis of mind**. Oxford: Oxford University Press.

Eccles, J.C. (1973). The cerebellum as a computer: Patterns in space and time. *Journal of Physiology (London)*, **229**, 1–32.

Eccles, J.C. (1977). An instruction-selection theory of learning in the cerebellar cortex *Brain Research*, **127**, 327–352.

Eccles, J.C., Faber, D.S., Murphy, J.T., Sabah, N.H., and Táboríková, H. (1971). Afferent volleys in limb nerves influencing impulse discharge in cerebellar cortex, II: In Purkinje cells. *Experimental Brain Research*, **13**, 36– 53.

Eccles, J.C., Ito, M., and Szentágothai, J. (1967). **The cerebellum as a neuronal machine.** New York: Springer-Verlag.

Eccles, J.C., Sabah, N.H., Schmidt, R.F., and Táboríková, H. (1972). Integration by Purkinje cells of mossy and climbing fiber inputs from cutaneous mechanoreceptors. *Experimental Brain Research*, **15**, 498–520.

Eckmiller, R. and Westheimer, G. (1983). Compensation of oculomotor deficits in monkeys with neonatal cerebellar ablations. *Experimental Brain Research*, **49**, 315–326.

Edelman, G.M. (1987). **Neural Darwinism.** New York: Basic Books.

Edwards, S.B. (1980). The deep cell layers of the superior colliculus: Their reticular characteristics and structural organization. In J.A. Hobson and M.A. Brazier (Eds.), **The reticular formation revisited: Specifying for a non-specific system.** New York: Raven Press.

Ellias, S.A. and Grossberg, S. (1975). Pattern formation, contrast control, and oscillations in the short term memory of shunting on-center off-surround networks. *Biological Cybernetics*, **20**, 69–98.

Enroth-Cugell, C. and Robson, J.G. (1966). The contrast sensitivity of retinal ganglion cells of the cat. *Journal of Physiology*, **187**, 517–552.

Epstein, W. (Ed.) (1977). **Stability and constancy in visual perception: Mechanisms and processes.** New York: Wiley and Sons.

Evarts, E.V. (1968). Relation of pyramidal tract activity to force exerted during voluntary movement. *Journal of Neurophysiology*, **31**, 14–27.

Evarts, E.V. and Fromm, C. (1978). The pyramidal tract neuron as summing point in a closed-loop control system in the monkey. In J.E. Desmedt (Ed.), **Cerebral motor control in man: Long loop mechanisms.** Basel, Switzerland: Karger, pp. 56–69.

Evarts, E.V. and Tanji, J. (1974). Gating of motor cortex reflexes by prior instruction. *Brain Research*, **71**, 479–494.

Feldman, A.G. (1974). Change in the length of the muscle as a consequence of a shift in equilibrium in the muscle-load system. *Biofizika*, **19**(3), 534–538.

Feldman, A.G. (1986). Once more on the equilibrium-point hypothesis (λ model) for motor control. *Journal of Motor Behavior*, **18**, 17–54.

Festinger, L., Burnham, C.A., Ono, H., and Bamber, D. (1967). Efference and the conscious experience of perception. *Journal of Experimental*

Psychology Monograph 74, (4, whole no. 637).

Fetters, L. and Todd, J. (1987). Quantitative assessment of infant reaching movements. *Journal of Motor Behavior*, in press.

Fitts, P.M. (1954). The information capacity of the human motor system in controlling the amplitude of movement. *Journal of Experimental Psychology*, **47**(6), 381–391.

Fitts, P.M. and Peterson, J.R. (1964). Information capacity of discrete motor responses. *Journal of Experimental Psychology*, **67**(2), 103–112.

Flash, T. and Hogan, N. (1985). The coordination of arm movements: An experimentally confirmed mathematical model. *Journal of Neuroscience*, **5**(7), 1688–1703.

Foley, J.P. (1940). An experimental investigation of the effect of prolonged inversion of the visual field in the rhesus monkey (Macaca mulatta). *Journal of Genetic Psychology*, **56**, 21–51.

Freund, H.-J. and Büdingen, H.J. (1978). The relationship between speed and amplitude of the fastest voluntary contractions of human arm muscles. *Experimental Brain Research*, **31**, 1–12.

Frost, B.J. and Nakayama, K. (1983). Single visual neurons code opposing motion independent of direction. *Science*, **220**, 744–745.

Fuchs, A.F. and Becker, W. (Eds.) (1981). **Progress in oculomotor research: Developments in neuroscience**, Vol. 12. New York: Elsevier/North-Holland.

Fuchs, A.F. and Kimm, J. (1975). Unit activity in vestibular nucleus of the alert monkey during horizontal angular acceleration and eye movement. *Journal of Neurophysiology*, **38**, 1140–1161.

Fujita, M. (1982a). Adaptive filter model of the cerebellum. *Biological Cybernetics*, **45**, 195–206.

Fujita, M. (1982b). Simulation of adaptive modification of the vestibulo-ocular reflex with an adaptive filter model of the cerebellum. *Biological Cybernetics*, **45**, 207–214.

Gellman, R., Gibson, A.R., and Houk, J.C. (1985). Inferior olivary neurons in the awake cat: Detection of contact and passive body displacement. *Journal of Neurophysiology*, **54**, 40–60.

Georgopoulos, A.P. (1986). On reaching. *Annual Review of Neuroscience*, **9**, 147–170.

Georgopoulos, A.P., Kalaska, J.F., Caminiti, R., and Massey, J.T. (1982). On the relations between the direction of two-dimensional arm movements and cell discharge in primate motor cortex. *Journal of Neuroscience*, **2**, 1527–1537.

Georgopoulos, A.P., Kalaska, J.F., Crutcher, M.D., Caminiti, R., and Massey, J.T. (1984). The representation of movement direction in the motor cortex: Single cell and population studies. In G.M. Edelman, W.E. Goll, and W.M. Cowan (Eds.), **Dynamic aspects of neocortical function**. Neurosciences Research Foundation, 501–524.

Georgopoulos, A.P., Kalaska, J.F., and Massey, J.T. (1981). Spatial trajectories and reaction times of aimed movements: Effects of practice, uncertainty, and change in target location. *Journal of Neurophysiology*, **46**, 725–743.

Georgopoulos, A.P., Kettner, R.E., and Schwartz, A.B. (1988). Primate motor cortex and free arm movements to visual targets in three-dimensional space, II: Coding of the direction of movement by a neuronal population. *Journal of Neuroscience*, **8**, 2928–2937.

Georgopoulos, A.P., Schwartz, A.B., and Kettner, R.E. (1986). Neuronal population coding of movement direction. *Science*, **233**, 1416–1419.

Ghez, C. and Martin, J.H. (1982). The control of rapid limb movement in the cat, III: Agonist–antagonist coupling. *Experimental Brain Research*, **45**, 115–125.

Ghez, C. and Vicario, D. (1978). The control of rapid limb movement in the cat, II: Scaling of isometric force adjustments. *Experimental Brain Research*, **33**, 191–202.

Gielen, C.C.A.M., van den Heuvel, P.J.M., and van Gisbergen, J.A.M. (1984). Coordination of fast eye and arm movements in a tracking task. *Experimental Brain Research*, **56**, 154–161.

Gilbert, P.F.C. and Thach, W.T. (1977). Purkinje cell activity during motor learning. *Brain Research*, **128**, 309–328.

Gisbergen, J.A.M. van, Robinson, D.A., and Gielen, S. (1981). A quantitative analysis of generation of saccadic eye movements by burst neurons. *Journal of Neurophysiology*, **45**, 417–442.

Goldberg, M.E. (1980). Cortical mechanisms in the visual instantiation of movement. *Experimental Brain Research*, **41**, A32–A33.

Goldberg, M.E. and Bushnell, M.C. (1981). Role of the frontal eye fields in visually guided saccades. In A.F. Fuchs and W. Becker (Eds.), **Progress in oculomotor research: Developments in neuroscience**, Vol. 12. New York: Elsevier/North-Holland.

Gordon, J. and Ghez, C. (1984). EMG patterns in antagonist muscles during isometric contraction in man: Relations to response dynamics. *Experimental Brain Research*, **55**, 167–171.

Gordon, J. and Ghez, C. (1987a). Control strategies determining the accuracy of targeted force impulses, I: Pulse height control. *Experimental Brain Research*, in press.

Gordon, J. and Ghez, C. (1987b). Trajectory control in targeted force impulses, III: Compensatory adjustments for initial errors. *Experimental Brain Research*, in press.

Gouras, P. (1981). Oculomotor system. In E.R. Kandel and J.H. Schwartz (Eds.), **Principles of neural science**. New York: Elsevier/North-Holland.

Granit, R. (1962). **Receptors and sensory perception**. New Haven: Yale University Press.

Grillner, S. (1975). Locomotion in vertebrates: Central mechanisms and reflex interaction. *Physiological Review*, **55**, 247–304.

Grobstein, P. (1987). Between the retinotopic projection and directed movement: Topography of a sensorimotor interface. *Brain, Behavior, and Evolution*, in press.

Grobstein, P., Comer, C., and Kostyk, S.K. (1981). Frog prey capture behavior: Between sensory maps and directed motor output. In J.-P. Ewert, R.R. Capranica, and D.J. Ingle (Eds.), **Advances in vertebrate neuuroethology**. New York: Plenum Press.

Grossberg, S. (1964). **The theory of embedding fields with applications to psychology and neurophysiology**. New York: Rockefeller Institute for Medical Research.

Grossberg, S. (1968a). Some physiological and biochemical consequences of psychological postulates. *Proceedings of the National Academy of Sciences*, **60**, 758–765.

Grossberg, S. (1968b). Some nonlinear networks capable of learning a spatial pattern of arbitrary complexity. *Proceedings of the National Academy of Sciences*, **59**, 368–372.

Grossberg, S. (1969a). On learning of spatiotemporal patterns by networks with ordered sensory and motor components, I: Excitatory components of the cerebellum. *Studies in Applied Mathematics*, **48**, 105–132.

Grossberg, S. (1969b). On the production and release of chemical transmitters and related topics in cellular control. *Journal of Theoretical Biology*, **22**, 325–364.

Grossberg, S. (1969c). On learning and energy-entropy dependence in recurrent and nonrecurrent signed networks. *Journal of Statistical Physics*, **1**, 319–350.

Grossberg, S. (1969d). Some networks that can learn, remember, and reproduce any number of complicated space-time patterns, I. *Journal of Mathematics and Mechanics*, **19**, 53–91.

Grossberg, S. (1970). Neural pattern discrimination. *Journal of Theoretical Biology*, **27**, 291–337.

Grossberg, S. (1972a). Neural expectation: Cerebellar and retinal analogs of cells fired by learnable or unlearned pattern classes. *Kybernetik*, **10**, 49–57.

Grossberg, S. (1972b). Pattern learning by functional-differential neural networks with arbitrary path weights. In K. Schmitt (Ed.), **Delay and functional-differential equations and their applications**. New York: Academic Press.

Grossberg, S. (1972c). A neural theory of punishment and avoidance, II: Quantitative theory. *Mathematical Biosciences*, **15**, 253–285.

Grossberg, S. (1973). Contour enhancement, short-term memory, and constancies in reverberating neural networks. *Studies in Applied Mathematics*, **52**, 217–257.

References

Grossberg, S. (1974). Classical and instrumental learning by neural networks. In R. Rosen and F. Snell (Eds.), **Progress in theoretical biology**, Vol. 3. New York: Academic Press.

Grossberg, S. (1975). A neural model of attention, reinforcement, and discrimination learning. *International Review of Neurobiology*, **18**, 263–327.

Grossberg, S. (1976a). Adaptive pattern classification and universal recoding, I: Parallel development and coding of neural feature detectors. *Biological Cybernetics*, **23**, 121–134.

Grossberg, S. (1976b). Adaptive pattern classification and universal recoding, II: Feedback, expectation, olfaction, and illusions. *Biological Cybernetics*, **23**, 187–202.

Grossberg, S. (1978a). A theory of human memory: Self-organization and performance of sensory-motor codes, maps, and plans. In R. Rosen and F. Snell (Eds.), **Progress in theoretical biology**, Vol. 5. New York: Academic Press.

Grossberg, S. (1978b). Communication, memory, and development. In R. Rosen and F. Snell (Eds.), **Progress in theoretical biology**, Vol. 5. New York: Academic Press.

Grossberg, S. (1978c). Behavioral contrast in short-term memory: Serial binary memory models or parallel continuous memory models? *Journal of Mathematical Psychology*, **17**, 199–219.

Grossberg, S. (1980). How does a brain build a cognitive code? *Psychological Review*, **87**, 1–51.

Grossberg, S. (Ed.) (1981). **Mathematical psychology and psychophysiology**. Providence, RI: American Mathematical Society.

Grossberg, S. (1982a). **Studies of mind and brain: Neural principles of learning, perception, development, cognition, and motor control**. Boston: Reidel Press.

Grossberg, S. (1982b). Processing of expected and unexpected events during conditioning and attention: A psychophysiological theory. *Psychological Review*, **89**, 529–572.

Grossberg, S. (1982c). A psychophysiological theory of reinforcement, drive, motivation, and attention. *Journal of Theoretical Neurobiology*, **1**, 286–369.

Grossberg, S. (1983). The quantized geometry of visual space: The coherent computation of depth, form, and lightness. *The Behavioral and Brain Sciences*, **6**, 625–692.

Grossberg, S. (1984). Some psychophysiological and pharmacological correlates of a developmental, cognitive, and motivational theory. In R. Karrer, J. Cohen, and P. Tueting (Eds.), **Brain and information: Event related potentials**. New York: New York Academy of Sciences.

Grossberg, S. (1985a). (Published as 1987b.)

Grossberg, S. (1985b). (Published as 1987c.)

Grossberg, S (1986a). The adaptive self-organization of serial order in behavior: Speech, language, and motor control. In E.C. Schwab and H.C. Nusbaum (Eds.), **Pattern recognition by humans and machines, Vol. 1: Speech perception**. New York: Academic Press.

Grossberg, S. (1986b). Adaptive compensation to changes in the oculomotor plant. In E. Keller and D. Zee (Eds.), **Adaptive processes in the visual and oculomotor systems**. Elmsford, NY: Pergamon Press.

Grossberg, S. (1987a). Cooperative self-organization of multiple neural systems during adaptive sensory-motor control. In D.M. Guthrie (Ed.), **Aims and methods in neuroethology**. Manchester: Manchester University Press.

Grossberg, S. (Ed.) (1987b). **The adaptive brain, I: Cognition, learning, reinforcement, and rhythm**. Amsterdam: Elsevier/North-Holland.

Grossberg, S. (Ed.), (1987c). **The adaptive brain, II: Vision, speech, language, and motor control**. Amsterdam: Elsevier/North-Holland.

Grossberg, S. (1987d). Competitive learning: From interactive activation to adaptive resonance. *Cognitive Science*, **11**, 23–63.

Grossberg, S. and Kuperstein, M. (1986). **Neural dynamics of adaptive sensory-motor control: Ballistic eye movements**. Amsterdam: Elsevier/North-Holland.

Grossberg, S. and Levine, D.S. (1975). Some developmental and attentional biases in the contrast enhancement and short term memory of recurrent neural networks. *Journal of Theoretical Biology*, **53**, 341–380.

Grossberg, S. and Mingolla, E. (1985a). Neural dynamics of form perceptioni: Boundary completion, illusory figures, and neon color spreading. *Psychological Review*, **92**, 173–211.

Grossberg, S. and Mingolla, E. (1985b). Neural dynamics of perceptual grouping: Textures, boundaries, and emergent segmentations. *Perception and Psychophysics*, **38**, 141–171.

Grossberg, S. Stone, G.O. (1986a). Neural dynamics of word recognition and recall: Attentional priming, learning, and resonance. *Psychological Review*, **93**, 46–74.

Grossberg, S. and Stone, G.O. (1986b). Neural dynamics of attention switching and temporal order information in short term memory. *Memory and Cognition*, **14**, 451–468.

Groves, P.M., Fenster, G.A., Tepper, J.M., Nakamura, S., and Young, S.J. (1981). Changes in dopaminergic terminal excitability induced by amphetamine and hatoperidol. *Brain Research*, **221**, 425–431.

Groves, P.M. and Tepper, J.M. (1983). Neuronal mechanisms of action of amphetamine. In I. Creese (Ed.), **Stimulants: Neurochemical, behavioral, and clinical perspectives**. New York: Raven Press.

Guitton, D. (1981). On the participation of the feline "prefrontal eye field" in the control of eye and head movements. In A.F. Fuchs and W. Becker (Eds.), **Progress in oculomotor research: Developments in neuroscience**, Vol. 12. New York: Elsevier/North-Holland.

Guitton, D., Crommelinck, M., and Roucoux, A. (1980). Stimulation of the superior colliculus in the alert cat: Eye movements and neck EMG activity evoked when the head is restrained. *Experimental Brain Research*, **39**, 63–73.

Guthrie, B.L., Porter, J.D., and Sparks, D.L. (1983). Corollary discharge provides accurate eye position information to the oculomotor system. *Science*, **221**, 1193–1195.

Hallett, P.E. and Lightstone, A.D. (1976). Saccadic eye movements to flashed targets. *Vision Research*, **16**, 107–114.

Hawkins, R.D., Abrams, T.W., Carew, T.J., and Kandel, E.R. (1983). A cellular mechanism of classical conditioning in *Aplysia*: Activity-dependent amplification of presynaptic facilitation. *Science*, **219**, 400–405.

Hebb, D.O. (1949). **The organization of behavior**. New York: Wiley and Sons.

Helmholtz, H. von (1866). **Handbuch der Physiologischen Optik**. Leipzig: Voss.

Hepp, K., Henn, V., Jaeger, J., and Waespe, W. (1981). Oculomotor pathways through the cerebellum. In A.F. Fuchs and W. Becker (Eds.), **Progress in oculomotor research: Developments in neuroscience**, Vol. 12. New York: Elsevier/North-Holland.

Hikosaka, O. and Wurtz, R.H. (1983). Visual and oculomotor functions of monkey substantia nigra pars reticulata, IV: Relation of substantia nigra to superior colliculus. *Journal of Neurophysiology*, **49**, 1285–1301.

Hodgkin, A.L. (1964). **The conduction of the nervous impulse**. Liverpool: Liverpool University.

Hofsten, C. von (1979). Development of visually directed reaching: The approach phase. *Journal of Human Movement Studies*, **5**, 160–178.

Hofsten, C. von (1982). Eye-hand coordination in the newborn. *Developmental Psychology*, **18**(3), 450–461.

Hogan, N. (1984). An organizing principle for a class of voluntary movements. *Journal of Neuroscience*, **4**(11), 2745–2754.

Hollerbach, J.M. (1982). Computers, brain, and the control of movement. *Trends in Neuroscience*, **5**, 189–192.

Hollerbach, J.M. (1984). Dynamic scaling of manipulator trajectories. *Journal of Dynamic Systems, Measurement, and Control*, **106**, 102–106.

Hollerbach, J.M., Moore, S.P., and Atkeson, C.G. (1986). Workspace effect in arm movement kinematics derived by joint interpolation. In G. Gantchev, B. Dimitrov, and P. Gatev (Eds.), **Motor control**. Plenum Press.

Holmes, G. (1938). The cerebral integration of ocular movements. *British Medical Journal*, **2**, 107–112.

Holst, E. von and Mittelstaedt, H. (1950). The reafference principle: Interaction between the central nervous system and the periphery. *Naturwissenschaften*, **37**, 464–476.

Horak, F.B. and Anderson, M.E. (1984a). Influence of globus pallidus on arm movements in monkeys, I: Effects of kainic acid-induced lesions. *Journal of Neurophysiology*, **52**, 290–304.

Horak, F.B. and Anderson, M.E. (1984b). Influence of globus pallidus on arm movements in monkeys, II: Effects of stimulation. *Journal of Neurophysiology*, **52**, 305–322.

Houck, J. and Henneman, E. (1967). Responses of Golgi tendon organs to active contractions of the soleus muscle of the cat. *Journal of Neurophysiology*, **30**, 466–481.

Houk, J.C. and Rymer, W.Z. (1981). Neural control of muscle length and tension. In **Handbook of physiology: The nervous system II**. Bethesda, MD: American Physiological Society, pp.257–322.

Howarth, C.I. and Beggs, W.D.A. (1971). The relationship between speed and accuracy of movement aimed at a target. *Acta Psychologica*, **35**, 207–218.

Howarth, C.I. and Beggs, W.D.A. (1981). Discrete movements. In D. Holding (Ed.), **Human skills**. New York: Wiley and Sons, pp.91–117.

Huerta, M.F. and Harting, J.K. (1984). Connectional organization of the superior colliculus. *Trends in Neuroscience*, **7**, 286–289.

Humphrey, D.R. and Reed, D.J. (1983). Separate cortical systems for control of joint movement and joint stiffness: Reciprocal activation and coactivation of antagonist muscles. In J.E. Desmedt (Ed.), **Motor control mechanisms in health and disease**. New York: Raven Press, pp.347–372.

Hunt, R.K. and Jacobson, M. (1972). Specification of positional information in retinal ganglion cells of *Xenopus*: Stability of the specified state. *Proceedings of the National Academy of Sciences USA*, **69**, 2860–2864.

Hunt, R.K. and Jacobson, M. (1973a). Specification of positional information in retinal ganglion cells of *Xenopus*: Assays for analysis of the unspecified state. *Proceedings of the National Academy of Sciences USA*, **70**, 507–511.

Hunt, R.K. and Jacobson, M. (1973b). Neuronal locus specificity: Altered pattern of spatial deployment in fused fragments of embryonic *Xenopus* eyes. *Science*, **180**, 509–511.

Hyvärinen, J. (1982). Posterior parietal lobe of the primate brain. *Physiological Reviews*, **62**, 1060–1129.

Ito, M. (1974). The control mechanism of cerebellar motor systems. In F.O. Schmidt and F.G. Worden (Eds.), **The neurosciences third study program**. Cambridge, MA: MIT Press.

Ito, M. (1982). Cerebellar control of the vestibulo-ocular reflex—around the flocculus hypothesis. *Annual Review of Neuroscience*, **5**, 275–296.

Ito, M. (1984). **The cerebellum and neural control**. New York: Raven Press.

Ito, M., Sakurai, M., and Tongroach, P. (1982). Climbing fibre induced depression of both mossy fibre responsiveness and glutamate sensitivity of cerebellar Purkinje cells. *Journal of Physiology*, **324**, 113–134.

Ito, M., Shiida, T., Yagi, N., and Yamamoto, M. (1974). Visual influence on rabbit horizontal vestibulo-ocular reflex presumably effected via the cerebellar flocculus. *Brain Research*, **65**, 170–174.

Jagacinski, R.J. and Monk, D.L. (1985). Fitts' Law in two dimensions with hand and hand movements. *Journal of Motor Behavior*, **17**(1), 77–95.

Jeannerod, M. (1984). The timing of natural prehension movements. *Journal of Motor Behavior*, **16**(3), 235–254.

Kalaska, J.F., Caminiti, R., and Georgopoulos, A.P. (1983). Cortical mechanisms related to the direction of two-dimensional arm movements: Relations in parietal area 5 and comparison with motor cortex. *Experimental Brain Research*, **51**, 247–260.

Kandel, E.R. and Schwartz, J.H. (1981). **Principles of neural science**. New York: Elsevier/North-Holland.

Kandel, E.R. and Schwartz, J.H. (1982). Molecular biology of learning: Modulation of transmitter release. *Science*, **218**, 433–443.

Kasamatsu, T. and Pettigrew, J.D. (1976). Depletion of brain catecholamines: Failure of ocular dominance shift after monocular occlusion in kittens. *Science*, **194**, 206–209.

Katz, B. (1966). **Nerve, muscle, and synapse**. New York: McGraw-Hill.

Keele, S.W. (1981). Behavioral analysis of movement. In V.B. Brooks (Ed.), **Handbook of physiology**, Section 1, Volume 2: *Motor Control*. Bethesda, MD: American Physiological Society, pp.1391–1414.

Keele, S.W. (1982). Component analysis and conceptions of skill. In J.A.S. Kelso (Ed.), **Human motor behavior**. Hillsdale, NJ: Erlbaum, pp.143–159.

Keele, S.W. and Posner, M.I. (1968). Processing of visual feedback in rapid movements. *Journal of Experimental Psychology*, **77**, 155–158.

Keller, E.L. (1974). Participation of the medial pontine reticular formation in eye movement generation in monkey. *Journal of Neurophysiology*, **37**, 316–332.

Keller, E.L. (1979). Colliculoreticular organization of the oculomotor system. In R. Granit and O. Pompeiano (Eds.), **Progress in brain research: Reflex control of posture and movement**, 725–734.

Keller, E.L. (1980). Oculomotor specificity within subdivisions of the brainstem reticular formation. In J.A. Hobson and M. Brazier (Eds.),

The reticular formation revisited. New York: Raven Press, 227–240.

Keller, E.L. (1981). Brain stem mechanisms in saccadic control. In A.F. Fuchs and W. Becker (Eds.), **Progress in oculomotor research: Developments in neuroscience**, Vol. 12. New York: Elsevier/North-Holland.

Keller, E.L. and Kamath, B.Y. (1975). Characteristics of head rotation and eye movement related neurons in alert monkey vestibular nucleus. *Brain Research*, **100**, 182–187.

Kelso, J.A.S. (1982). **Human motor behavior**. Hillsdale, NJ: Erlbaum.

Kelso, J.A.S. and Holt, K.G. (1980). Exploring a vibratory systems analysis of human movement production. *Journal of Neurophysiology*, **28**, 45–52.

Kelso, J.A.S., Southard, D.L., and Goodman, D. (1979). On the nature of human interlimb coordination. *Science*, **203**, 1029–1031.

Kerr, B. and Langolf, G.D. (1977). Speed of aimed movements. *Quarterly Journal of Experimental Psychology*, **29**, 475–481.

Kettner, R.E., Schwartz, A.B., and Georgopoulos, A.P. (1988). Primate motor cortex and free arm movements to visual targets in three-dimensional space, III: Positional gradients and population coding of movement direction from various movement origins. *Journal of Neuroscience*, **8**, 2938–2947.

Knight, A.A. and Dagnall, P.R. (1967). Precision in movements. *Ergonomics*, **10**, 327–330.

Knudsen, E.I. (1983). Early auditory experience aligns the auditory map of space in the optic tectum of the barn owl. *Science*, **222**, 939–942.

Knudsen, E.I. (1984). The role of auditory experience in the development and maintenance of sound localization. *Trends in Neuroscience*, **7**, 326–330.

Knudsen, E.I. (1985). Experience alters the spatial tuning of auditory units in the optic tectum during a sensitive period in the barn owl. *Journal of Neuroscience*, **5**, 3094–3109.

Knudsen, E.I. and Knudsen, P.F. (1985). Vision guides the adjustment of auditory localization in young barn owls. *Science*, **230**, 545–548.

Konishi, M. (1984). Spatial receptive fields in the auditory system. In L. Bolis, R.D. Keynes, and S.H.P. Maddrell (Eds.), **Comparative physiology of sensory systems**. Cambridge, England: Cambridge University Press.

Kowler, E. (1982). Characteristics and visual consequences of saccades used to scan displays. Presentation at the 1982 AFOSR Technical Meeting, Sarasota, Florida.

Kuperstein, M. (1987). Adaptive visual-motor coordination in multijoint robots using parallel architecture. In **Proceedings of the IEEE international conference on robotics and automation**, Raleigh, North Carolina, March 31—April 3, 1987.

Kuperstein, M. (1988a). An adaptive neural model for mapping invariant target position. *Behavioral Neuroscience*, **102**, 148–162.

Kuperstein, M. (1988b). Neural model of adaptive hand-eye coordination for single postures. *Science*, **239**, 1308–1311.

Kuperstein, M. and Eichenbaum, H. (1985). Unit activity, evoked potentials, and slow waves in the rat hippocampus and olfactory bulb recorded with a 24-channel microelectrode. *Neuroscience*, in press.

Kurtzberg, D. and Vaughan, H.G. Jr. (1982). Topographic analysis of human cortical potentials preceding self-initiated and visually triggered saccades. *Brain Research*, **243**, 1–9.

Lanman, J., Bizzi, E., and Allum, J. (1978). The coordination of eye and head movement during smooth pursuit. *Brain Research*, **153**, 39–53.

Latto, R. and Cowey, A. (1971). Fixation changes after frontal eye-field lesions in monkeys. *Brain Research*, **30**, 25–36.

Lestienne, F. (1979). Effects of inertial load and velocity on the braking process of voluntary limb movements. *Experimental Brain Research*, **35**, 407–418.

Levine, D.S. and Grossberg, S. (1976). Visual illusions in neural networks: Line neutralization, tilt aftereffect, and angle expansion. *Journal of Theoretical Biology*, **61**, 477–504.

Llinás, R. (1969). Neuronal operations in cerebellar transactions. In F.O. Schmitt (Ed.), **The neurosciences second study program**. New York: Rockefeller University Press.

Llinás, R. and Wolfe, J.W. (1977). Functional linkage between the electrical activity in the vermal cerebellar cortex and saccadic eye movements. *Experimental Brain Research*, **29**, 1–14.

Luschei, E.S. and Fuchs, A.F. (1972). Activity of brain stem neurons during eye movements of alert monkeys. *Journal of Neurophysiology*, **35**, 445– 461.

Lynch, J.C. (1980). The functional organization of posterior parietal association cortex. *Behavioral and Brain Sciences*, **3**, 485–534.

Marr, D. (1969). A theory of cerebellar cortex. *Journal of Physiology (London)*, **202**, 437–470.

Marteniuk, R.G. and MacKenzie, C.L. (1980). A preliminary theory of two-hand co-ordinated control. In G.E. Stelmach and J. Requin (Eds.), **Tutorials in motor behavior**. Amsterdam: Elsevier/North-Holland, pp.185–197.

Massey, J.T., Schwartz, A.B., and Georgopoulos, A.P. (1985). On information processing and performing a movement sequence. In C. Fromm and H. Heuver (Eds.), **Generation and modulation of action patterns**, Experimental Brain Research Supplement.

Mays, L.E. and Sparks, D.L. (1980). Saccades are spatially, not retinocentrically, coded. *Science*, **208**, 1163–1165.

Mays, L.E. and Sparks, D.L. (1981). The localization of saccade targets using a combination of retinal and eye position information. In A.F. Fuchs and W. Becker (Eds.), **Progress in oculomotor research: Developments in neuroscience**, Vol. 12. New York: Elsevier/North-Holland.

McCormick, D.A. and Thompson, R.F. (1984). Cerebellum: Essential movement in the classically conditioned eyelid response. *Science*, **223**, 296–299.

Meredith, M.A. and Stein, B.E. (1983). Interactions among converging sensory inputs in the superior colliculus. *Science*, **221**, 389–391.

Meyer, D.E., Keith-Smith, J.E., and Wright, C.E. (1982). Models for the speed and accuracy of aimed movements. *Psychological Review*, **89**, 449–482.

Miles, F.A. (1974). Single unit firing patterns in the vestibular nuclei related to voluntary eye movements and passive head movement in conscious monkeys. *Brain Research*, **71**, 215–224.

Miles, F.A., Braitman, D.J., and Dow, B.M. (1980). Long-term adaptive changes in primate vestibuloocular reflex, IV: Electrophysiological observations in flocculus of adapted monkeys. *Journal of Neurophysiology*, **43**, 1477– 1493.

Miles, F.A., Fuller, J.H., Braitman, D.J., and Dow, B.M. (1980). Long-term adaptive changes in primate vestibuloocular reflex, III: Electrophysiological observations in flocculus of normal monkeys. *Journal of Neurophysiology*, **43**, 1437–1474.

Milner, B. and Petrides, M. (1984). Behavioural effects of frontal-lobe lesions in man. *Trends in Neuroscience*, **7**, 403–407.

Morasso, P. (1981). Spatial control of arm movements. *Experimental Brain Research*, **42**, 223–227.

Motter, B.C. and Mountcastle, V.B. (1981). The functional properties of the light-sensitive neurons of the posterior parietal cortex studied in waking monkeys: Foveal sparing and opponent vector organization. *Journal of Neuroscience*, **1**, 3–26.

Mountcastle, V.B. (1957). Modality and topographic properties of single neurons of cat's somatic sensory cortex. *Journal of Neurophysiology*, **20**, 408–434.

Mountcastle, V.B. (1978). Brain mechanisms for directed attention. *Journal of the Royal Society of Medicine*, **71**, 14–28.

Mountcastle, V.B., Andersen, R.A., and Motter, B.C. (1981). The influence of attentive fixation upon the excitability of the light-sensitive neurons of the posterior parietal cortex. *Journal of Neuroscience*, **1**, 1218–1235.

Murphy, B.J., Haddad, G.M., and Steinman, R.M. (1974). Simple forms and fluctuations in the line of sight: Implications for motor theories of form processing. *Perception and Psychophysics*, **16**, 557–563.

Nemire, K. and Bridgeman, B. (1987). Oculomotor and skeletal motor systems share one map of visual space. *Vision Research*, **27**, 393–400.

Nichols, T.R. (1985). Is "the Mass-Spring Model" a testable hypothesis? *Journal of Motor Behavior*, **17**(4), 499–500.

Niedzwiecki, D.M., Mailman, R.B., and Cubeddu, L.X. (1984). Greater potency of mesoridazine and sulforidazine compared with the parent compound, thioridazine, on striatal dopamine autoreceptors. *Journal of Pharmacology and Experimental Therapeutics*, **228**, 636–639.

Optican, L.M. and Miles, F.A. (1979). Visually induced adaptive changes in oculomotor control signals. *Society for Neuroscience Abstracts*, **5**, 380.

Optican, L.M. and Robinson, D.A. (1980). Cerebellar-dependent adaptive control of primate saccadic system. *Journal of Neurophysiology*, **44**, 1058–1076.

Oscarsson, O. (1975). Spatial distribution of climbing and mossy fibre inputs into the cerebellar cortex. In **Proceedings of the 7th international neurobiology meeting on afferent and intrinsic organization of laminated structures in the brain**, Göttingen.

Pearson, J.C., Sullivan, W.E., Gelfand, J.J., and Peterson, R.M. (1987). A computational map approach to sensory fusion. **Proceedings of the AOG/AAAIC 87 joint conference on merging tomorrow's technology with defense readiness requirements.**

Peck, C.K., Schlag-Rey, M., and Schlag, J. (1980). Visuo-oculomotor properties of cells in the superior colliculus of the alert cat. *Journal of Comparative Neurology*, **194**, 97–116.

Pellionisz, A. and Llinás, R. (1980). Tensorial approach to the geometry of brain function: Cerebellar coordination via a metric tensor. *Neuroscience*, **5**, 1125–1136.

Pellionisz, A. and Llinás, R. (1982). Tensor theory of brain function: The cerebellum as a space-time metric. In S. Amari and M. Arbib (Eds.), **Competition and cooperation in neural networks**. New York: Springer-Verlag.

Pettigrew, J.D. and Kasamatsu, T. (1978). Local perfusion of noradrenaline maintains visual cortical plasticity. *Nature*, **271**, 761–763.

Piaget, J. (1963). **The origins of intelligence in children**. New York: Norton.

Polit, A. and Bizzi, E. (1978). Processes controlling arm movements in monkeys. *Science*, **201**, 1235–1237.

Ratliff, F. (1965). **Mach bands: Quantitative studies on neural networks in the retina**. New York: Holden-Day.

Raybourn, M.S. and Keller, E.L. (1977). Colliculoreticular organization in primate oculomotor system. *Journal of Neurophysiology*, **40**, 861–878.

Robinson, D.A. (1970). Oculomotor unit behavior in the monkey. *Journal of Neurophysiology*, **35**, 393–404.

Robinson, D.A. (1973). Models of the saccadic eye movement control system. *Kybernetik*, **14**, 71–83.

Robinson, D.A. (1975). Oculomotor control signals. In G. Lennerstrand and P. Bach-y-Rita (Eds.), **Basic mechanisms of ocular motility and their clinical implications**. Oxford: Pergamon Press.

Robinson, D.A. (1981). Control of eye movements. In J.M. Brookhart, V.B. Mountcastle, V.B. Brooks, and S.R. Geiger (Eds.), **Handbook of physiology**, Vol. II. Bethesda, MD: American Physiological Society.

Robinson, D.A. (1981). Models of the mechanics of eye movements. In B.L. Zuber (Ed.), **Models of oculomotor behavior and control**. Boca Raton, FL: CRC Press.

Robinson, D.A. (1982). Plasticity in the oculomotor system. *Federation Proceedings*, **41**, 2153–2155.

Rodieck, R.W. and Stone, J. (1965). Analysis of receptive fields of cat retinal ganglion cells. *Journal of Neurophysiology*, **28**, 833–849.

Ron, S. and Robinson, D.A. (1973). Eye movements evoked by cerebellar stimulation in the alert monkey. *Journal of Neurophysiology*, **36**, 1004–1021.

Ruffini, A. (1898). On the minute anatomy of the neuro-muscular spindles of the cat, and on their physiological significance. *Journal of Physiology*, **23**, 190–208.

Saint-Cyr, J.A. and Woodward, D.J. (1980). A topographic analysis of limbic and somatic inputs to the cerebellar cortex in the rat. *Experimental Brain Research*, **40**, 13–22.

Sakata, H., Shibutani, H., and Kawano, K. (1980). Spatial properties of visual fixation neurons in posterior parietal association cortex of the monkey. *Journal of Neurophysiology*, **43**, 1654–1672.

Sakitt, B. (1980). A spring model and equivalent neural network for arm posture control. *Biological Cybernetics*, **37**, 227–234.

Salapatek, P., Aslin, R.N., Simonson, J., and Pulos, E. (1980). Infant saccadic eye movements in visible and previously visible targets. *Child Development*, **51**, 1090–1094.

Saltzman, E.L. and Kelso, J.A.S. (1983). Skilled actions: A task dynamics approach. Haskins Laboratories Status Report on Speech Research, SR-76, 3–50.

Schiller, P.H. (1970). The discharge characteristics of single units in the oculomotor and abducens nuclei of the unanesthetized monkey. *Experimental Brain Research*, **10**, 347–362.

Schiller, P.H. and Koerner, F. (1971). Discharge characteristics of single units in superior colliculus of the alert rhesus monkey. *Journal of Neurophysiology*, **34**, 920–936.

Schiller, P.H. and Sandell, J.H. (1983). Interactions between visually and electrically elicited saccades before and after superior colliculus and frontal eye field ablations in the rhesus monkey. *Experimental Brain Research*, **49**, 381–392.

References

Schiller, P.H., Sandell, J.H., and Maunsell, J.H.R. (1984). The effect of superior colliculus and frontal eye field lesions on saccadic latency in the monkey. *Society for Neuroscience Abstracts*, **10**, 21.9.

Schiller, P.H. and Stryker, M. (1972). Single-unit recording and stimulation in superior colliculus of the alert rhesus monkey. *Journal of Neurophysiology*, **35**, 915–924.

Schiller, P.H., True, S.D., and Conway, J.L. (1979). Paired stimulation of the frontal eye fields and the superior colliculus of the rhesus monkey. *Brain Research*, **179**, 162–164.

Schlag, J. and Schlag-Rey, M. (1981). The thalamic internal medullary lamina and gaze control in cat and monkey. In A.F. Fuchs and W. Becker (Eds.), **Progress in oculomotor research: Developments in neuroscience**, Vol. 12. New York: Elsevier/North-Holland.

Schlag, J., Schlag-Rey, M., Peck, C.K., and Joseph, J.P. (1980). Visual responses of thalamic neurons depending on the direction of gaze and position of targets in space. *Experimental Brain Research*, **40**, 170–184.

Schlag-Rey, M. and Schlag, J. (1983). Saccade-related pause-rebound cells in central thalamus of monkeys. *Society for Neuroscience Abstracts*, **9**, 1087.

Schmidt, E.M., Jost, R.G., and Davis, K.K. (1975). Reexamination of the force relationship of cortical cell discharge patterns with conditioned wrist movements. *Brain Research*, **83**, 213–223.

Schmidt, R.A. (1982). **Motor control and learning**. Champaign, IL: Human Kinetics Press.

Schmidt, R.A., Zelaznik, H.N., and Frank, J.S. (1978). Sources of inaccuracy in rapid movement. In G.E. Stelmach (Ed.), **Information processing in motor control and learning**. New York: Academic Press, 183–203.

Schwartz, E.L. (1980). Computational anatomy and functional architecture of striate cortex: A spatial mapping approach to perceptual coding. *Vision Research*, **20**, 645–669.

Schwartz, A.B., Kettner, R.E., and Georgopoulos, A.P. (1988). Primate motor cortex and free arm movements to visual targets in three-dimensional space, I: Relations between single cell discharge and direction of movement. *Journal of Neuroscience*, **8**, 2913–2927.

Scudder, C.A. (1988). A new local feedback model of the saccadic burst generator. *Journal of Neurophysiology*, **59**, 1455–1475.

Shebilske, W. (1977). Visuomotor coordination in visual direction and position constancies. In W. Epstein (Ed.), **Stability and constancy in visual perception: Mechanisms and processes**. New York: Wiley and Sons.

Sherrington, C.S. (1894). On the anatomical constitution of nerves of skeletal muscles, with remarks on recurrent fibres in the ventral spinal nerve-root. *Journal of Physiology*, **17**, 211–258.

Siever, L. and Sulser, F. (1984). Regulations of amine neurotransmitter systems: Implication for the major psychiatric syndromes and their treatment. *Psychopharmacology Bulletin*, **20**, 500–504.

Simpson, J.I., Soodak, R.E., and Hess, R. (1979). The accessory optic system and its relation to the vestibulocerebellum. In R. Granit and P. Pompeiano (Eds.), **Reflex control of posture and movement**. Amsterdam: Elsevier/North-Holland.

Singer, W. (1983). Neuronal activity as a shaping factor in the self-organization of neuron assemblies. In E. Basar, H. Flohr, H. Haken, and A.J. Mandell (Eds.), **Synergetics of the brain**. New York: Springer-Verlag.

Skavenski, A.A., Haddad, G.M., and Steinman, R.M. (1972). The extraretinal signal for the visual perception of direction. *Perception and Psychophysics*, **11**, 287.

Slotnick, R.S. (1969). Adaptation to curvature distortion. *Journal of Experimental Psychology*, **81**, 441–448.

Smith, K.U. (1966). Cybernetic theory and analysis of learning. In E.A. Bilodeau (Ed.), **Acquisition of skill**. New York: Academic Press.

Soechting, J.F. and Lacquaniti, F. (1981). Invariant characteristics of a pointing movement in man. *Journal of Neuroscience*, **1**(7), 710–720.

Sparks, D.L. (1978). Functional properties of neurons in the monkey superior colliculus: Coupling of neuronal activity and saccade onset. *Brain Research*, **156**, 1–16.

Sparks, D.L. and Jay, M. (1987). The role of the primate superior colliculus in sensorimotor integration. In M.A. Arbib and A.R. Hanson (Eds.), **Vision, brain, and cooperative computation**. Cambridge, MA: MIT Press, 109–128.

Sparks, D.L. and Mays, L.E. (1981). The role of the monkey superior colliculus in the control of saccadic eye movements: A current perspective. In A.F. Fuchs and W. Becker (Eds.), **Progress in oculomotor research**. New York: Elsevier/North-Holland.

Sperling, G. and Sondhi, M.M. (1968). Model for visual luminance distribution and flicker detection. *Journal of the Optical Society of America*, **58**, 1133–1145.

Steinbach, M.J. and Smith, D.R. (1981). Spatial localization after strabismus surgery: Evidence for inflow. *Science*, **213**, 1407–1408.

Steinman, R.M. (1965). Effect of target size, luminance, and color on monocular fixation. *Journal of the Optical Society of America*, **55**, 1158–1165.

Steinman, R.M. (1976). The role of eye movements in maintaining a phenomenally clear and stable world. In R.A. Monty and J.M. Senders (Eds.), **Eye movements and psychological processes**. Hillsdale, NJ: Erlbaum.

Stratton, G.M. (1897). Vision without inversion of the retinal image. *Psychological Review*, **4**, 341–360, 463–481.

Stricker, E.M. and Zigmond, M.J. (1976). Brain catecholamines and the lateral hypothalamic syndrome. In D. Novin, W. Wyrwicka, and G. Bray (Eds.), **Hunger: Basic mechanisms and clinical implications**. New York: Raven Press.

Sullivan, W.E. and Konishi, M. (1984). Segregation of stimulus phase and intensity coding in the cochlear nucleus of the barn owl. *Journal of Neuroscience*, **4**, 1787–1799.

Suzuki, H. and Azuma, M. (1977). Prefrontal neuronal activity during gazing at a light spot in the monkey. *Brain Research*, **126**, 497–508.

Szentágothai, J. (1968). Structuro-functional considerations of the cerebellar network. *Proceedings IEEE*, **56**, 960–968.

Takahashi, T., Moiseff, A., and Konishi, M. (1984). Time and intensity cues are processed independently in the auditory system of the owl. *Journal of Neuroscience*, **4**, 1781–1786.

Tanji, J. and Evarts, E.V. (1976). Anticipatory activity of motor cortex units in relation to direction of an intended movement. *Journal of Neurophysiology*, **39**, 1062–1068.

Taylor, J.G. (1962). **The behavioral basis of perception**. New Haven, CT: Yale University Press.

Tepper, J.M., Young, S.J., and Groves, P.M. (1984). Autoreceptor mediated changes in dopaminergic terminal excitability effects of increases in impulse flow. *Brain Research*, **309**, 309–316.

Traub, R.D. and Wong, R.K.S. (1983). Synchronized burst discharge in disinhibited hippocampal slice, II: Model of cellular mechanism. *Journal of Neurophysiology*, **49**, 459–471.

Vilis, T. and Hore, J. (1986). A comparison of disorders in saccades and in fast and accurate elbow flexions during cerebellar dysfunction. In H.J. Freund, U. Büttner, B. Cohen, and J. Noth (Eds.), **The oculomotor and skeletal motor systems: Differences and similarities**. New York: Elsevier.

Vilis, T., Snow, R., and Hore, J. (1983). Cerebellar saccadic dysmetria is not equal in the two eyes. *Experimental Brain Research*, **51**, 343–350.

Viviani, P. and Terzuolo, C. (1980). Space-time invariance in learned motor skills. In Stelmach, G.E. and Requin, J. (Eds.), **Tutorials in Motor Behavior**. Amsterdam: North-Holland.

Waespe, W., Büttner, U., and Henn, V. (1981). Visual-vestibular interaction in the flocculus of the alert monkey, I: Input activity. *Experimental Brain Research*, **43**, 337–348.

Walters, E.T. and Bryne, J.H. (1983). Associative conditioning of single sensory neurons suggests a cellular mechanism for learning. *Science*, **219**, 405–408.

Weber, R.B. and Daroff, R.B. (1972). Corrective movements following refixation saccades: Type and control system analysis. *Vision Research*, **12**, 467–475.

Welch, R.B. (1978). **Perceptual modification: Adapting to altered sensory environments**. New York: Academic Press.

Welford, A.T., Norris, A.H., and Schock, N.W. (1969). Speed and accuracy of movement and their changes with age. In W.G. Koster (Ed.), **Attention and performance II**. Amsterdam: North-Holland, pp.3–15.

Whittington, D.A. (1980). The role of preoculomotor brainstem neurons in coordinated eye-head movements. Ph.D. Thesis, Massachusetts Institute of Technology.

Wilson, H.R. and Bergen, J.R. (1979). A four mechanism model for spatial vision. *Vision Research*, **19**, 19–32.

Woodworth, R.S. (1899). The accuracy of voluntary movement. *Psychological Review*, **3**, 1–114.

Wurtz, R.H. and Albano, J.E. (1980). Visual-motor function of the primate superior colliculus. *Annual Review of Neuroscience*, **3**, 189–226.

Wurtz, R.H., Goldberg, M.E., and Robinson, D.L. (1982). Brain mechanisms of visual attention. *Scientific American*, 124–135.

Wurtz, R.H. and Mohler, C.W. (1976). Enhancement of visual responses in monkey striate cortex and frontal eye fields. *Journal of Neurophysiology*, **39**, 766–772.

Yarbus, A.L. (1967). **Eye movements and vision**. New York: Plenum Press.

Yin, T.C.T. and Mountcastle, V.B. (1977). Visual input to the visuomotor mechanisms of the monkey's parietal lobe. *Science*, **197**, 1381–1383.

Young, L.R. (1981). The sampled data model and foveal dead zone for saccades. In B.L. Zuber (Ed.), **Models of oculomotor behavior and control**. Boca Raton, FL: CRC Press.

Young, L.R. and Stark, L. (1963). Variable feedback experiments testing a sampled data model for eye tracking movements. *IEEE Transactions of the Professional Technical Group on Human Factors in Electronics*, **4**, 38–51.

Zee, D.S., Optican, L.M., Cook, J.D., Robinson, D.A., and Engel, W.K. (1976). Slow saccades in spinocerebellar degeneration. *Archives of Neurology*, **33**, 243–251.

Zelaznik, H.N., Hawkins, B., and Kisselburgh, K. (1983). Rapid visual feedback processing in single-aiming movements. *Journal of Motor Behavior*, **15**, 217–236.

Zelaznik, H.N., Schmidt, R.A., and Gielen, S.C.A.M. (1987). Kinematic properties of rapid aimed head movements. *Journal of Motor Behavior*, in press.

Zingale, C.M. and Kowler, E. (1987). Planning sequences of saccades. *Vision Research*, **27**, 1327–1341.

Zipser, D. and Andersen, R.A. (1988). A back propagation programmed network that simulates response properties of a subset of posterior parietal neurons. *Nature*, **331**, 679–684.

Zuber, B.L. (Ed.) (1981). **Models of oculomotor behavior and control.** Boca Raton, FL: CRC Press.

AUTHOR INDEX

ABOUT THE AUTHORS

Stephen Grossberg

Stephen Grossberg is Wang Professor of Cognitive and Neural Systems at Boston University, where he founded and is the Director of the Center for Adaptive Systems and the graduate program in Cognitive and Neural Systems. He also organized the Boston Consortium for Behavioral and Neural Studies, which includes investigators from six Boston-area institutions. He founded and was first President of the International Neural Network Society, and is co-editor-in-chief of the Society's journal, *Neural Networks*.

During the past few decades, he and his colleagues at the Center for Adaptive Systems have pioneered and developed a number of the fundamental principles, mechanisms, and architectures that form the foundation for contemporary neural network research. These investigations include contributions to content-addressable memory; associative learning; biological vision and multidimensional image processing; cognitive information processing; adaptive pattern recognition; speech and language perception, learning, and production; adaptive robotics; conditioning and attention; development; biological rhythms; certain mental disorders; and their substrates in neurophysiological and anatomical mechanisms.

A hallmark of this work is its focus upon the design principles and mechanisms which enable the behavior of individuals to adapt successfully in real-time to unexpected environmental changes. The core models pioneered by this approach and which are embedded in these neural network theories include models which go under such names as competitive learning, adaptive resonance theory, masking fields, gated dipole opponent processes, associative outstars and instars, associative avalanches, associative spatial maps, nonlinear cooperative-competitive feedback networks, boundary contour and feature contour systems, adaptive vector encoders, and vector integration to endpoint circuits. Such models have been used both to analyse and predict a wide range of interdisciplinary data about mind and brain, as well as to suggest novel architectures for technological applications.

Grossberg received his graduate training at Stanford University and Rockefeller University, and was a Professor at M.I.T. before assuming his present position at Boston University.

Michael Kuperstein

Michael Kuperstein received his Ph.D. from M.I.T. in Psychology and Brain Science in 1982. He invented a 24-channel microelectrode for neural recording called PRONG and was the first to implement a neural robot in 1987. He has founded and is president of three companies: Network Instruments, which manufactures the PRONG; Neurogen Laboratories, which does research in neural networks; and Neurogen, which manufactures neural network devices in robotics and pattern recognition.